The Misery Journal
Finding Patterns in Your Aches & Pains

First Edition Published in 2020 by Laughing Wu Media, Salem, MA

laughingwu.com

© 2022, jeanie marie mossa kraft, MS, L.Ac., and Norman R. Kraft, MS, L.Ac.,

All Rights Reserved.

ISBN: 978-1-7357792-2-5

No part of this publication may be reproduced, stored in a retrieval system, or transmitted in any form or by any means, electronic, mechanical, photocopying, recording or otherwise, without the prior written permission of the copyright owner.

Warning and Disclaimer

The information presented here is not intended to substitute for any treatment that may have been prescribed by your physician. The information is given in good faith, but the authors cannot be held responsible for any error or omission, nor can they be held in any way responsible for treatment given on the basis of information contained herein. This book is also not a substitute for common sense. If you are in doubt concerning any aspect of this book, consult with your physician.

About the Authors

Jeanie Mossa is the founder of Four Paws Acupuncture, a veterinary acupuncture practice north of Boston. She is an acupuncturist (L.Ac.) with over 25 years of experience treating animals and humans with holistic medicine. She holds a masters degree (MS) in Traditional Oriental Medicine from Pacific College of Oriental Medicine and has completed the Animal Acupuncture certification program at New England School of Acupuncture. She is a former faculty member of the Canadian College of Oriental Medicine (Toronto, Canada). She has written and illustrated six books and created several online classes. Jeanie lives in Salem MA with her husband and their menagerie of magical creatures.

Norman R. Kraft is a writer, photographer and retired acupuncturist. He holds a masters degree (MS) in Traditional Oriental Medicine from Pacific College of Oriental Medicine and has served in administrator and faculty roles at acupuncture colleges in San Diego, New York and Toronto. He also holds a Licentiate in Sacred Theology (STL) and a Doctorate in Theology (ThD). He is the author of Ogdoadic Magick (Weiser), has co-authored another four books and written several articles on the application of Traditional Chinese Medicine to psychiatric issues. He maintains his photography portfolio at normankraft.com

Other books by jeanie mossa and Norman Kraft:

- Barkopaedia
- The Woof & Warp of Canine Pain
- The Screaming Uterus Syndrome
- Whispers of the O'Fae, Art & Affirmations for the Wounded Inner Child.
- Dr. Calamari's Guide to the Herbs, Minerals and Bugs of China.
- Ogdoadic Magick

Find these books and others at laughingwu.com

Classes by jeanie mossa:

Online Classes for People & Their Pets

Holistic Therapies, Alternative Medicine & Magical Realms

https://www.udemy.com/user/jeanie-mossa/

The Misery Journal

"We can't learn without pain." - Aristotle

Pain Sucks! When we experience aches, throbbing and pain, it seems like pure misery, and it consumes us. Our every waking thought becomes the mantra OUCH. However, all pain serves a purpose. What message is our body trying to tell us? Do we continue each day in a constant loop of agony? Ignore it and hope it leaves? Turn into one of those cranky people that perpetually complain? Become another Dr. House addicted to Vicodin? Eventually, we all reach a point where we actually want to do something about it. We know we can't live our whole lives like this. The discomfort may lead us to try to ease symptoms through medication, alternative medicine, holistic therapies, or lifestyle changes. That's a good start, as pain teaches us to be responsible for our own bodies and our own state of mind.

The **Misery Journal** is a daily tool to discover patterns in your aches and pains. Many types of pain have patterns when we look at the big picture. Does it hurt at 3am every morning? Does it hurt more with cold weather, or hot weather? Does movement make it worse? Are there foods that make it worse? These and many similar patterns to be found in our daily lives can give us, and your doctor, a much better idea of what's going on with you.

We are both acupuncturists and herbalists with more than 25 years of experience each. Treating pain has been the most common complaint we have heard over the past decades from our patients, both human and animals. As practitioners trained in Traditional Chinese Medicine, we were taught to look for patterns in the symptoms and pain in the body. We also learned to treat the whole body, not just the specific area of pain or illness. For instance, you may see an acupuncturist for back pain. As much as it might be the back pain that brought you in, your back is not separate from the rest of your body. Back pain is often a symptom of something larger going on, an imbalance in your body. Your practitioner most probably will do what is needed to relieve the discomfort while also treating various other organs and parts of your body at the same time. He or she may also recommend herbs, supplements and life-style changes to help manage the symptoms. Your back pain may decrease, and you may find that your sleep, digestion or mood improves as well.

There are several factors which cause pain. Besides traumatic causes such as illness or injury, other reasons can be related to things such as weather conditions, food allergies, alcohol consumption, stress, various body positions, strenuous exercise, hormonal cycles and more.

For instance, you may notice that your arthritic knees hurt more during hot damp weather and using an ice pack helps relieve it. Maybe your neck and back pain are worse after eating a large meal of pasta smothered with tomato sauce and bread. Gluten and tomato can both be food triggers that exacerbate pain. Having a glass of wine with sulfites may cause flare ups. Bending or sitting the wrong way could set off a week of laying on the couch with a heating pad. Your neuropathy may flare up during cold or windy weather. Women may experience more pain during ovulation or during menses. All these puzzle pieces may add up eventually.

By tracking your pain level along with other various influences, you and your healthcare provider may determine a better approach to managing and relieving it. These revelations may also give you insight on things to avoid, use with caution or inspire you to be aware of conditions that may exacerbate your pain so that you can avoid them or be prepared. If you know that pain

The Misery Journal

is going to strike after that big pasta meal you now have the choice to avoid it, suffer through it or find a natural remedy to ease the symptoms afterwards!

How to Use This Book

You will need a few highlighters or colored pens to mark the areas you are experiencing pain. You will also need to be honest with yourself. It's okay to record that Vodka tonic with potato skins in your journal! It may be a waste of ink, or it just might show up as a puzzle piece. Sometimes we just need to know what exactly the cause of our discomfort is.

Each day in the journal consists of two pages. The first page is for you to track and record your pain level, areas of discomfort and various factors that may aggravate your symptoms. The second page is dedicated to things that help reduce your ache such as therapies, remedies, and healthy habits. This is to help you track those various modalities that are working and as a reminder. Is it time for you to see your chiropractor, get an acupuncture treatment, buy more herbs or take a day off from work? These pages may also be shared with your health care practitioners for their recommendations.

Recording Your Daily Pain Level 1 -10

On a scale from 1 to 10, 1 is the least amount of pain you experience and 10 is the most extreme pain you have ever experienced. Giving birth is beyond 10!

It is recommended to track your pain every day. Do you have the same pain level each day? Maybe Monday mornings your back ache seems a bit more severe. Does it change with the weather, time of day or night, your stress level or when you bend or exercise? Do your aches seem more extreme during a full moon? Is there a correlation to your misery and food allergies such as gluten or soy? Is there a time you have no pain at all? How does your pain vary over weeks and months? These are the insights this book was created to help you discover.

Recording Times of Day and/or Night You Experience Pain

Recording the times of day and night your pain appears is very helpful, especially if you are seeing an acupuncturist or holistic practitioner. For instance, in Traditional Chinese Medicine every two hours the energy (aka Qi) in your body travels through a different organ. This is known as the Chinese Body Clock. Depending on the time your pain manifests or is the most extreme may determine which organ meridian for your practitioner to treat. An example would be your discomfort shows around 5 – 7 pm which is Kidney time. Your practitioner would then also use that information to treat the symptoms associated with that organ as well as recommending herbs, foods, or supplements to help strengthen it.

Record You Main Emotion for the Day

Research has shown that stress, anger, and grief can intensify pain and deplete the immune system. Once you have identified that emotional stress is the cause, what will you do to remedy it? Hint – therapy, laughter, meditation, kitchen dancing, EFT Tapping and music may help.

The Misery Journal

Record the Weather Every Day

It's no secret that weather can cause various symptoms. By tracking the weather along with your pain level, you can be prepared to expect an increase of pain when those pesky storms, cold snaps and humidity show up. Please consult with your holistic health care practitioner for recommendations for herbs, supplements and foods that help relieve pain during cold, hot, dry, windy, and muggy weather.

Record the Type of Pain

Recording if you pain is stabbing, throbbing, fixed, etc. will help your doctor or holistic practitioner make a better diagnosis.

Record Your Sleep Each Night

There is a section on the first page to record the quality of your sleep in general terms. Pain often makes for restless nights, and it can be helpful to track if your sleep is worse on Sunday night, but better on Friday night, or other similar patterns.

Record Your Daily Food Intake

Keeping track of what you eat each day may provide a pain pattern. It may also help you become aware of everything that you consume and perhaps will aid in weight loss. Excess weight can also cause pain in the back, knees and hips. Certain foods that we eat everyday may cause pain triggers. A few of these but not limited to are:

- Gluten – known to exacerbate arthritic pain and fibromyalgia pain.
- Nightshade Vegetables: Potato, Tomato, Eggplant, Zucchini, Bell Peppers, Peppers
- Alcohol (Beer and Vodka may contain gluten. Wine may contain sulfites.)
- Soy
- Corn
- Peanuts, Walnuts, and other nuts
- MSG
- Artificial sweeteners and flavorings

Women – Record Your Menstrual Cycle Day

Hormones can impact our emotions and pain levels. Tracking each day of your pain through your cycle may help you find a natural way to relieve it and may help ease the ache of any cramps or PMS.

Record Everything That Relieves Your Pain That Day

Record what helps to relieve your symptoms. Sometimes we need to be reminded that it is time to see the chiropractor, acupuncturist, massage therapist. Are there certain herbs, supplements, or liniments that you use daily? Does the pain return when you run out of supplements or oils? Does taking a hot bath, shower or using a heating pad help reduce pain or would you prefer an ice pack? All this information is vital to finding a pattern and solution.

The Misery Journal

You may not believe in holistic medicine or natural remedies. That is okay! You can use this book for your own personal information and share it with your medical doctors so that they have a better picture of what is going on in your body.

Daily Astrological & Moon Phase

Feel free to skip this if you are not interested in astrology or the effect of the moon on our bodies. If you are fan of such things, you may find this info coincides with your pain, moods and symptoms.

Record at Least Three Things You Are Grateful for Today

Page two of each day includes a special gratitude section. This for you to jot down each night a few things you are thankful for. Keep it simple. For example: I am grateful for my cat purring. I am grateful for this warm cozy blanket. I am grateful for coffee.

Research has shown that keeping a gratitude journal helps to reduce stress, improve sleep and your mood. By taking the time to focus on the good things in your life you will naturally become more positive. Relax the mind and the body will follow!

Remember, this is your journal. Fill out the sections that apply to you, and don't worry about the others. Feel free to make notes in the margins. Feel free to note anything you feel might be important. While this journal can help your healthcare practitioner, you don't have to share the actual pages, just the insights.

When this journal becomes really useful is when you look back at your symptoms over time. This is when patterns emerge, when you view your pain over a week, or month.

We hope this 90 day journal helps you understand your aches and pains and move toward a better and healthier future. We wish you a healthy, happy, and pain-free journey!

Today's Day & Date

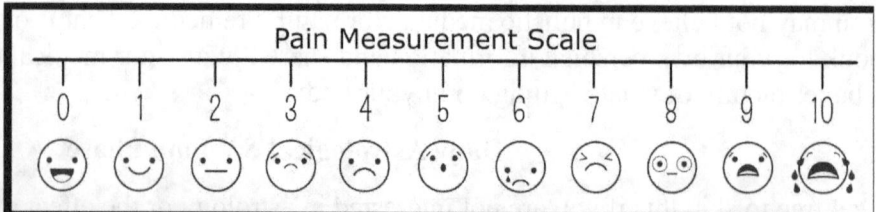

Highlight All Painful Areas

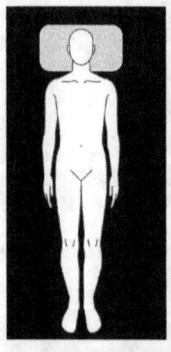 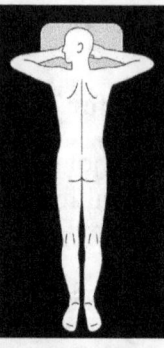 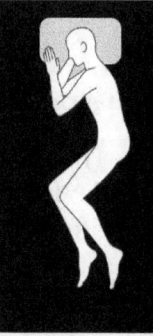 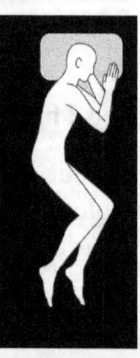

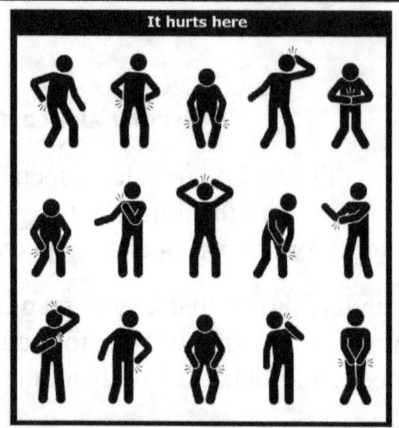
It hurts here

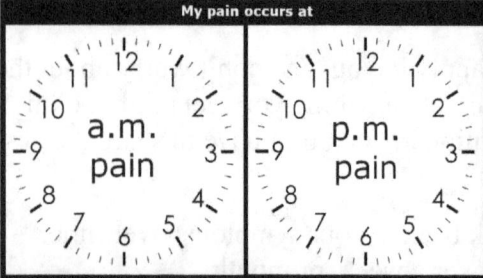
My pain occurs at — a.m. pain / p.m. pain

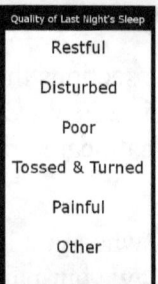

Quality of Last Night's Sleep
- Restful
- Disturbed
- Poor
- Tossed & Turned
- Painful
- Other

My mood today

My pain is
Hot
Burning
Cold
Stabbing
Throbbing
Fixed
Moving Traveling
Constant
On & Off

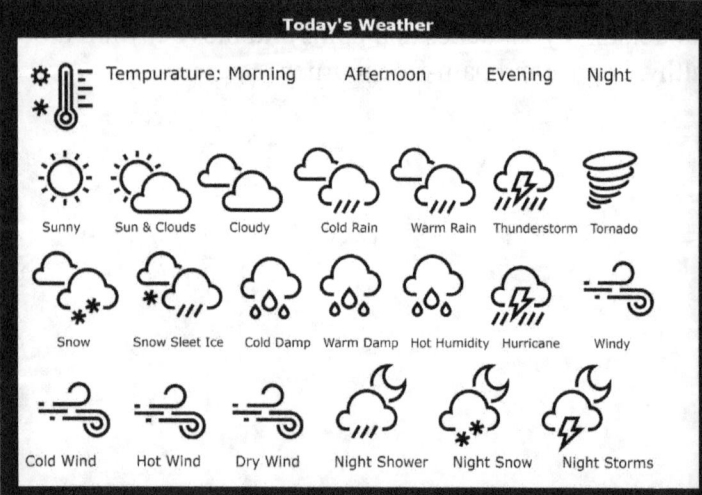
Today's Weather — Temperature: Morning, Afternoon, Evening, Night

Breakfast

Lunch

Dinner

Snacks

Alcohol

Food Allergy Triggers

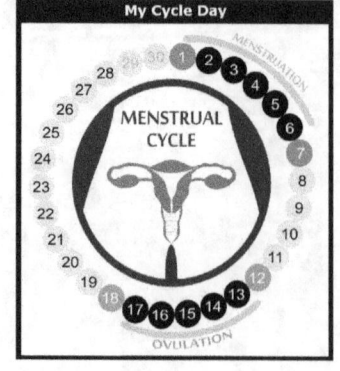
My Cycle Day

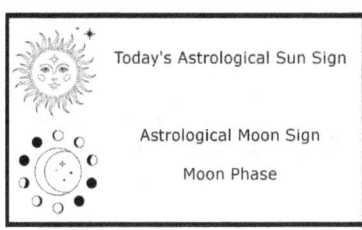

Today's Astrological Sun Sign

Astrological Moon Sign

Moon Phase

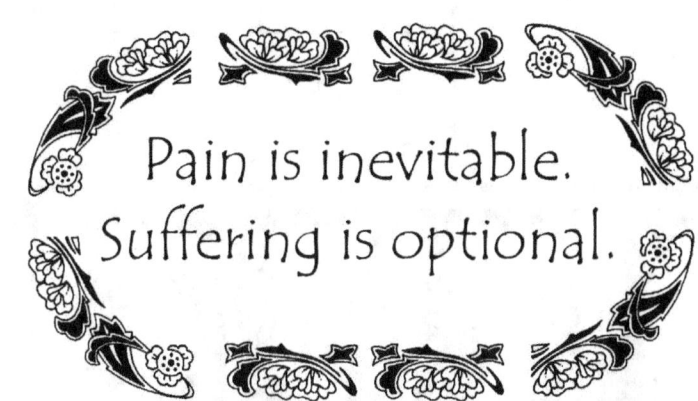

Pain is inevitable.
Suffering is optional.

Notes

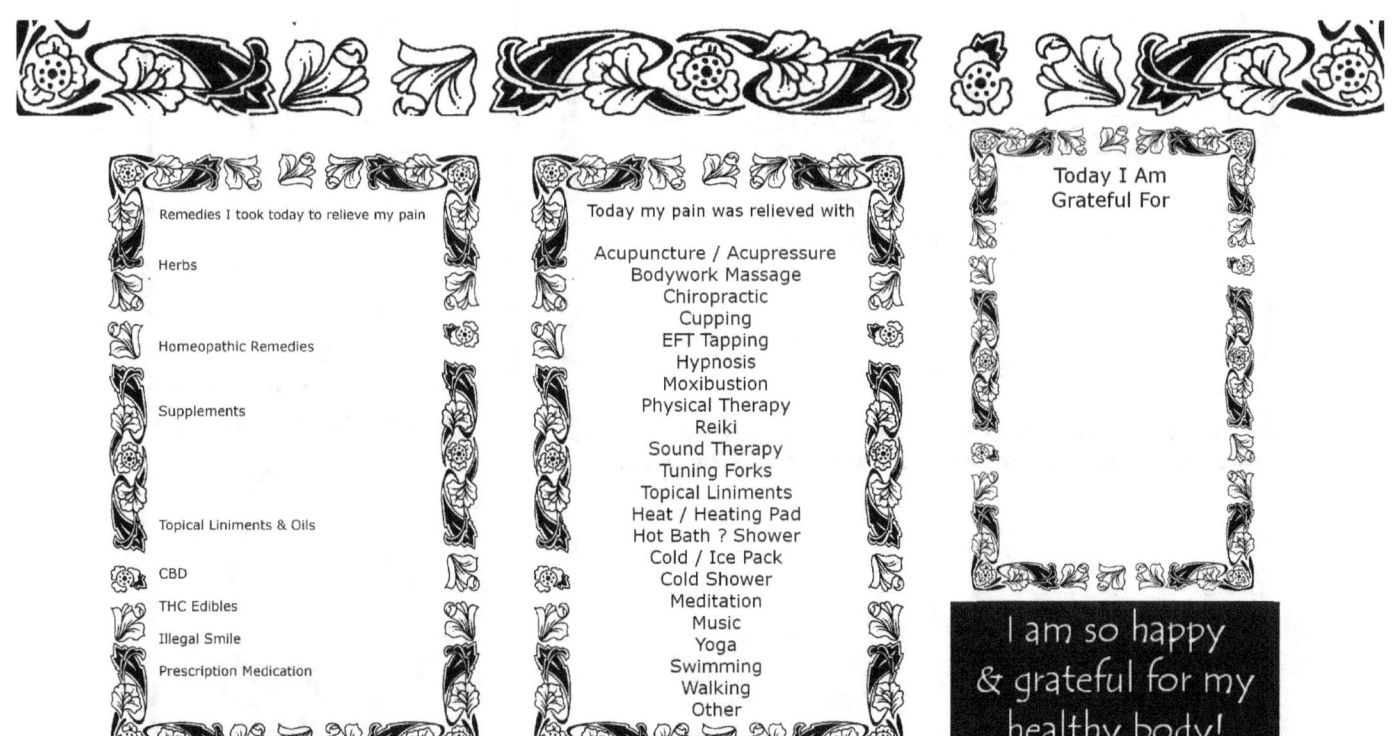

Remedies I took today to relieve my pain

Herbs

Homeopathic Remedies

Supplements

Topical Liniments & Oils

CBD

THC Edibles

Illegal Smile

Prescription Medication

Today my pain was relieved with

Acupuncture / Acupressure
Bodywork Massage
Chiropractic
Cupping
EFT Tapping
Hypnosis
Moxibustion
Physical Therapy
Reiki
Sound Therapy
Tuning Forks
Topical Liniments
Heat / Heating Pad
Hot Bath ? Shower
Cold / Ice Pack
Cold Shower
Meditation
Music
Yoga
Swimming
Walking
Other

Today I Am Grateful For

I am so happy & grateful for my healthy body!

Today's Day & Date

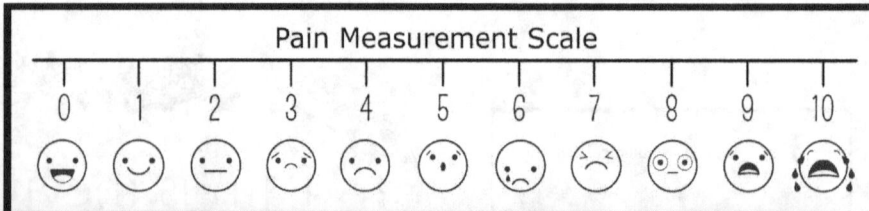

Highlight All Painful Areas

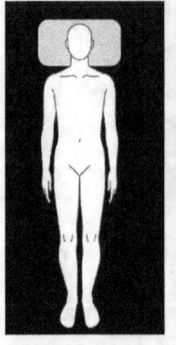 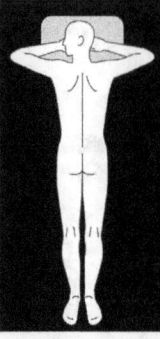 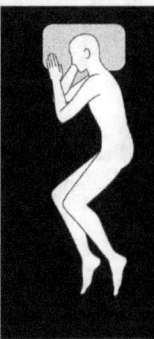 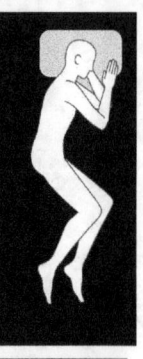

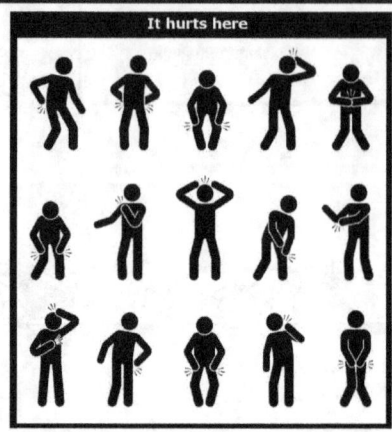
It hurts here

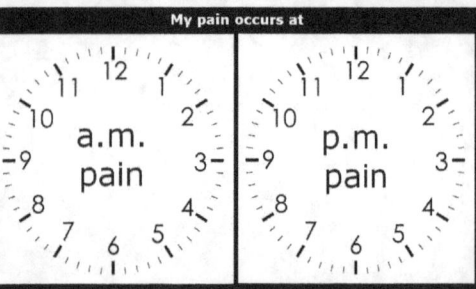

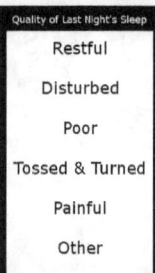

Quality of Last Night's Sleep
- Restful
- Disturbed
- Poor
- Tossed & Turned
- Painful
- Other

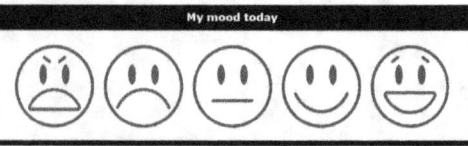
My mood today

My pain is
Hot
Burning
Cold
Stabbing
Throbbing
Fixed
Moving Traveling
Constant
On & Off

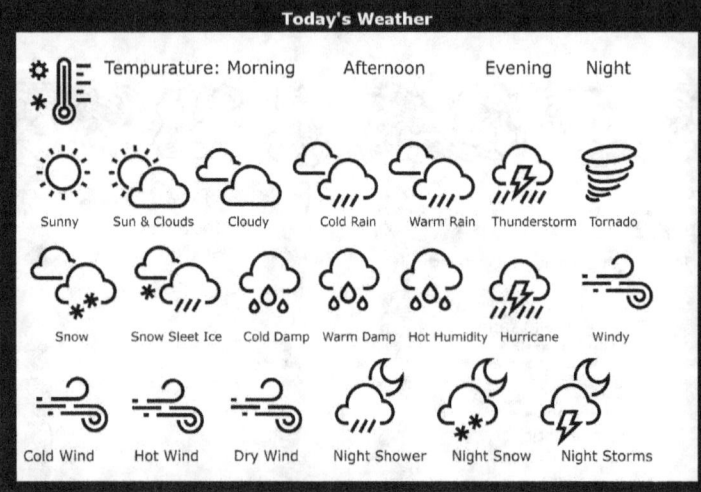

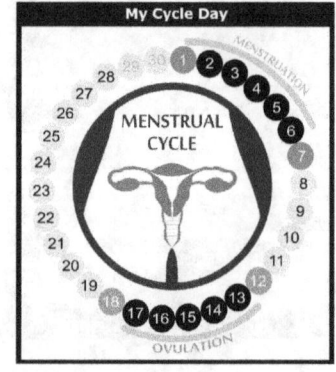
My Cycle Day

Breakfast

Lunch

Dinner

Snacks

Alcohol

Food Allergy Triggers

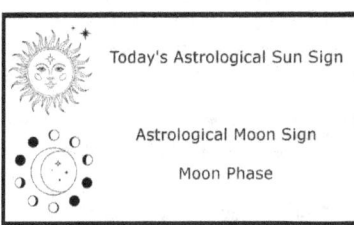

Today's Astrological Sun Sign

Astrological Moon Sign

Moon Phase

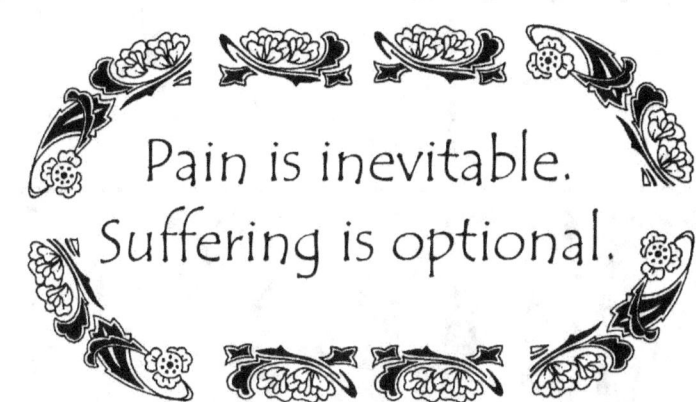

Pain is inevitable.
Suffering is optional.

Notes

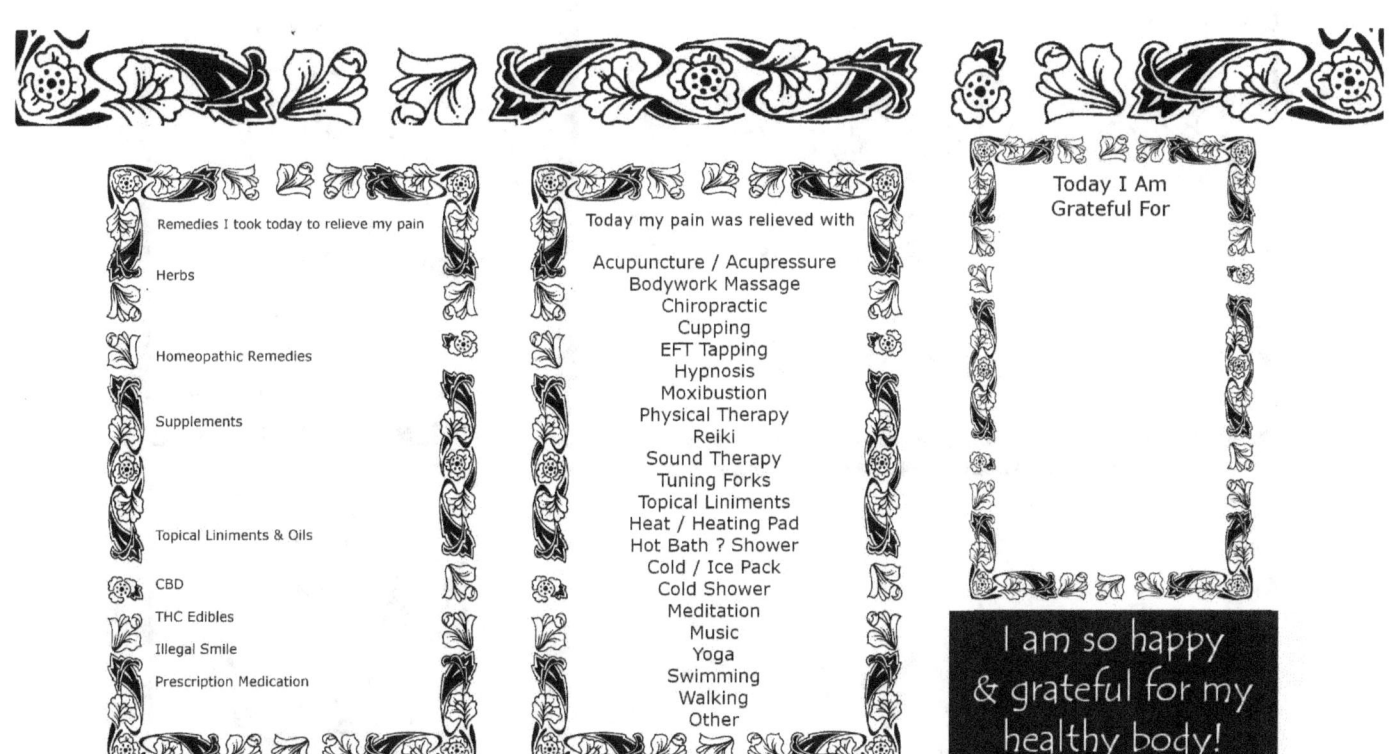

Remedies I took today to relieve my pain

Herbs

Homeopathic Remedies

Supplements

Topical Liniments & Oils

CBD

THC Edibles

Illegal Smile

Prescription Medication

Today my pain was relieved with

Acupuncture / Acupressure
Bodywork Massage
Chiropractic
Cupping
EFT Tapping
Hypnosis
Moxibustion
Physical Therapy
Reiki
Sound Therapy
Tuning Forks
Topical Liniments
Heat / Heating Pad
Hot Bath ? Shower
Cold / Ice Pack
Cold Shower
Meditation
Music
Yoga
Swimming
Walking
Other

Today I Am Grateful For

I am so happy & grateful for my healthy body!

Today's Day & Date

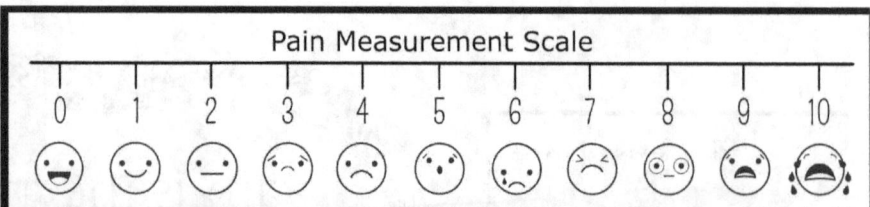

Highlight All Painful Areas

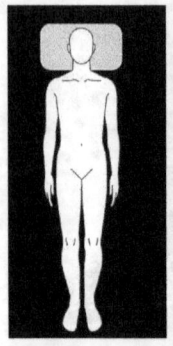 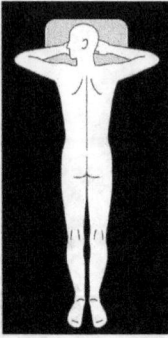 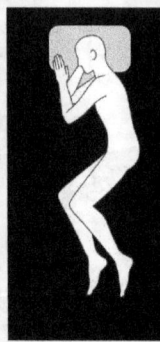 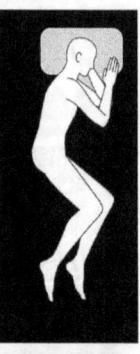

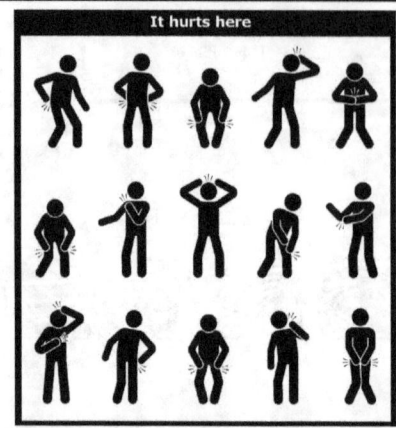
It hurts here

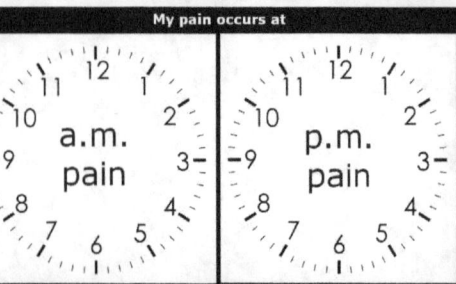
My pain occurs at — a.m. pain / p.m. pain

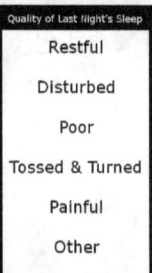

Quality of Last Night's Sleep
- Restful
- Disturbed
- Poor
- Tossed & Turned
- Painful
- Other

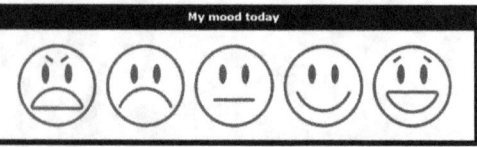
My mood today

My pain is
Hot
Burning
Cold
Stabbing
Throbbing
Fixed
Moving Traveling
Constant
On & Off

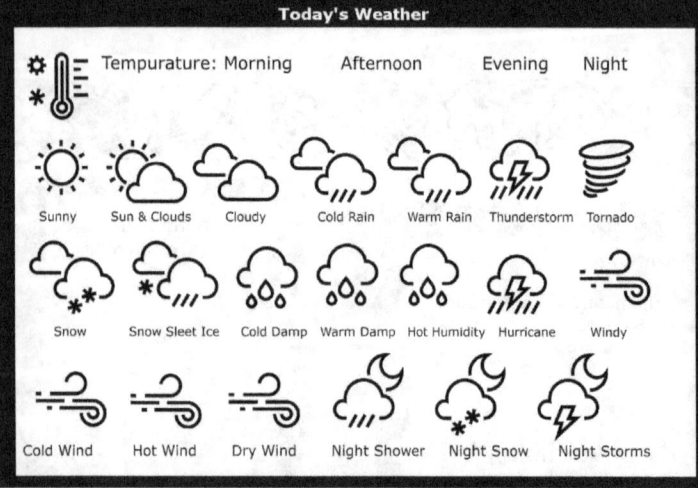
Today's Weather — Temperature: Morning, Afternoon, Evening, Night

Breakfast

Lunch

Dinner

Snacks

Alcohol

Food Allergy Triggers

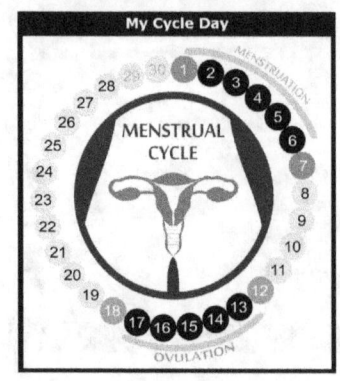
My Cycle Day

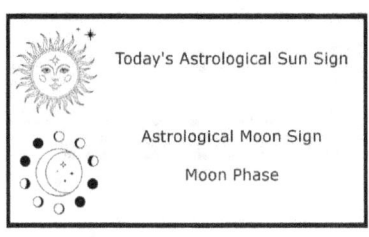

Today's Astrological Sun Sign

Astrological Moon Sign

Moon Phase

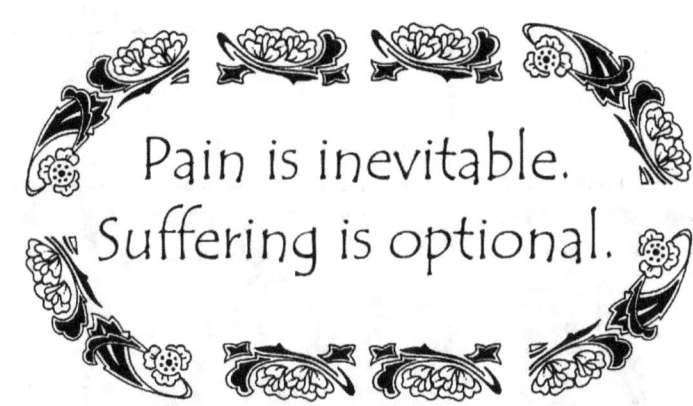

Pain is inevitable.
Suffering is optional.

Notes

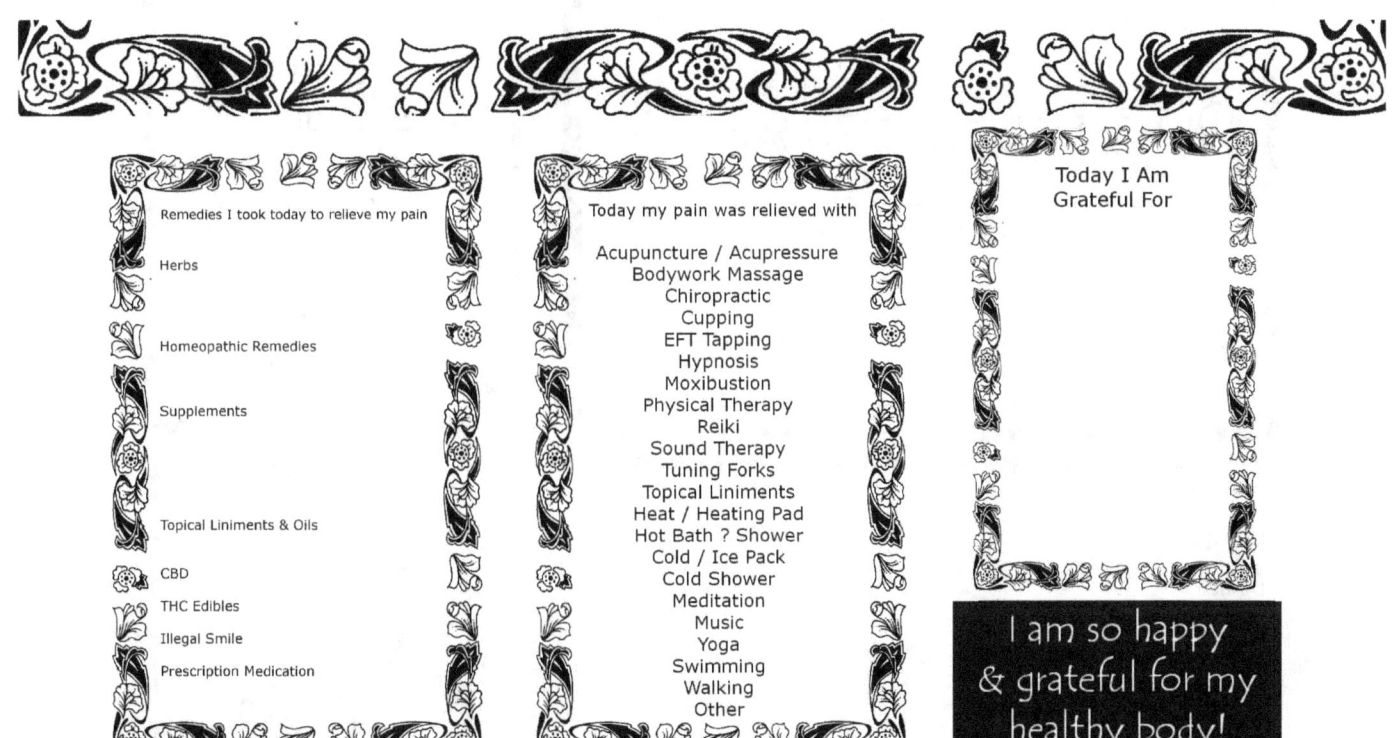

Remedies I took today to relieve my pain

Herbs

Homeopathic Remedies

Supplements

Topical Liniments & Oils

CBD
THC Edibles
Illegal Smile
Prescription Medication

Today my pain was relieved with

Acupuncture / Acupressure
Bodywork Massage
Chiropractic
Cupping
EFT Tapping
Hypnosis
Moxibustion
Physical Therapy
Reiki
Sound Therapy
Tuning Forks
Topical Liniments
Heat / Heating Pad
Hot Bath ? Shower
Cold / Ice Pack
Cold Shower
Meditation
Music
Yoga
Swimming
Walking
Other

Today I Am Grateful For

I am so happy & grateful for my healthy body!

Today's Day & Date

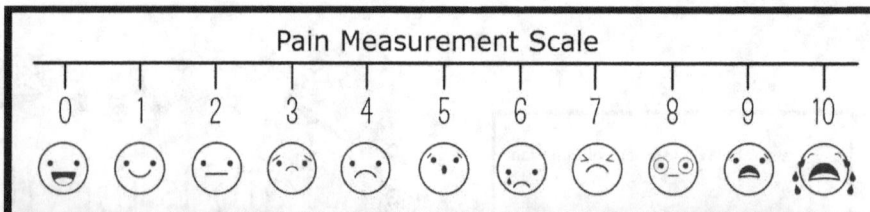

Highlight All Painful Areas

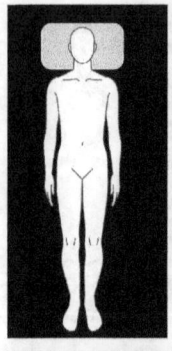 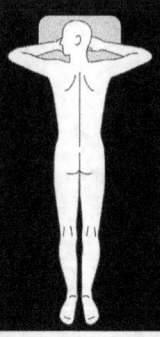 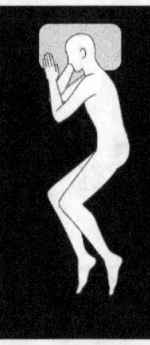 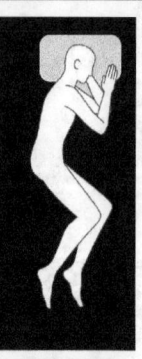

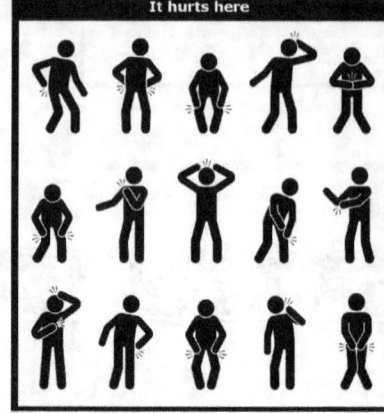
It hurts here

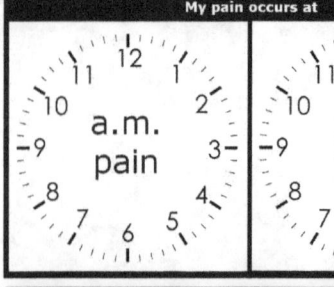
My pain occurs at — a.m. pain / p.m. pain

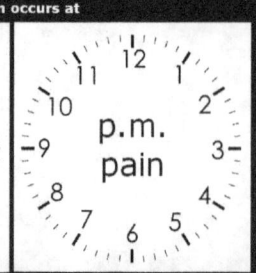
Quality of Last Night's Sleep
- Restful
- Disturbed
- Poor
- Tossed & Turned
- Painful
- Other

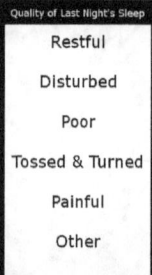
My mood today

My pain is
Hot
Burning
Cold
Stabbing
Throbbing
Fixed
Moving Traveling
Constant
On & Off

Today's Weather

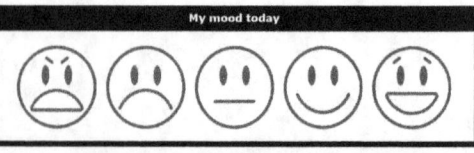
Tempurature: Morning   Afternoon   Evening   Night

Sunny | Sun & Clouds | Cloudy | Cold Rain | Warm Rain | Thunderstorm | Tornado
Snow | Snow Sleet Ice | Cold Damp | Warm Damp | Hot Humidity | Hurricane | Windy
Cold Wind | Hot Wind | Dry Wind | Night Shower | Night Snow | Night Storms

Breakfast

Lunch

Dinner

Snacks

Alcohol

Food Allergy Triggers

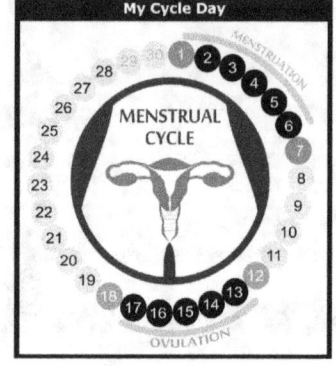
My Cycle Day

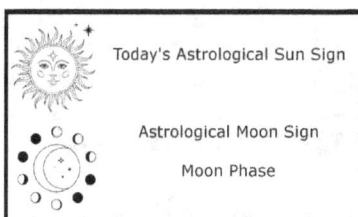

Today's Astrological Sun Sign

Astrological Moon Sign

Moon Phase

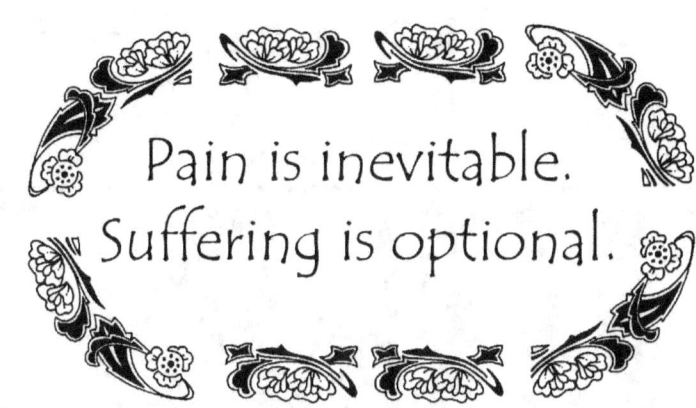

Pain is inevitable.
Suffering is optional.

Notes

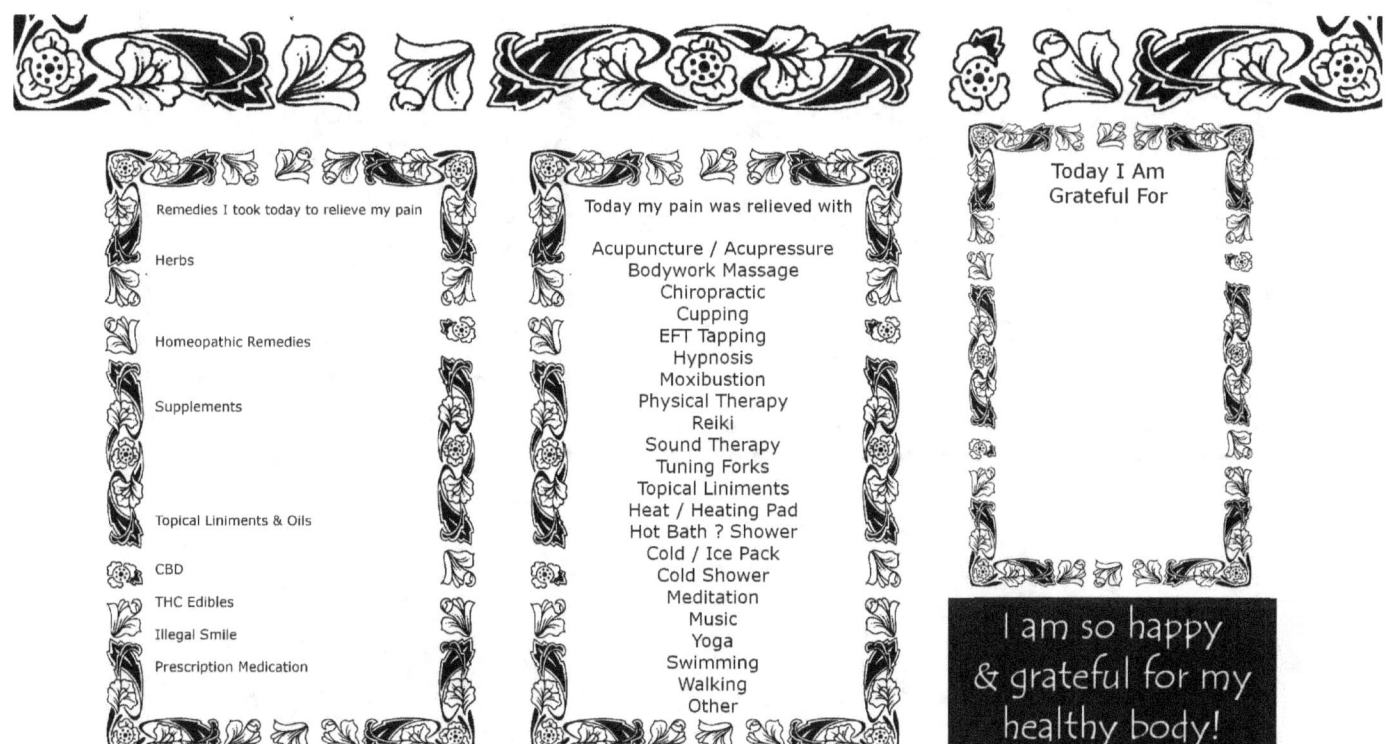

Remedies I took today to relieve my pain

Herbs

Homeopathic Remedies

Supplements

Topical Liniments & Oils

CBD

THC Edibles

Illegal Smile

Prescription Medication

Today my pain was relieved with

Acupuncture / Acupressure
Bodywork Massage
Chiropractic
Cupping
EFT Tapping
Hypnosis
Moxibustion
Physical Therapy
Reiki
Sound Therapy
Tuning Forks
Topical Liniments
Heat / Heating Pad
Hot Bath ? Shower
Cold / Ice Pack
Cold Shower
Meditation
Music
Yoga
Swimming
Walking
Other

Today I Am Grateful For

I am so happy & grateful for my healthy body!

Today's Day & Date

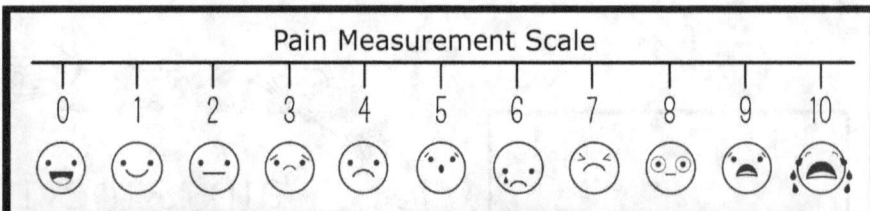

Highlight All Painful Areas

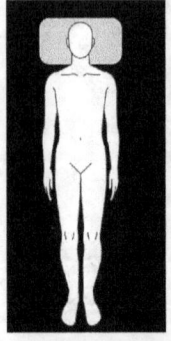 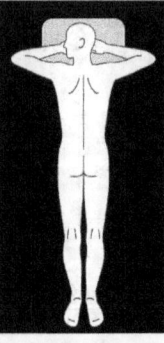 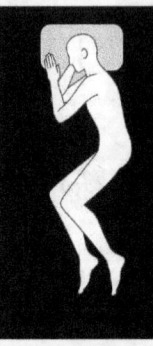 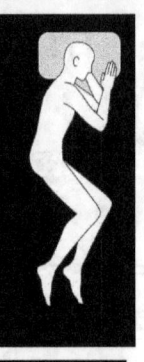

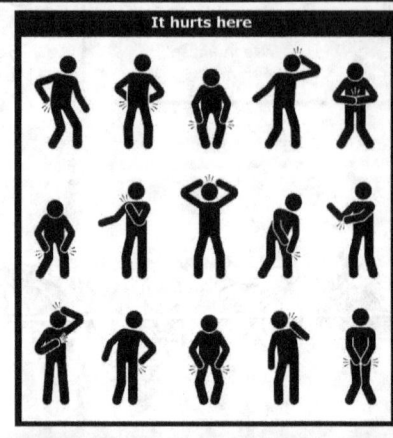

It hurts here

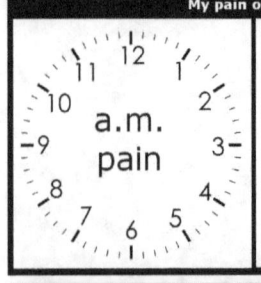 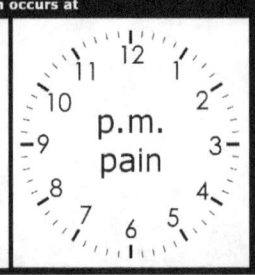 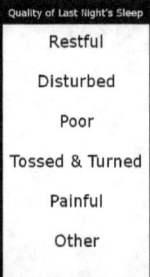

My pain occurs at — a.m. pain / p.m. pain

Quality of Last Night's Sleep
- Restful
- Disturbed
- Poor
- Tossed & Turned
- Painful
- Other

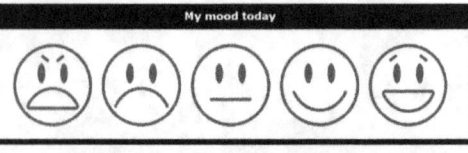

My mood today

My pain is

Hot
Burning
Cold
Stabbing
Throbbing
Fixed
Moving Traveling
Constant
On & Off

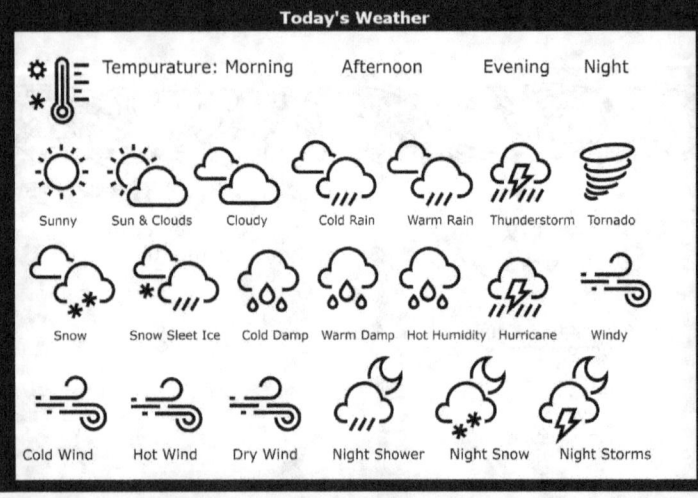

Today's Weather

Tempurature: Morning   Afternoon   Evening   Night

Sunny, Sun & Clouds, Cloudy, Cold Rain, Warm Rain, Thunderstorm, Tornado
Snow, Snow Sleet Ice, Cold Damp, Warm Damp, Hot Humidity, Hurricane, Windy
Cold Wind, Hot Wind, Dry Wind, Night Shower, Night Snow, Night Storms

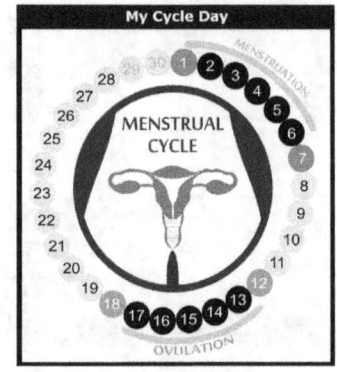

My Cycle Day

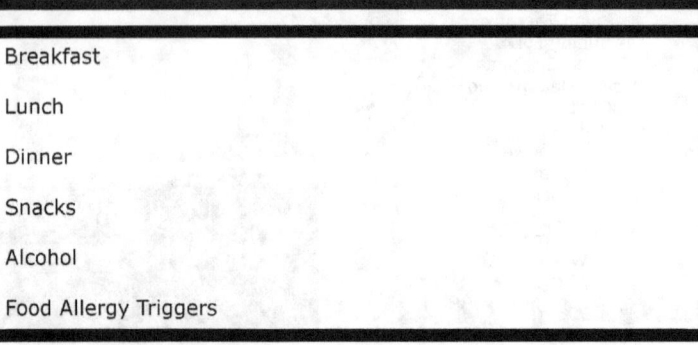

Breakfast

Lunch

Dinner

Snacks

Alcohol

Food Allergy Triggers

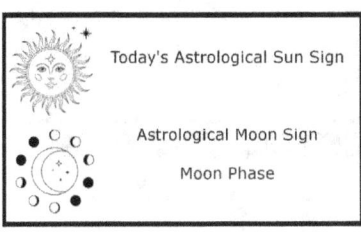

Today's Astrological Sun Sign

Astrological Moon Sign

Moon Phase

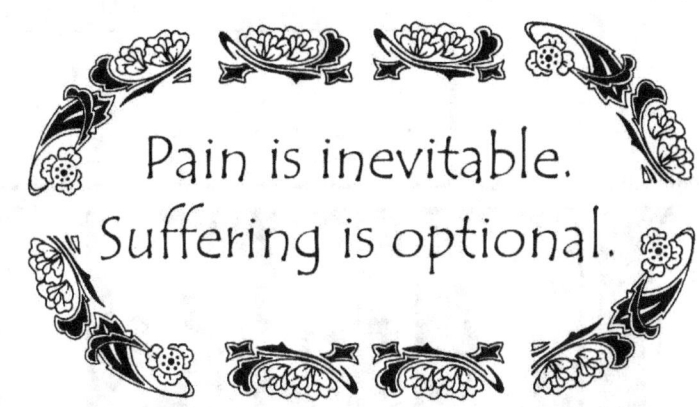

Pain is inevitable. Suffering is optional.

Notes

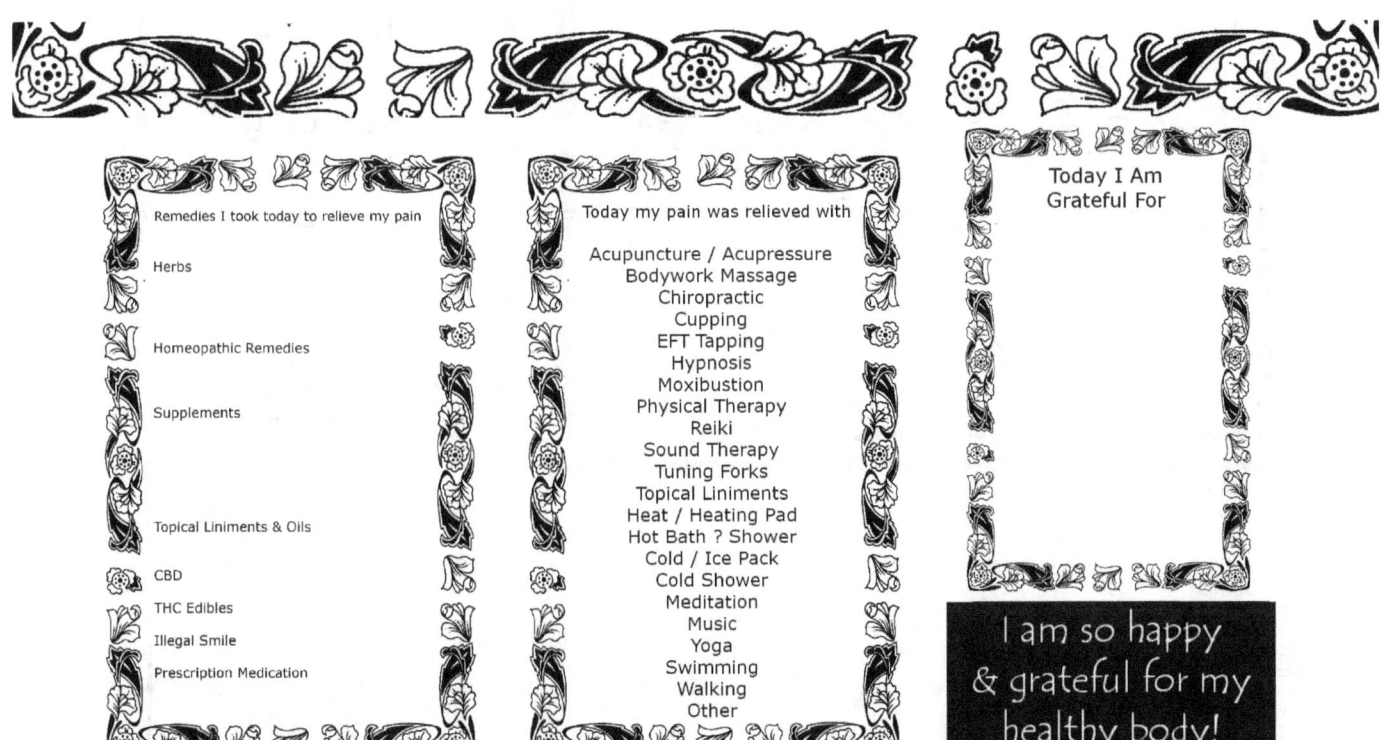

Remedies I took today to relieve my pain

Herbs

Homeopathic Remedies

Supplements

Topical Liniments & Oils

CBD

THC Edibles

Illegal Smile

Prescription Medication

Today my pain was relieved with

Acupuncture / Acupressure
Bodywork Massage
Chiropractic
Cupping
EFT Tapping
Hypnosis
Moxibustion
Physical Therapy
Reiki
Sound Therapy
Tuning Forks
Topical Liniments
Heat / Heating Pad
Hot Bath ? Shower
Cold / Ice Pack
Cold Shower
Meditation
Music
Yoga
Swimming
Walking
Other

Today I Am Grateful For

I am so happy & grateful for my healthy body!

Today's Day & Date

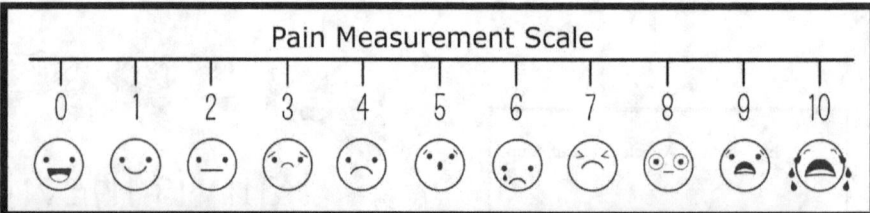

Highlight All Painful Areas

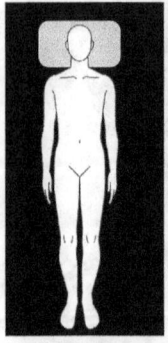 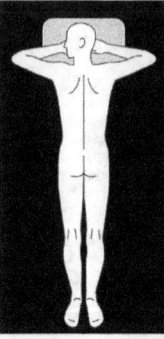 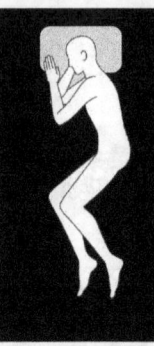 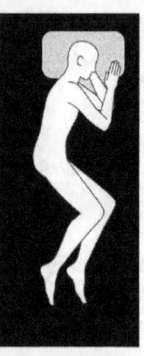

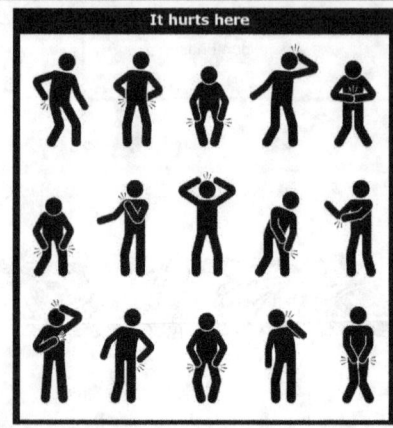

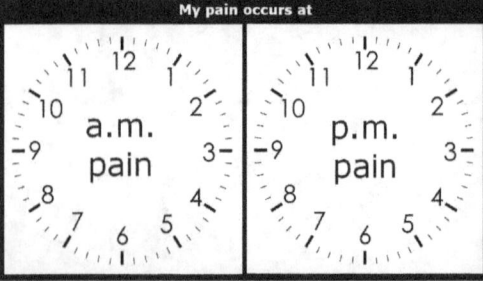

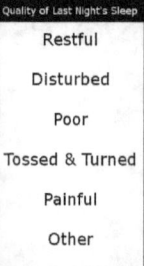

Quality of Last Night's Sleep
- Restful
- Disturbed
- Poor
- Tossed & Turned
- Painful
- Other

My pain is
Hot
Burning
Cold
Stabbing
Throbbing
Fixed
Moving Traveling
Constant
On & Off

Today's Weather

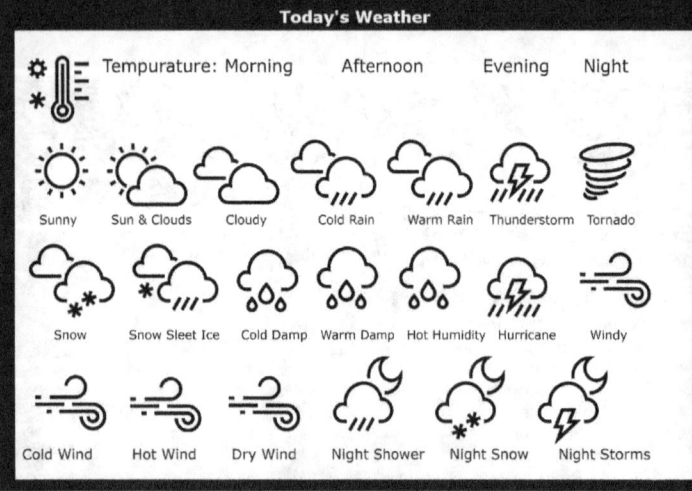

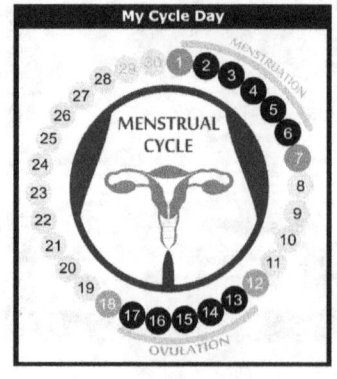

Breakfast

Lunch

Dinner

Snacks

Alcohol

Food Allergy Triggers

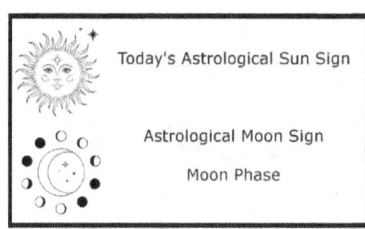

Today's Astrological Sun Sign

Astrological Moon Sign

Moon Phase

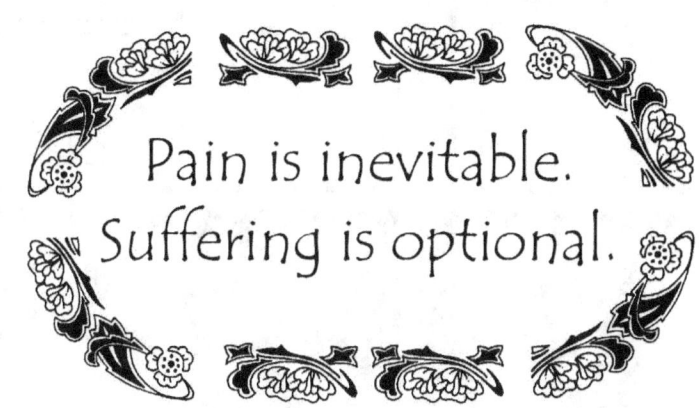

Pain is inevitable.
Suffering is optional.

Notes

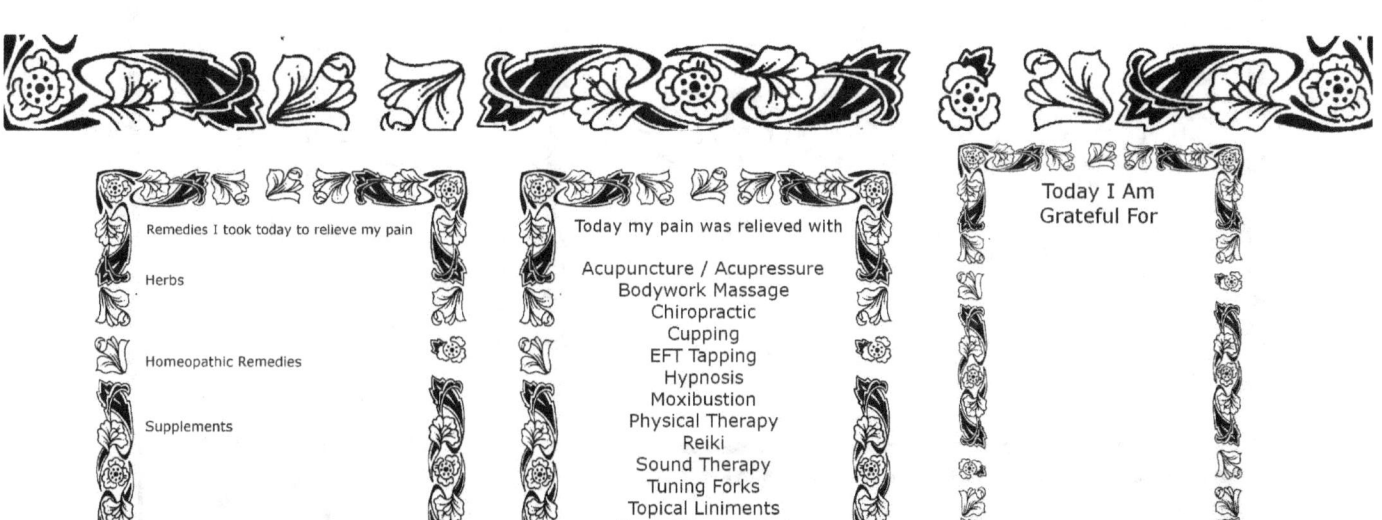

Remedies I took today to relieve my pain

Herbs

Homeopathic Remedies

Supplements

Topical Liniments & Oils

CBD

THC Edibles

Illegal Smile

Prescription Medication

Today my pain was relieved with

Acupuncture / Acupressure
Bodywork Massage
Chiropractic
Cupping
EFT Tapping
Hypnosis
Moxibustion
Physical Therapy
Reiki
Sound Therapy
Tuning Forks
Topical Liniments
Heat / Heating Pad
Hot Bath ? Shower
Cold / Ice Pack
Cold Shower
Meditation
Music
Yoga
Swimming
Walking
Other

Today I Am Grateful For

I am so happy & grateful for my healthy body!

Today's Day & Date

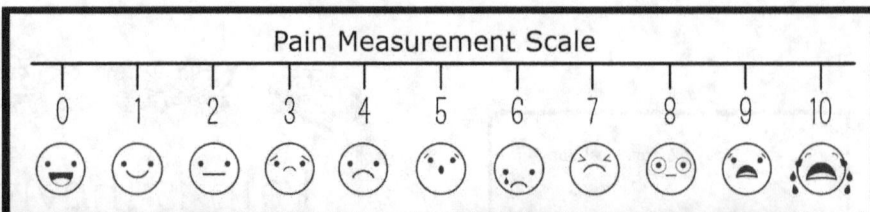

Highlight All Painful Areas

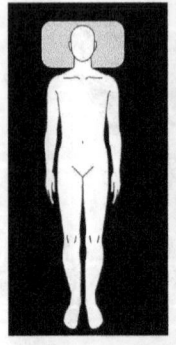 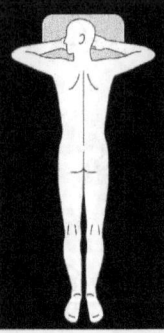 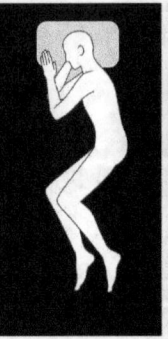 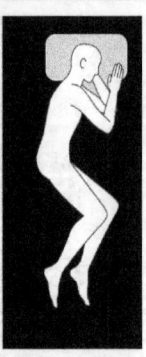

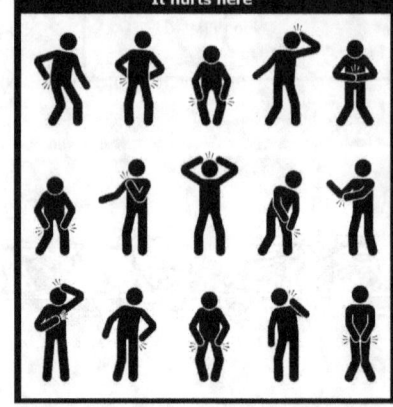
It hurts here

My pain occurs at

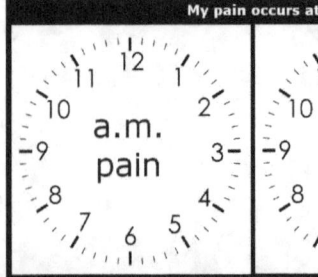

a.m. pain — p.m. pain

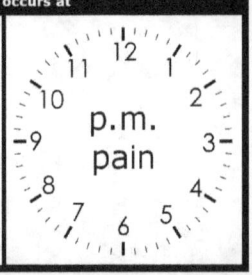

Quality of Last Night's Sleep
- Restful
- Disturbed
- Poor
- Tossed & Turned
- Painful
- Other

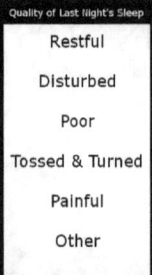
My mood today

My pain is
Hot
Burning
Cold
Stabbing
Throbbing
Fixed
Moving Traveling
Constant
On & Off

Today's Weather

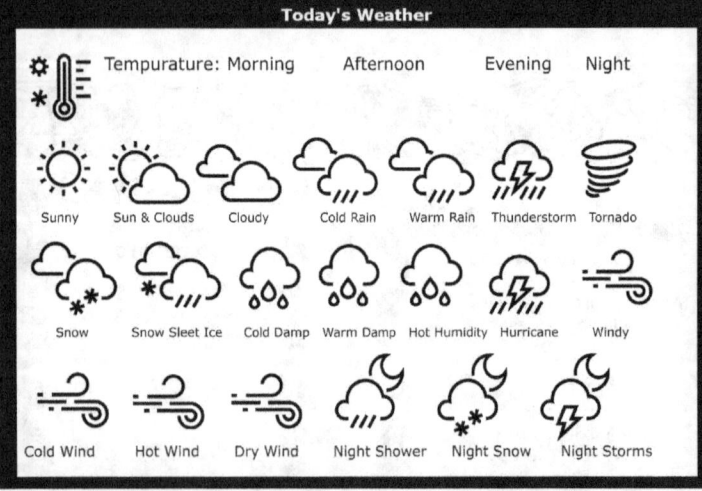

Temperature: Morning   Afternoon   Evening   Night

Sunny · Sun & Clouds · Cloudy · Cold Rain · Warm Rain · Thunderstorm · Tornado
Snow · Snow Sleet Ice · Cold Damp · Warm Damp · Hot Humidity · Hurricane · Windy
Cold Wind · Hot Wind · Dry Wind · Night Shower · Night Snow · Night Storms

Breakfast

Lunch

Dinner

Snacks

Alcohol

Food Allergy Triggers

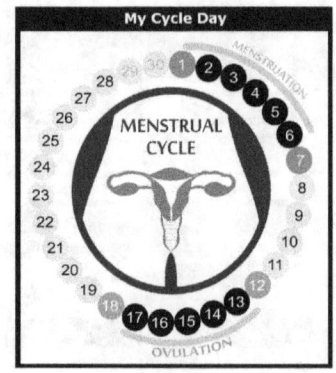
My Cycle Day

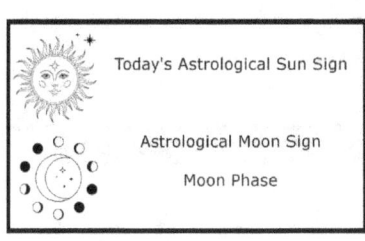

Today's Astrological Sun Sign

Astrological Moon Sign

Moon Phase

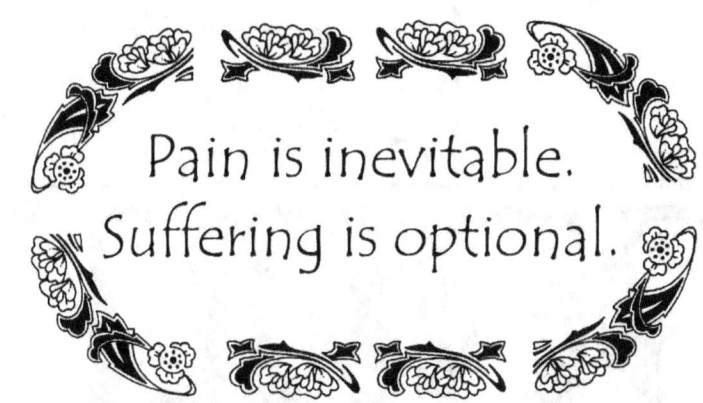

Pain is inevitable. Suffering is optional.

Notes

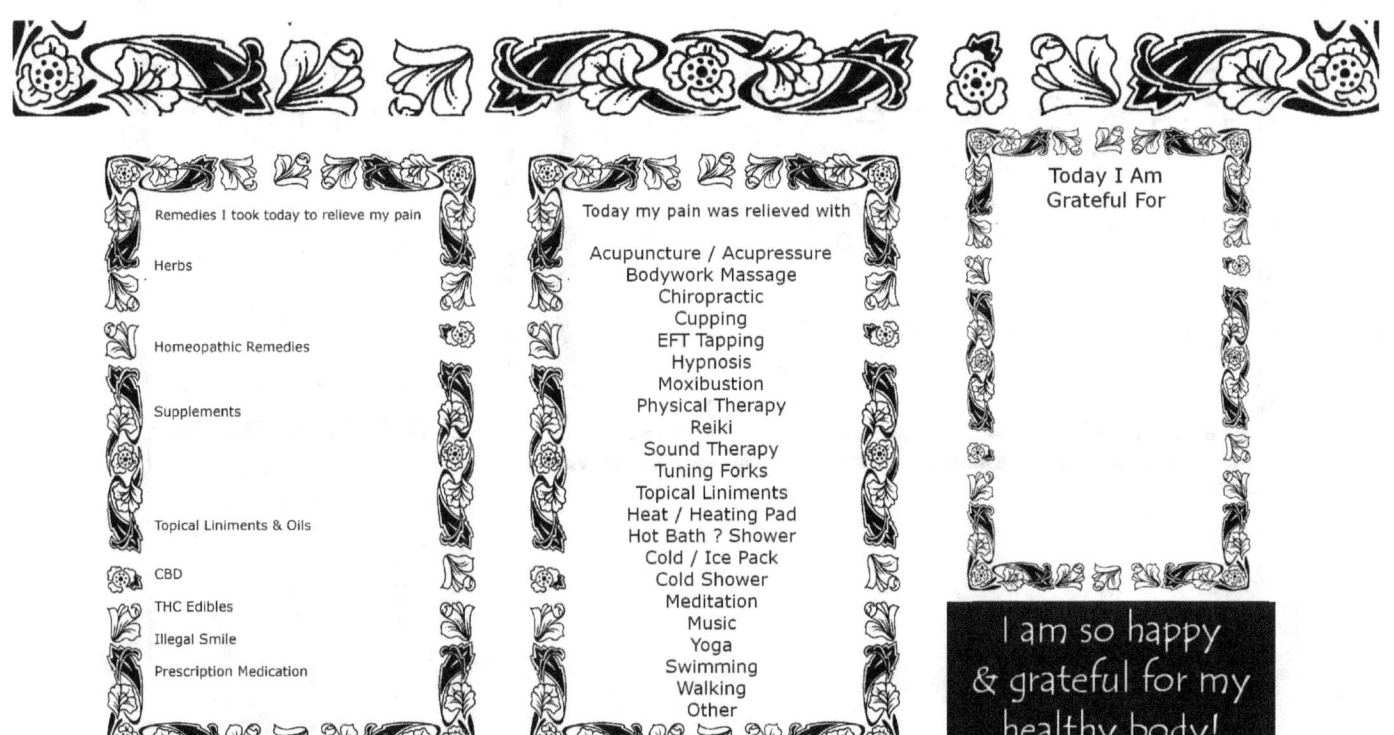

Remedies I took today to relieve my pain

Herbs

Homeopathic Remedies

Supplements

Topical Liniments & Oils

CBD

THC Edibles

Illegal Smile

Prescription Medication

Today my pain was relieved with

Acupuncture / Acupressure
Bodywork Massage
Chiropractic
Cupping
EFT Tapping
Hypnosis
Moxibustion
Physical Therapy
Reiki
Sound Therapy
Tuning Forks
Topical Liniments
Heat / Heating Pad
Hot Bath ? Shower
Cold / Ice Pack
Cold Shower
Meditation
Music
Yoga
Swimming
Walking
Other

Today I Am Grateful For

I am so happy & grateful for my healthy body!

Today's Day & Date

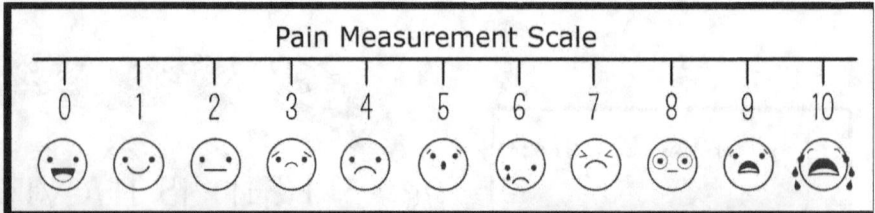

Highlight All Painful Areas

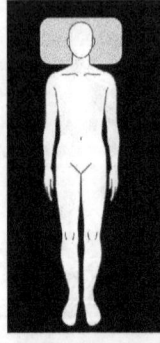 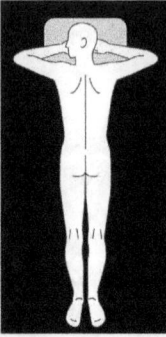 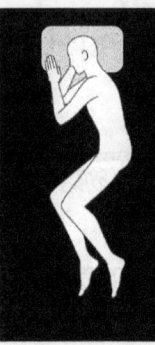 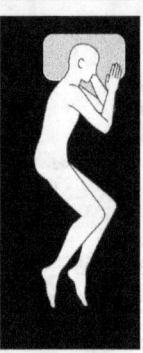

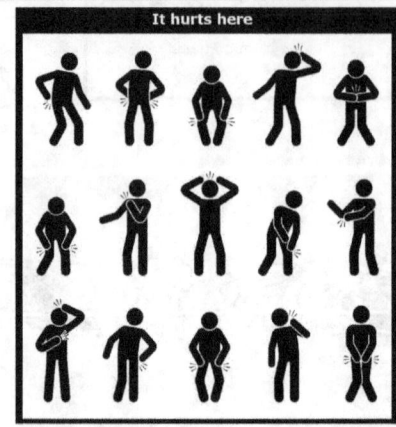
It hurts here

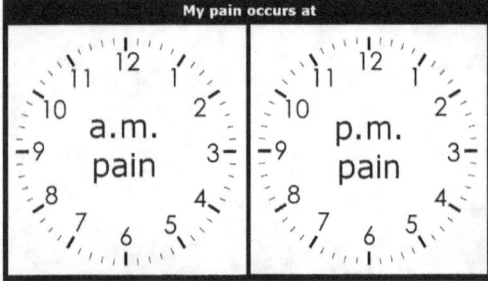
My pain occurs at — a.m. pain / p.m. pain

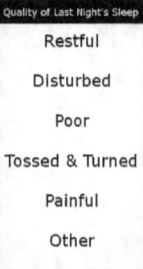
Quality of Last Night's Sleep
- Restful
- Disturbed
- Poor
- Tossed & Turned
- Painful
- Other

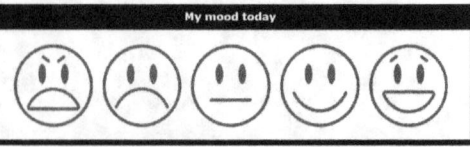
My mood today

My pain is
Hot
Burning
Cold
Stabbing
Throbbing
Fixed
Moving Traveling
Constant
On & Off

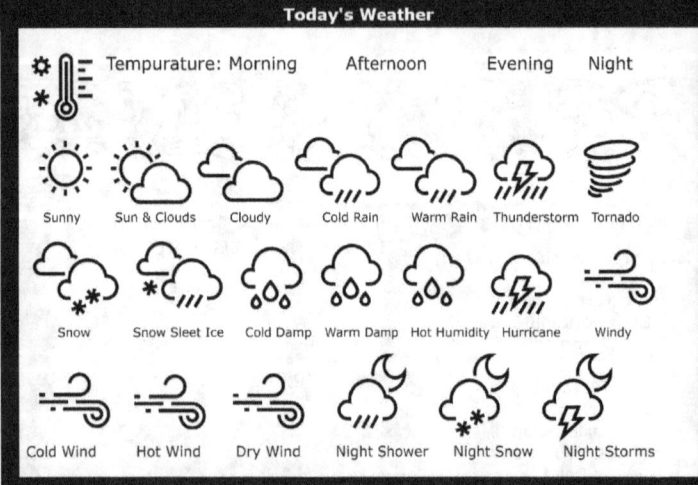
Today's Weather — Temperature: Morning, Afternoon, Evening, Night

Breakfast

Lunch

Dinner

Snacks

Alcohol

Food Allergy Triggers

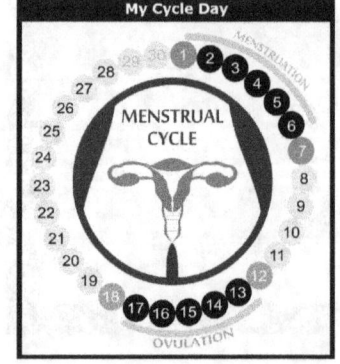
My Cycle Day

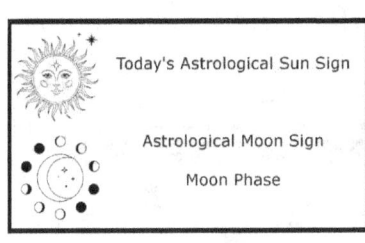

Today's Astrological Sun Sign

Astrological Moon Sign

Moon Phase

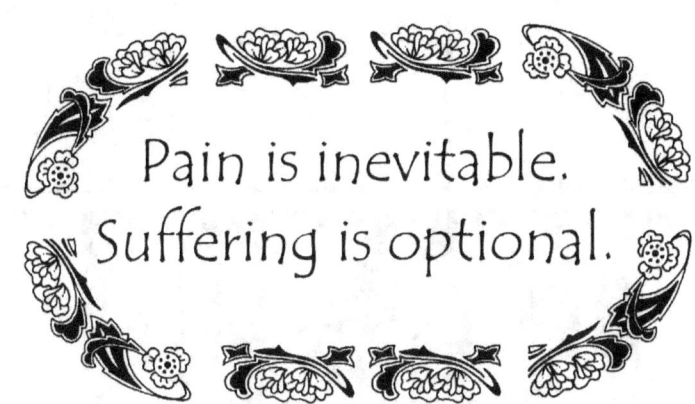

Pain is inevitable.
Suffering is optional.

Notes

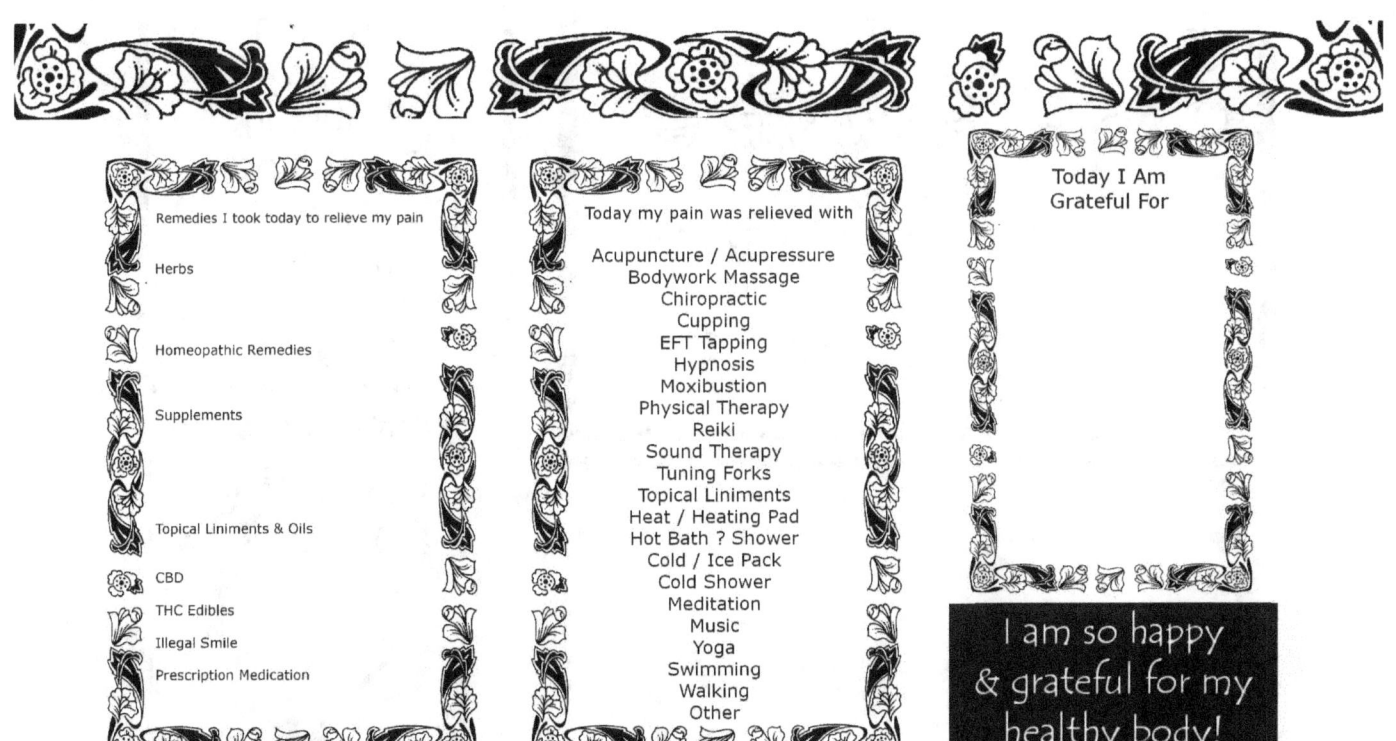

Remedies I took today to relieve my pain

Herbs

Homeopathic Remedies

Supplements

Topical Liniments & Oils

CBD

THC Edibles

Illegal Smile

Prescription Medication

Today my pain was relieved with

Acupuncture / Acupressure
Bodywork Massage
Chiropractic
Cupping
EFT Tapping
Hypnosis
Moxibustion
Physical Therapy
Reiki
Sound Therapy
Tuning Forks
Topical Liniments
Heat / Heating Pad
Hot Bath ? Shower
Cold / Ice Pack
Cold Shower
Meditation
Music
Yoga
Swimming
Walking
Other

Today I Am Grateful For

I am so happy & grateful for my healthy body!

Today's Day & Date

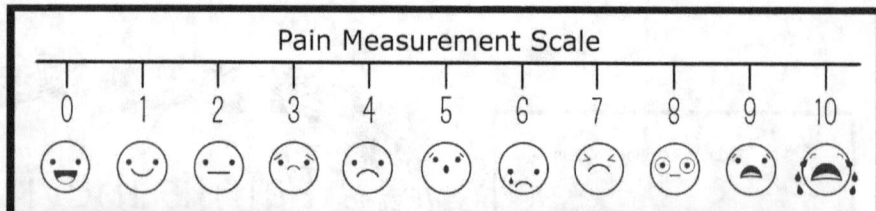

Highlight All Painful Areas

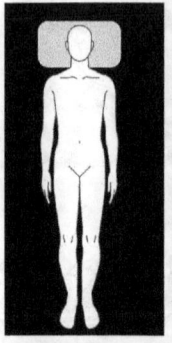
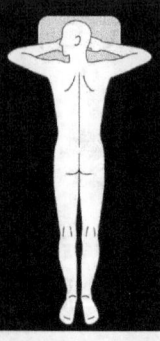
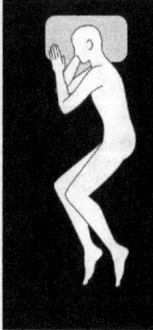
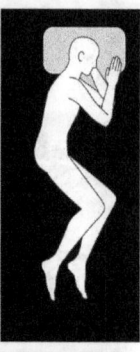

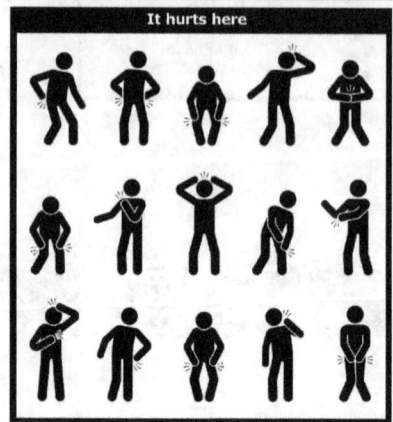

My pain occurs at

a.m. pain | p.m. pain

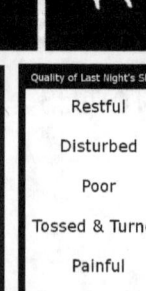

Quality of Last Night's Sleep
- Restful
- Disturbed
- Poor
- Tossed & Turned
- Painful
- Other

My pain is
Hot
Burning
Cold
Stabbing
Throbbing
Fixed
Moving Traveling
Constant
On & Off

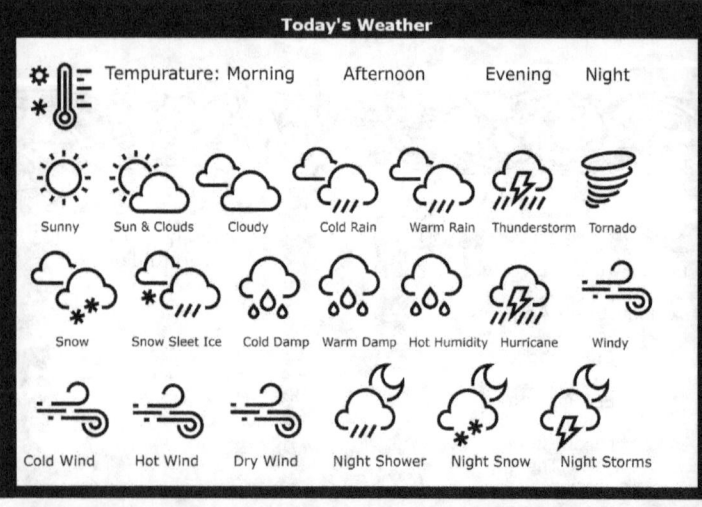

Breakfast

Lunch

Dinner

Snacks

Alcohol

Food Allergy Triggers

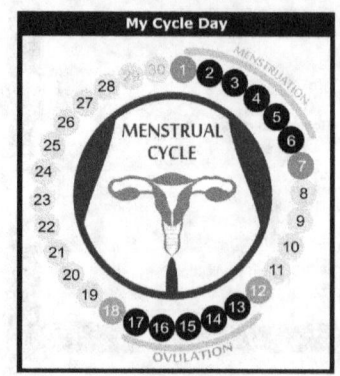

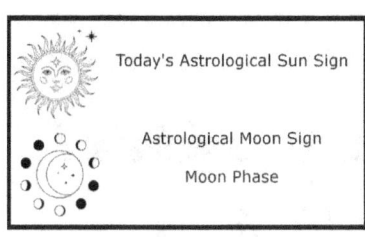

Today's Astrological Sun Sign

Astrological Moon Sign

Moon Phase

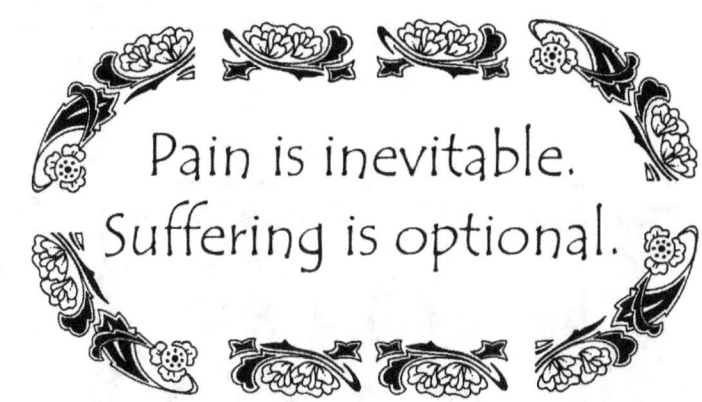

Pain is inevitable.
Suffering is optional.

Notes

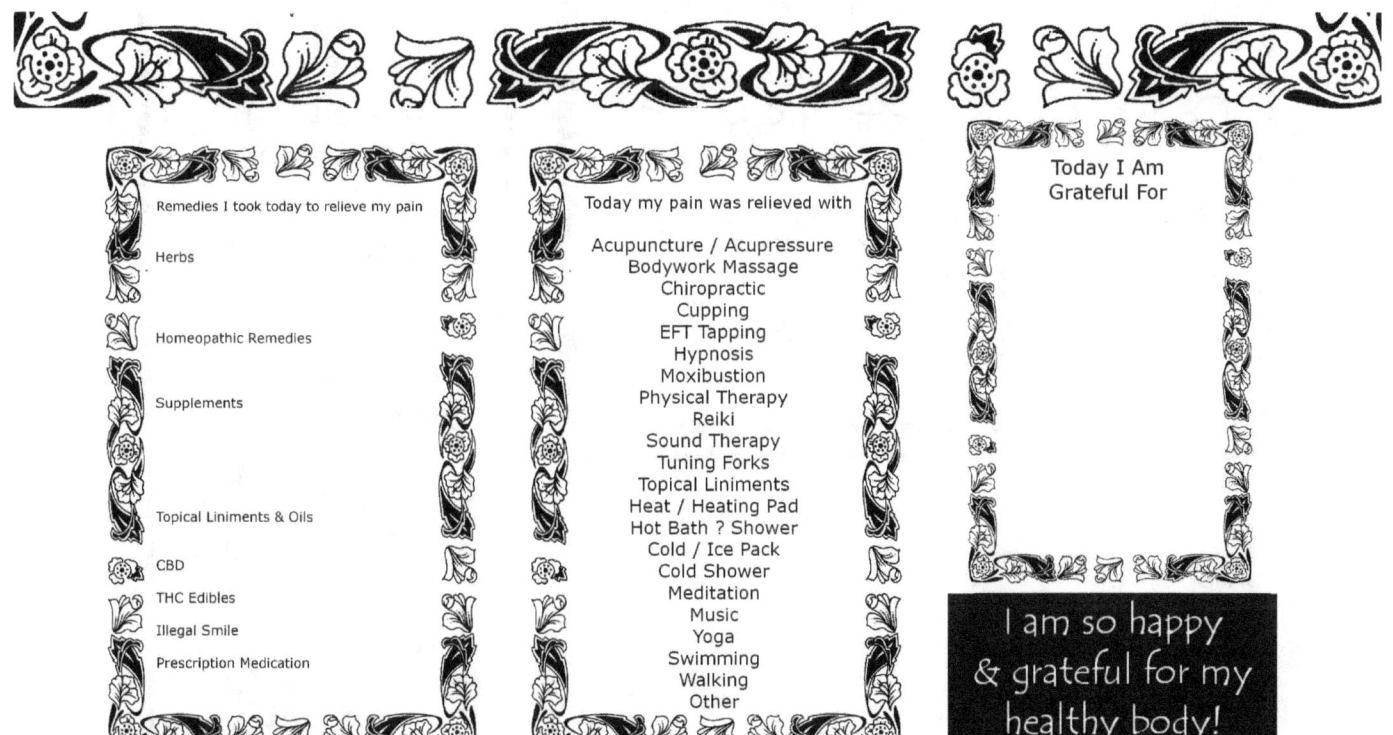

Remedies I took today to relieve my pain

Herbs

Homeopathic Remedies

Supplements

Topical Liniments & Oils

CBD
THC Edibles
Illegal Smile
Prescription Medication

Today my pain was relieved with

Acupuncture / Acupressure
Bodywork Massage
Chiropractic
Cupping
EFT Tapping
Hypnosis
Moxibustion
Physical Therapy
Reiki
Sound Therapy
Tuning Forks
Topical Liniments
Heat / Heating Pad
Hot Bath ? Shower
Cold / Ice Pack
Cold Shower
Meditation
Music
Yoga
Swimming
Walking
Other

Today I Am Grateful For

I am so happy & grateful for my healthy body!

Today's Day & Date

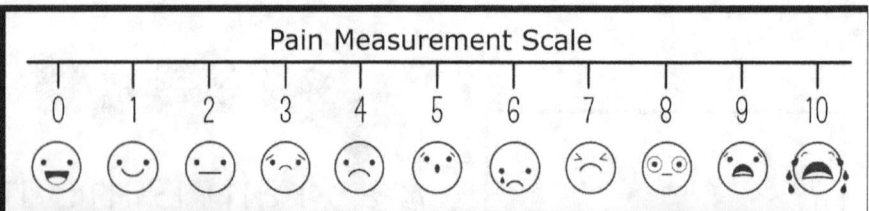

Highlight All Painful Areas

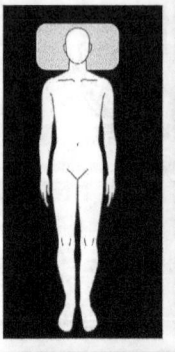 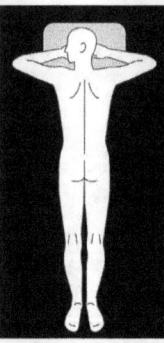 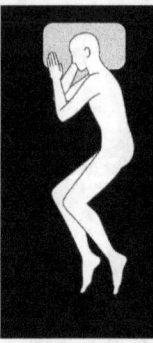 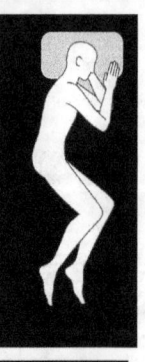

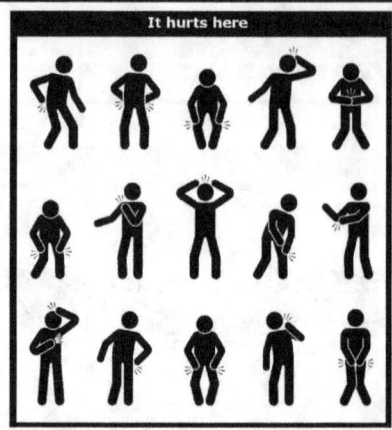

It hurts here

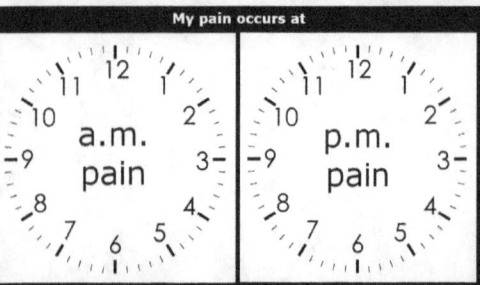

My pain occurs at — a.m. pain / p.m. pain

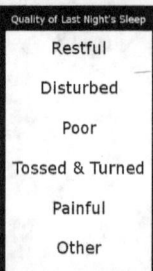

Quality of Last Night's Sleep
- Restful
- Disturbed
- Poor
- Tossed & Turned
- Painful
- Other

My mood today

My pain is

Hot
Burning
Cold
Stabbing
Throbbing
Fixed
Moving Traveling
Constant
On & Off

Today's Weather

Tempurature: Morning   Afternoon   Evening   Night

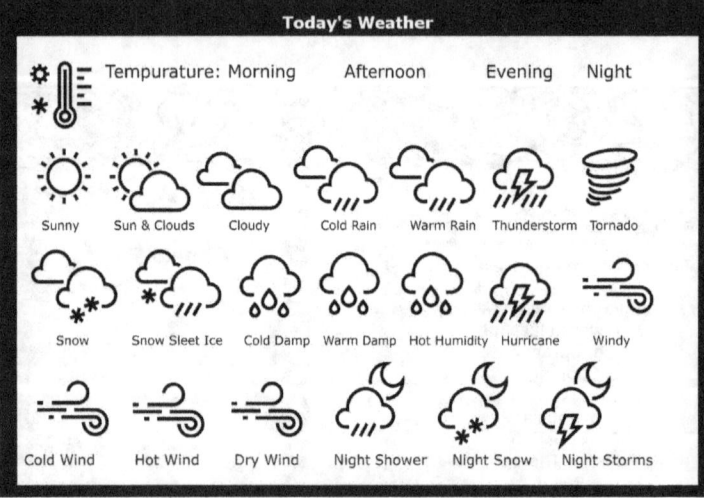

Breakfast

Lunch

Dinner

Snacks

Alcohol

Food Allergy Triggers

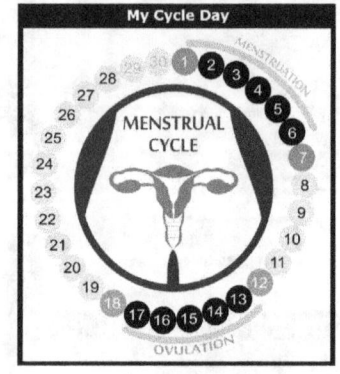

My Cycle Day

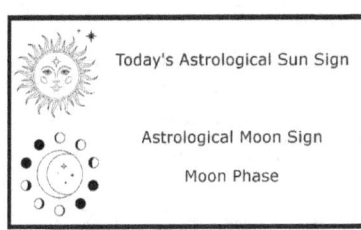

Today's Astrological Sun Sign

Astrological Moon Sign
Moon Phase

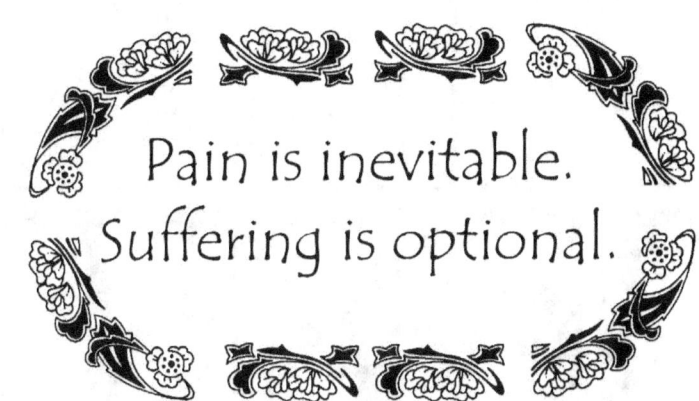

Pain is inevitable.
Suffering is optional.

Notes

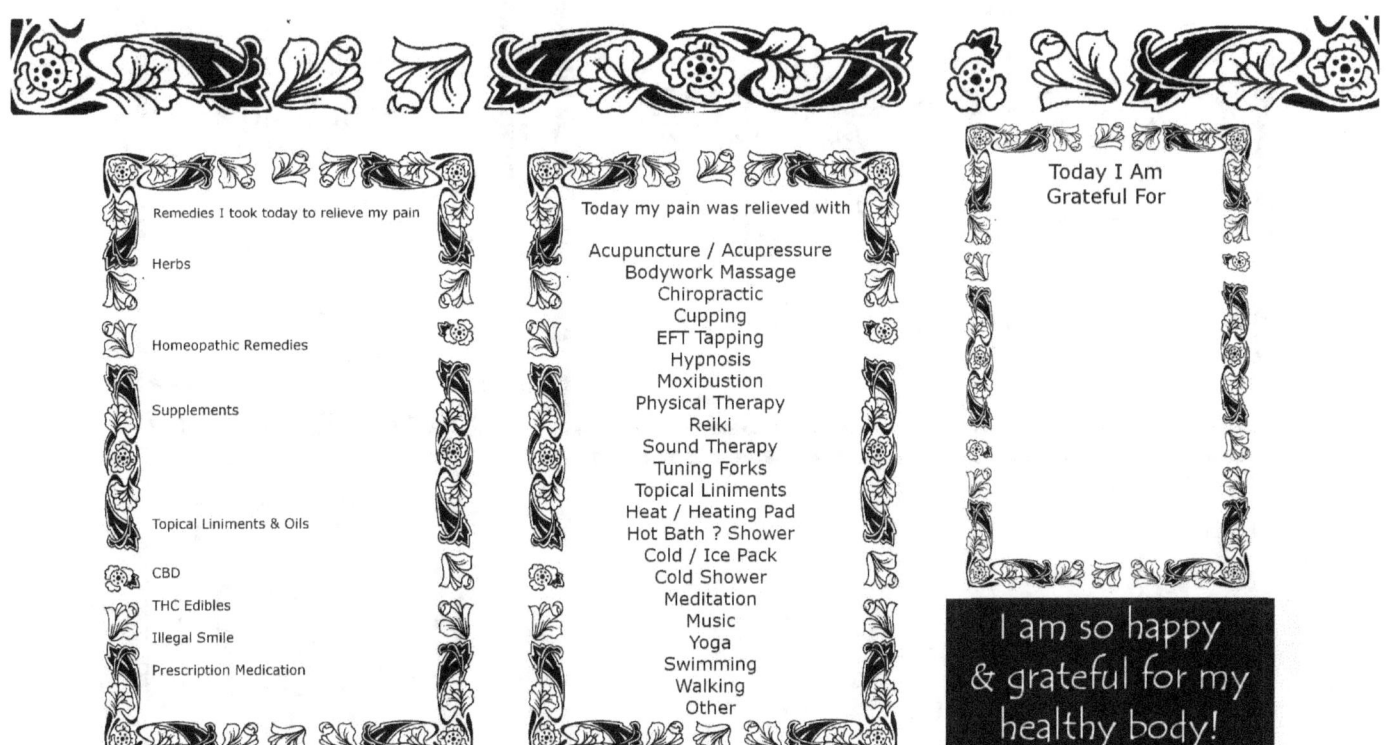

Remedies I took today to relieve my pain

Herbs

Homeopathic Remedies

Supplements

Topical Liniments & Oils

CBD
THC Edibles
Illegal Smile
Prescription Medication

Today my pain was relieved with

Acupuncture / Acupressure
Bodywork Massage
Chiropractic
Cupping
EFT Tapping
Hypnosis
Moxibustion
Physical Therapy
Reiki
Sound Therapy
Tuning Forks
Topical Liniments
Heat / Heating Pad
Hot Bath ? Shower
Cold / Ice Pack
Cold Shower
Meditation
Music
Yoga
Swimming
Walking
Other

Today I Am Grateful For

I am so happy & grateful for my healthy body!

Today's Day & Date

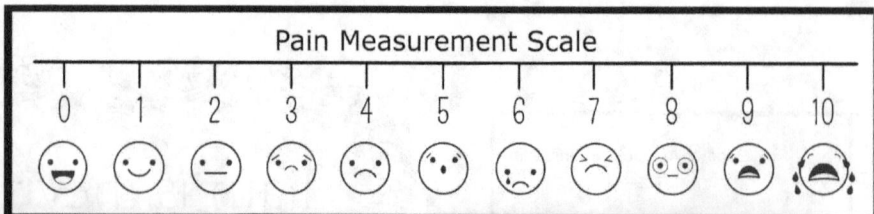

Highlight All Painful Areas

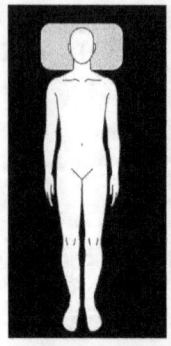 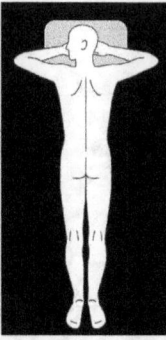 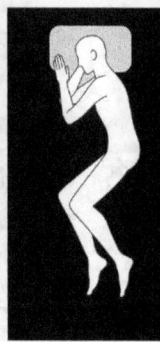 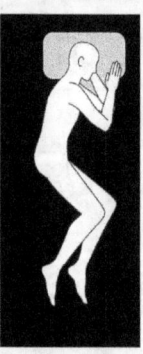

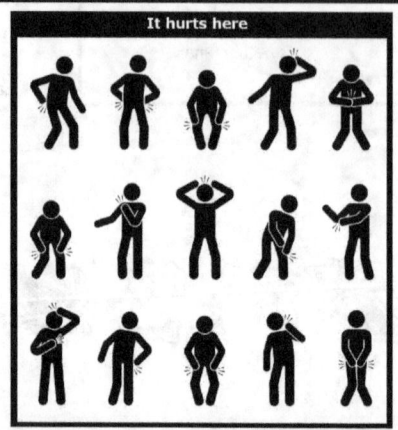
It hurts here

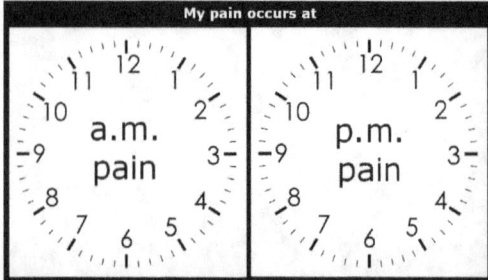
My pain occurs at — a.m. pain / p.m. pain

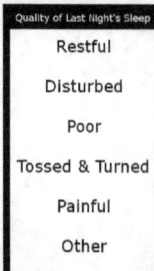

Quality of Last Night's Sleep
- Restful
- Disturbed
- Poor
- Tossed & Turned
- Painful
- Other

My mood today

My pain is
Hot
Burning
Cold
Stabbing
Throbbing
Fixed
Moving Traveling
Constant
On & Off

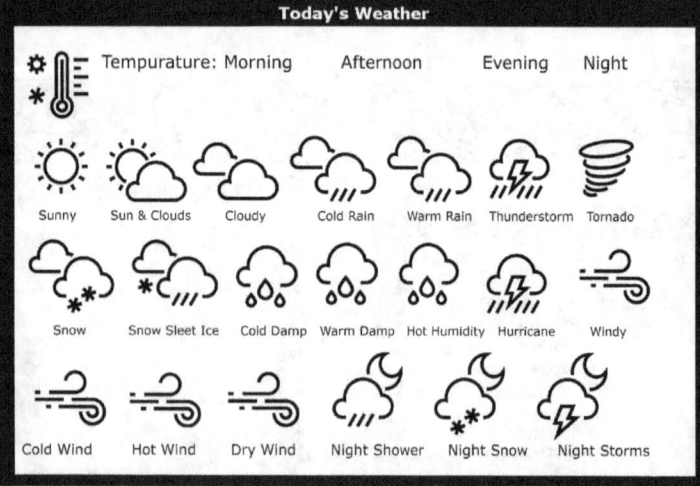
Today's Weather — Temperature: Morning, Afternoon, Evening, Night

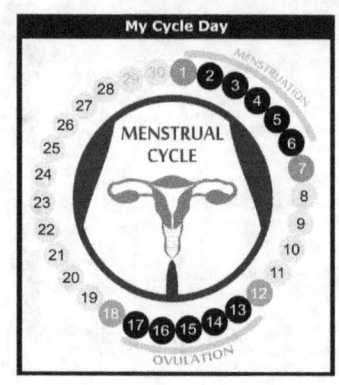
My Cycle Day

Breakfast

Lunch

Dinner

Snacks

Alcohol

Food Allergy Triggers

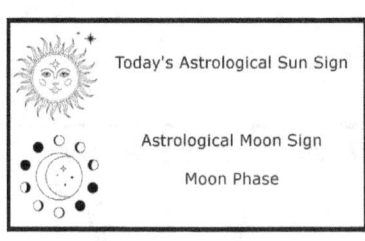

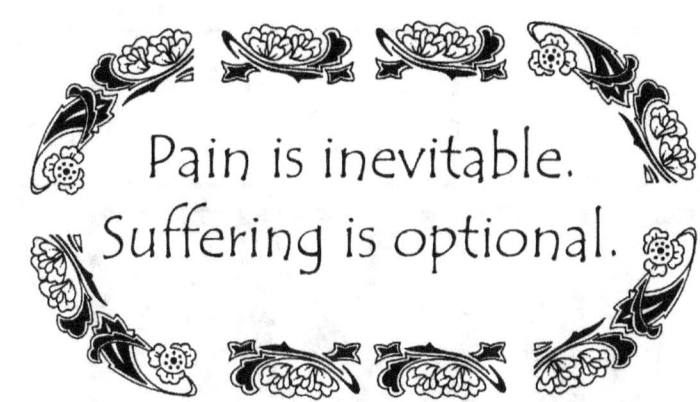

Today's Astrological Sun Sign

Astrological Moon Sign

Moon Phase

Pain is inevitable. Suffering is optional.

Notes

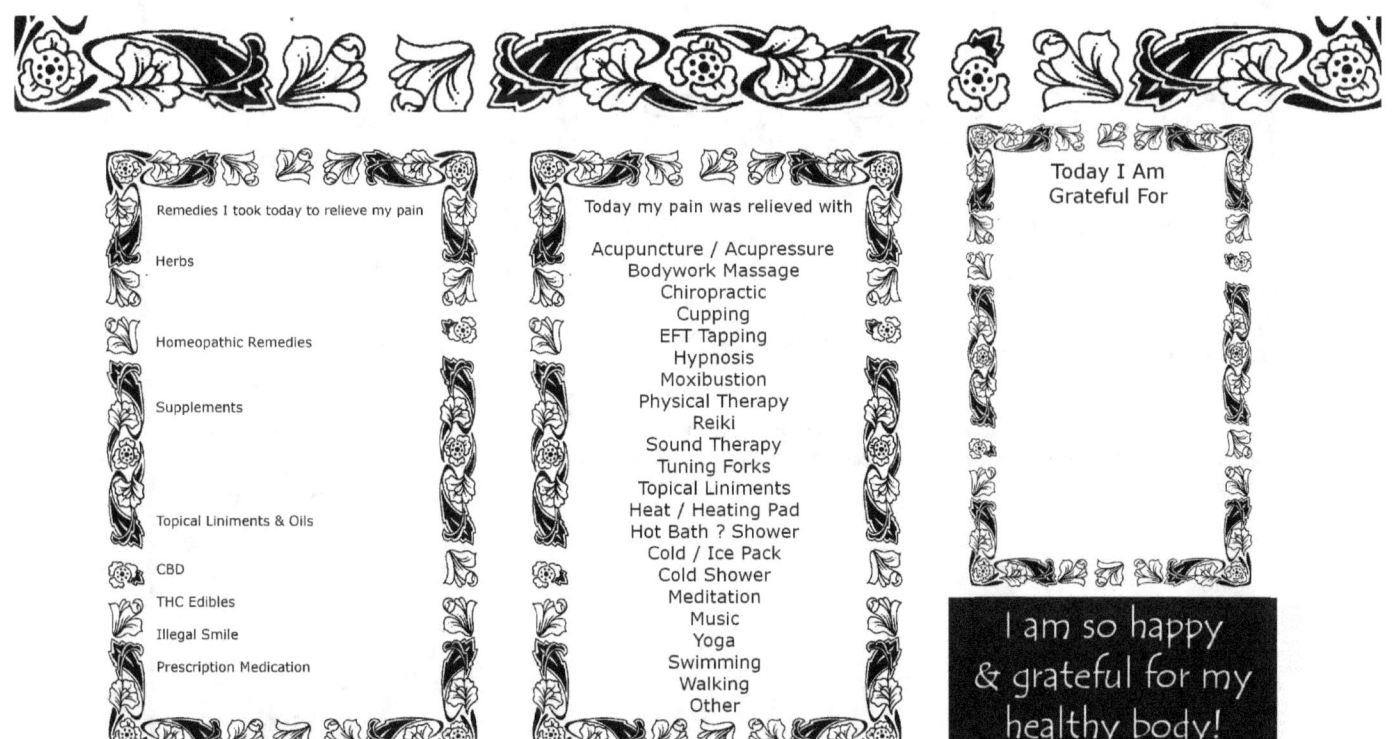

Remedies I took today to relieve my pain

Herbs

Homeopathic Remedies

Supplements

Topical Liniments & Oils

CBD

THC Edibles

Illegal Smile

Prescription Medication

Today my pain was relieved with

Acupuncture / Acupressure
Bodywork Massage
Chiropractic
Cupping
EFT Tapping
Hypnosis
Moxibustion
Physical Therapy
Reiki
Sound Therapy
Tuning Forks
Topical Liniments
Heat / Heating Pad
Hot Bath ? Shower
Cold / Ice Pack
Cold Shower
Meditation
Music
Yoga
Swimming
Walking
Other

Today I Am Grateful For

I am so happy & grateful for my healthy body!

Today's Day & Date

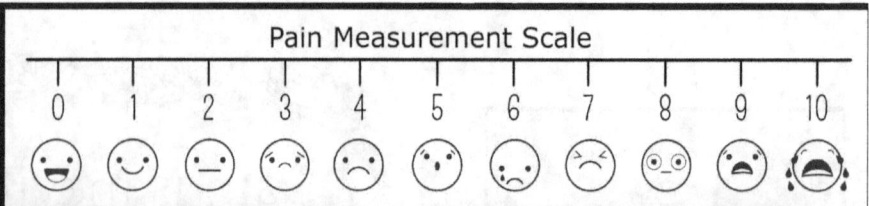

Highlight All Painful Areas

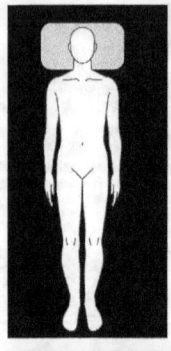 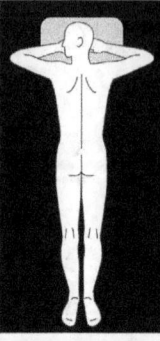 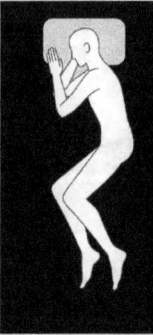 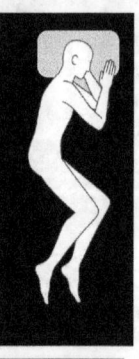

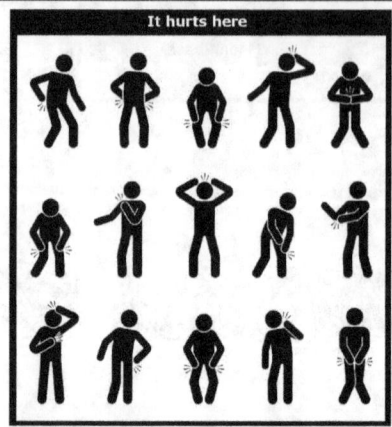
It hurts here

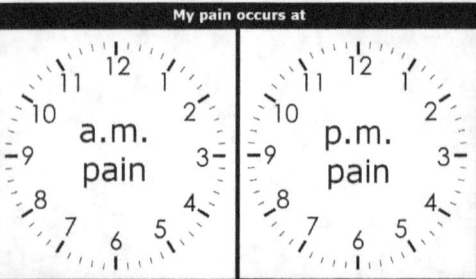
My pain occurs at — a.m. pain / p.m. pain

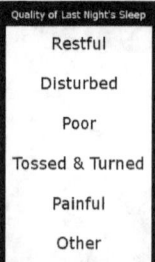
Quality of Last Night's Sleep
- Restful
- Disturbed
- Poor
- Tossed & Turned
- Painful
- Other

My mood today

My pain is
Hot
Burning
Cold
Stabbing
Throbbing
Fixed
Moving Traveling
Constant
On & Off

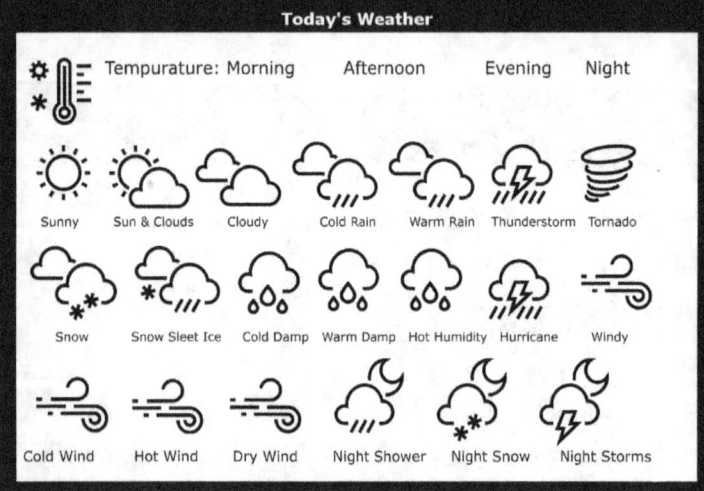
Today's Weather — Temperature: Morning, Afternoon, Evening, Night

Sunny, Sun & Clouds, Cloudy, Cold Rain, Warm Rain, Thunderstorm, Tornado, Snow, Snow Sleet Ice, Cold Damp, Warm Damp, Hot Humidity, Hurricane, Windy, Cold Wind, Hot Wind, Dry Wind, Night Shower, Night Snow, Night Storms

Breakfast

Lunch

Dinner

Snacks

Alcohol

Food Allergy Triggers

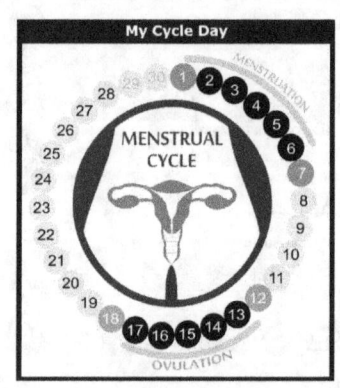
My Cycle Day

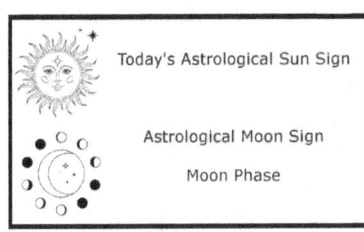

Today's Astrological Sun Sign

Astrological Moon Sign
Moon Phase

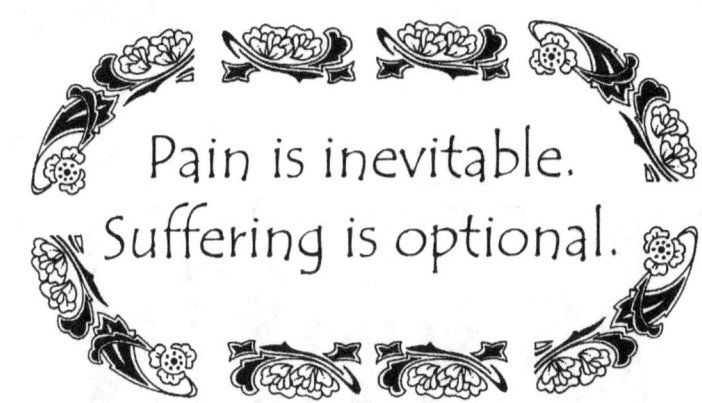

Pain is inevitable.
Suffering is optional.

Notes

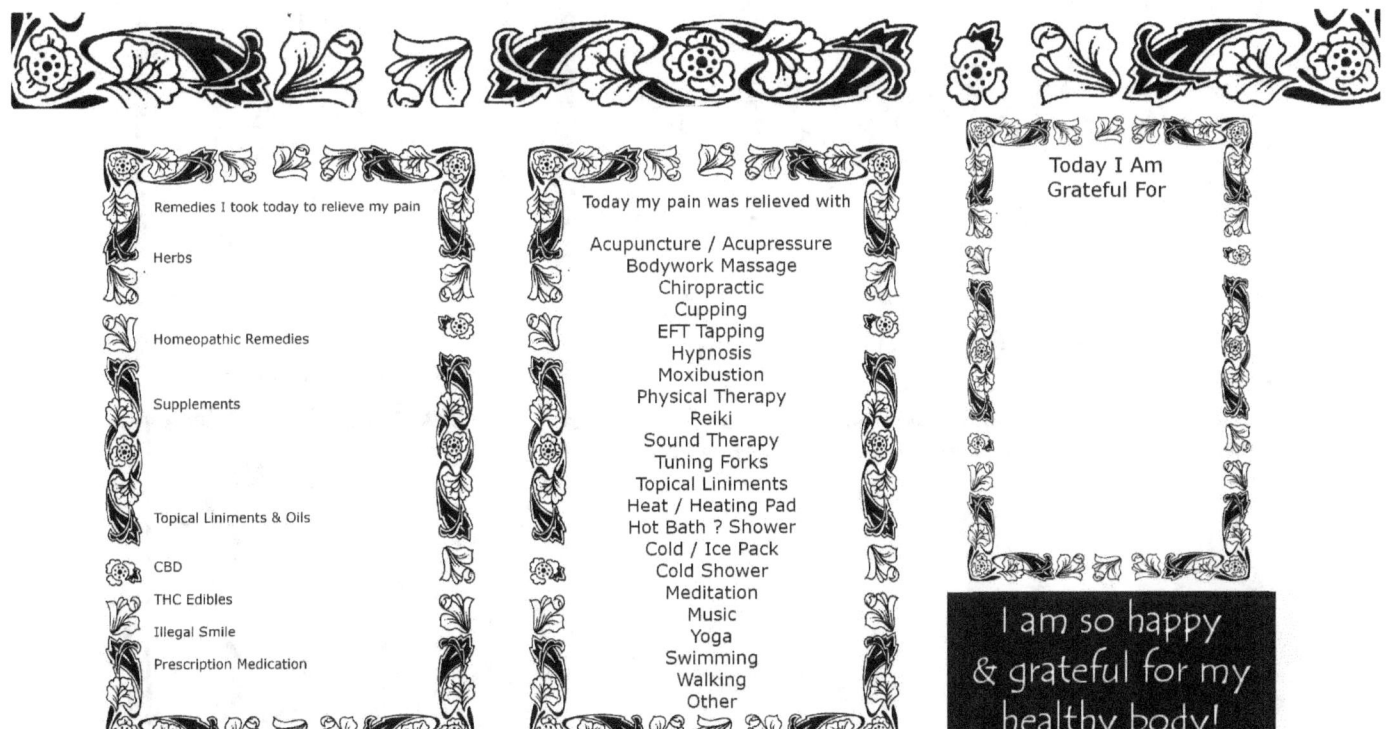

Remedies I took today to relieve my pain

Herbs

Homeopathic Remedies

Supplements

Topical Liniments & Oils

CBD
THC Edibles
Illegal Smile
Prescription Medication

Today my pain was relieved with

Acupuncture / Acupressure
Bodywork Massage
Chiropractic
Cupping
EFT Tapping
Hypnosis
Moxibustion
Physical Therapy
Reiki
Sound Therapy
Tuning Forks
Topical Liniments
Heat / Heating Pad
Hot Bath ? Shower
Cold / Ice Pack
Cold Shower
Meditation
Music
Yoga
Swimming
Walking
Other

Today I Am Grateful For

I am so happy & grateful for my healthy body!

Today's Day & Date

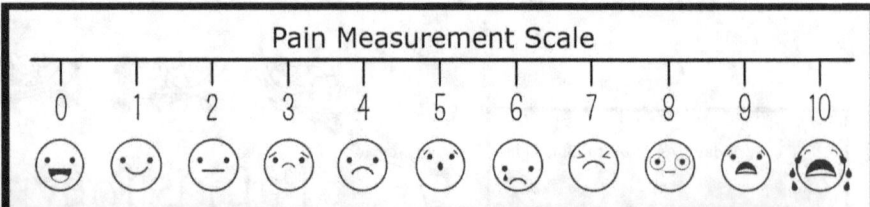

Highlight All Painful Areas

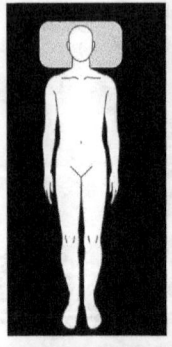 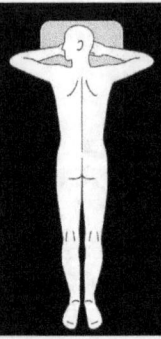 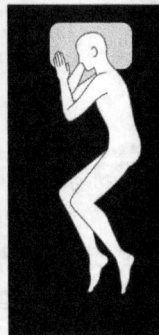 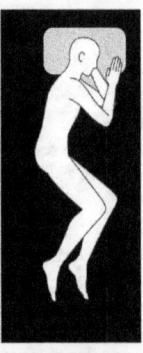

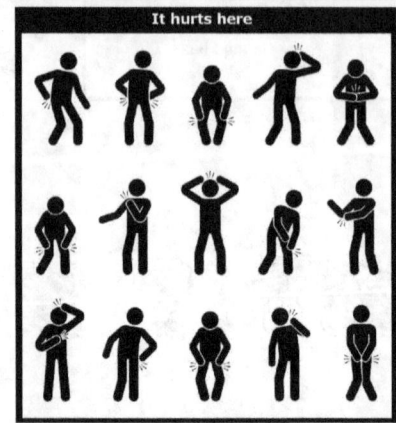
It hurts here

My pain occurs at

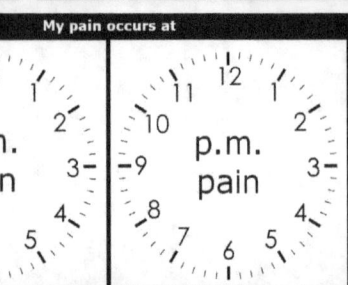

a.m. pain | p.m. pain

Quality of Last Night's Sleep
- Restful
- Disturbed
- Poor
- Tossed & Turned
- Painful
- Other

My mood today

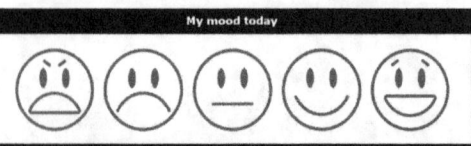

My pain is
Hot
Burning
Cold
Stabbing
Throbbing
Fixed
Moving Traveling
Constant
On & Off

Today's Weather

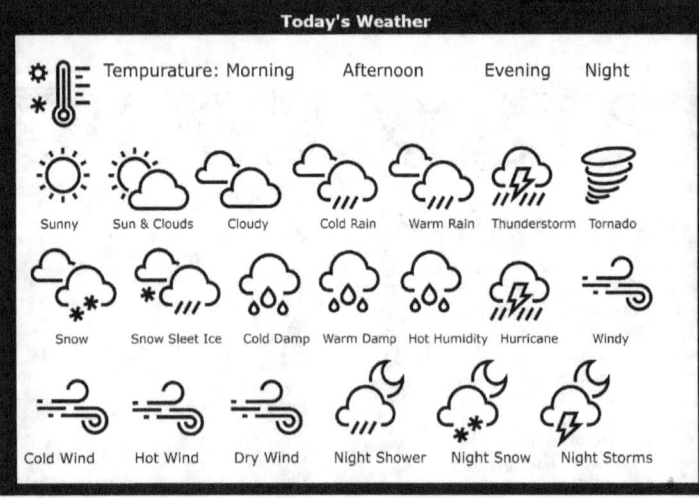

Temperature: Morning Afternoon Evening Night

Sunny | Sun & Clouds | Cloudy | Cold Rain | Warm Rain | Thunderstorm | Tornado
Snow | Snow Sleet Ice | Cold Damp | Warm Damp | Hot Humidity | Hurricane | Windy
Cold Wind | Hot Wind | Dry Wind | Night Shower | Night Snow | Night Storms

Breakfast

Lunch

Dinner

Snacks

Alcohol

Food Allergy Triggers

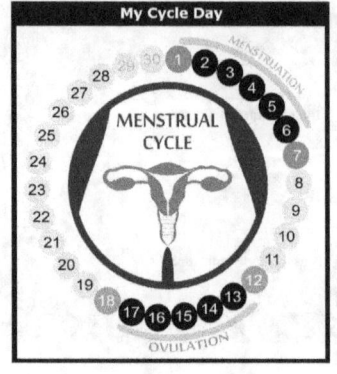

My Cycle Day

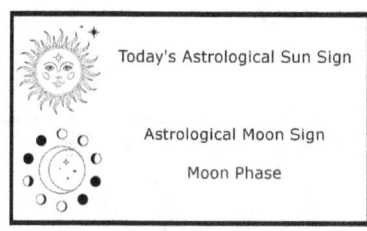

Today's Astrological Sun Sign

Astrological Moon Sign
Moon Phase

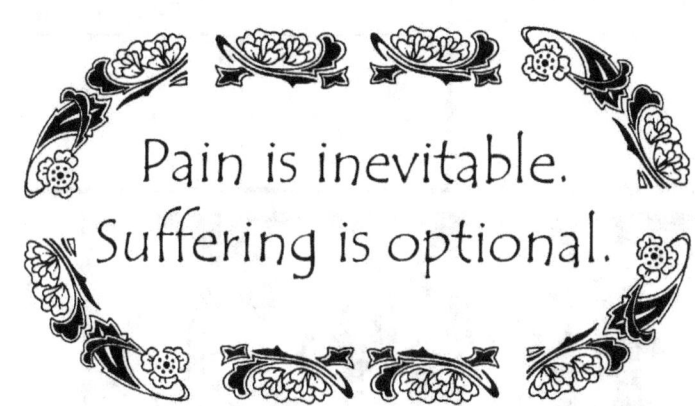

Pain is inevitable.
Suffering is optional.

Notes

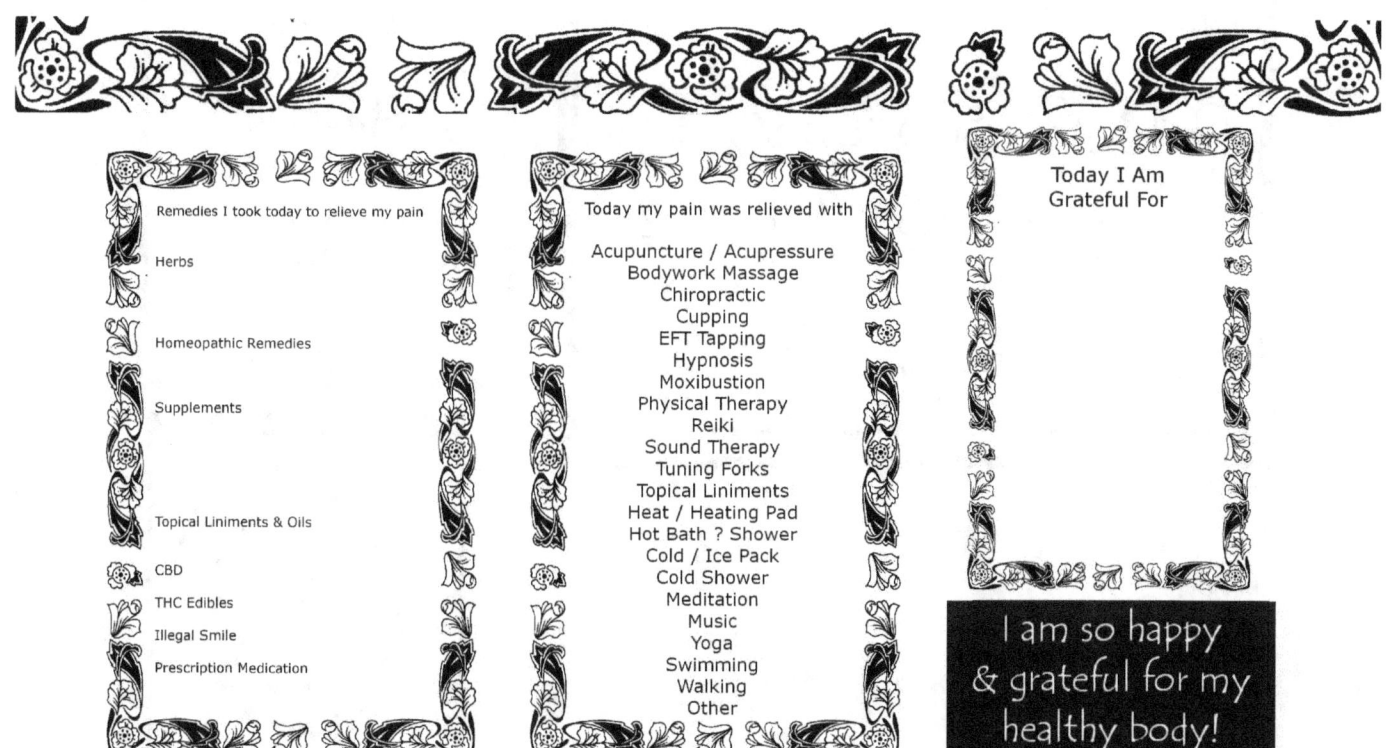

Remedies I took today to relieve my pain

Herbs

Homeopathic Remedies

Supplements

Topical Liniments & Oils

CBD

THC Edibles

Illegal Smile

Prescription Medication

Today my pain was relieved with

Acupuncture / Acupressure
Bodywork Massage
Chiropractic
Cupping
EFT Tapping
Hypnosis
Moxibustion
Physical Therapy
Reiki
Sound Therapy
Tuning Forks
Topical Liniments
Heat / Heating Pad
Hot Bath ? Shower
Cold / Ice Pack
Cold Shower
Meditation
Music
Yoga
Swimming
Walking
Other

Today I Am Grateful For

I am so happy & grateful for my healthy body!

Today's Day & Date

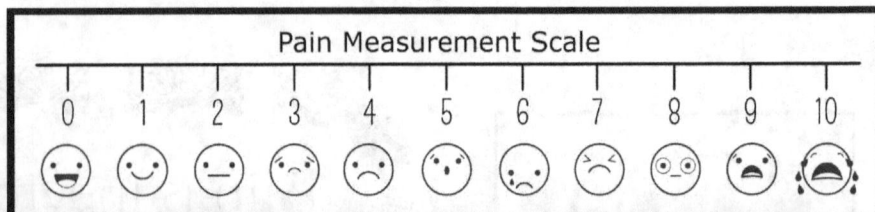

Highlight All Painful Areas

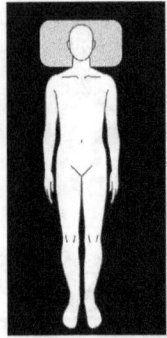 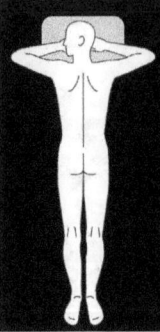 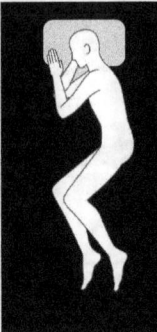 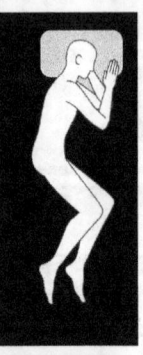

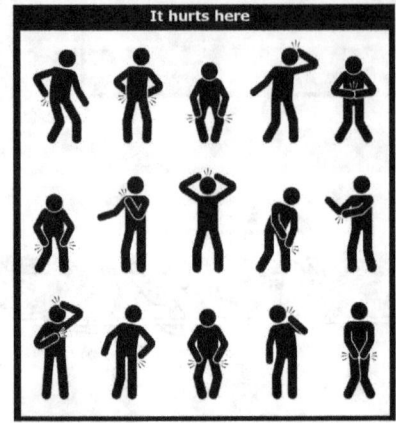
It hurts here

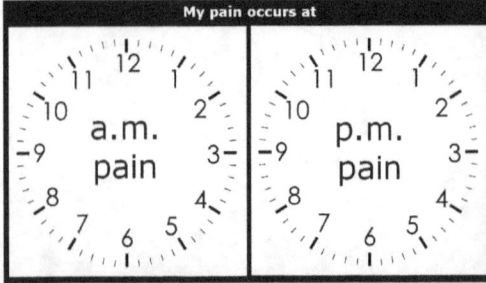
My pain occurs at — a.m. pain / p.m. pain

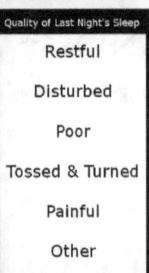
Quality of Last Night's Sleep
- Restful
- Disturbed
- Poor
- Tossed & Turned
- Painful
- Other

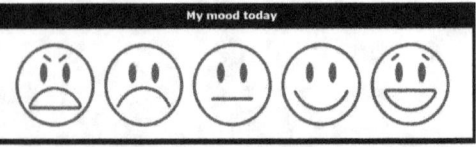
My mood today

My pain is
Hot
Burning
Cold
Stabbing
Throbbing
Fixed
Moving Traveling
Constant
On & Off

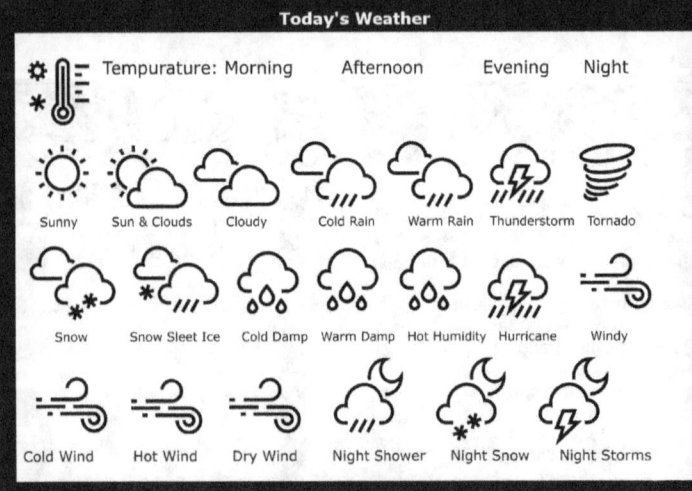
Today's Weather — Temperature: Morning, Afternoon, Evening, Night

Sunny, Sun & Clouds, Cloudy, Cold Rain, Warm Rain, Thunderstorm, Tornado
Snow, Snow Sleet Ice, Cold Damp, Warm Damp, Hot Humidity, Hurricane, Windy
Cold Wind, Hot Wind, Dry Wind, Night Shower, Night Snow, Night Storms

Breakfast

Lunch

Dinner

Snacks

Alcohol

Food Allergy Triggers

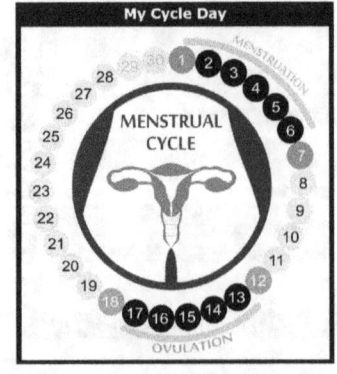
My Cycle Day

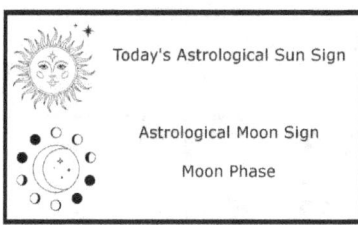

Today's Astrological Sun Sign

Astrological Moon Sign

Moon Phase

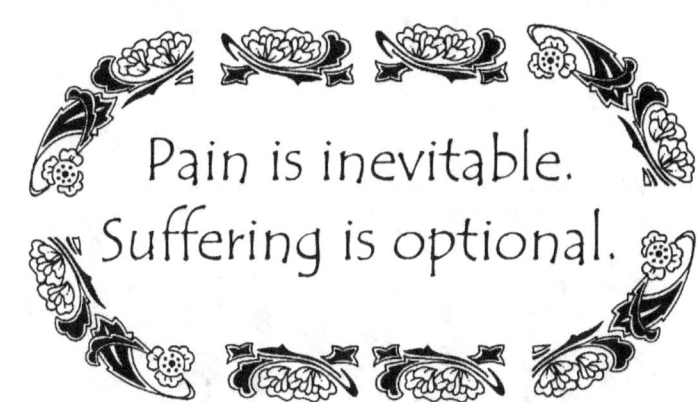

Pain is inevitable.
Suffering is optional.

Notes

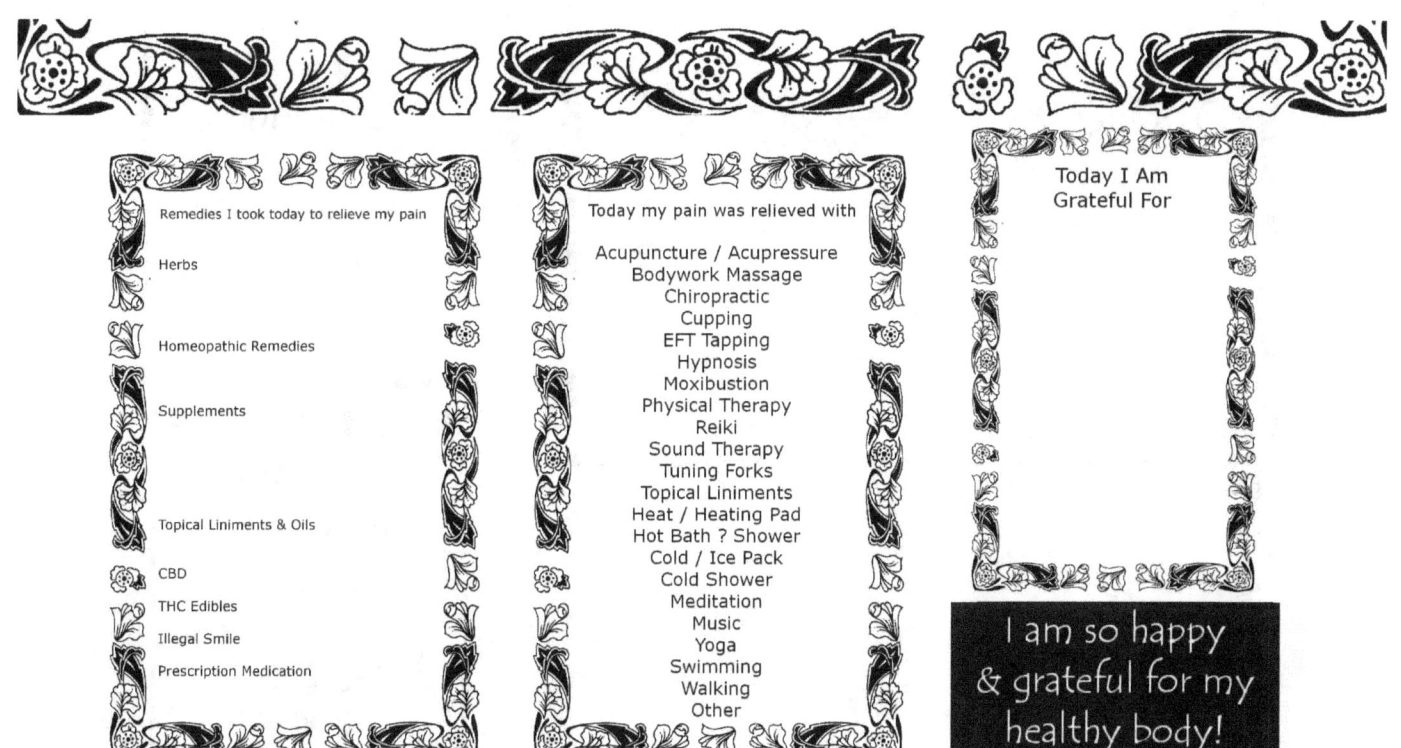

Remedies I took today to relieve my pain

Herbs

Homeopathic Remedies

Supplements

Topical Liniments & Oils

CBD
THC Edibles
Illegal Smile
Prescription Medication

Today my pain was relieved with

Acupuncture / Acupressure
Bodywork Massage
Chiropractic
Cupping
EFT Tapping
Hypnosis
Moxibustion
Physical Therapy
Reiki
Sound Therapy
Tuning Forks
Topical Liniments
Heat / Heating Pad
Hot Bath ? Shower
Cold / Ice Pack
Cold Shower
Meditation
Music
Yoga
Swimming
Walking
Other

Today I Am
Grateful For

I am so happy
& grateful for my
healthy body!

Today's Day & Date

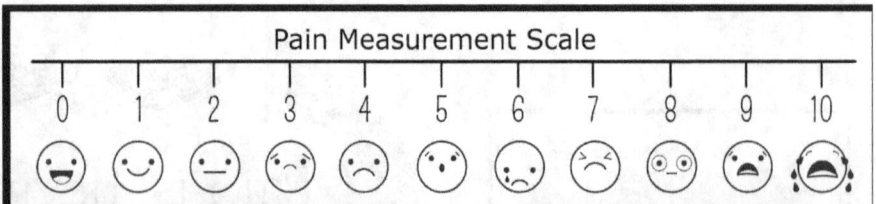

Highlight All Painful Areas

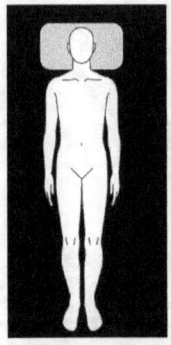 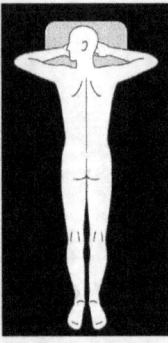 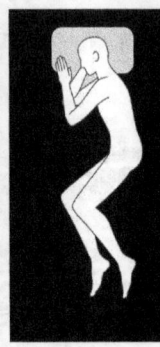 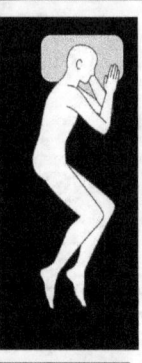

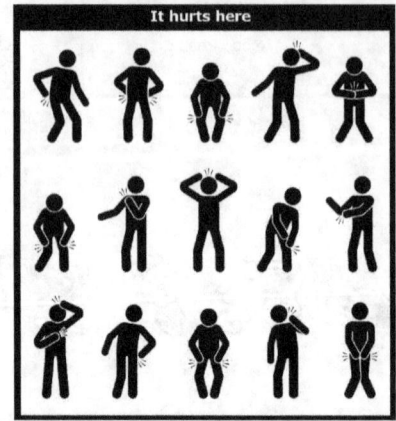

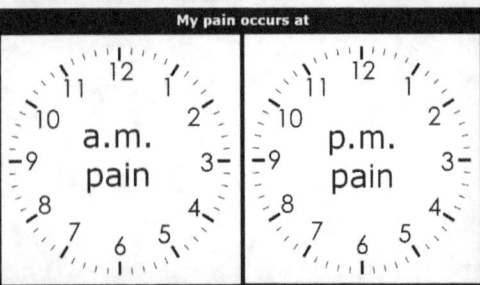

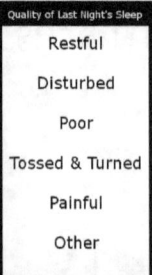

Quality of Last Night's Sleep
- Restful
- Disturbed
- Poor
- Tossed & Turned
- Painful
- Other

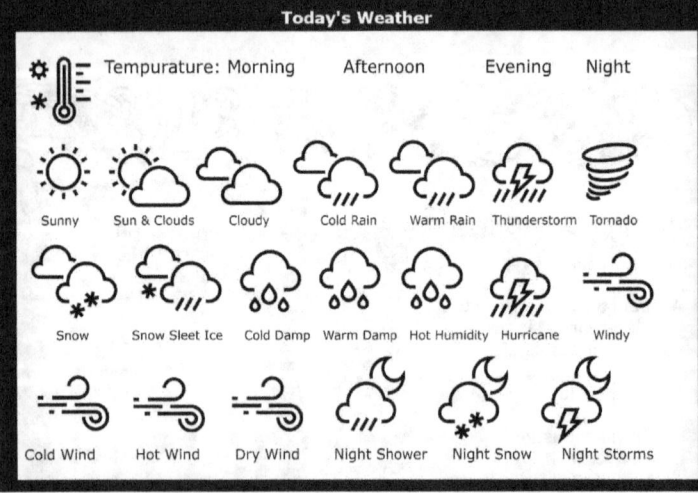

My pain is
Hot
Burning
Cold
Stabbing
Throbbing
Fixed
Moving Traveling
Constant
On & Off

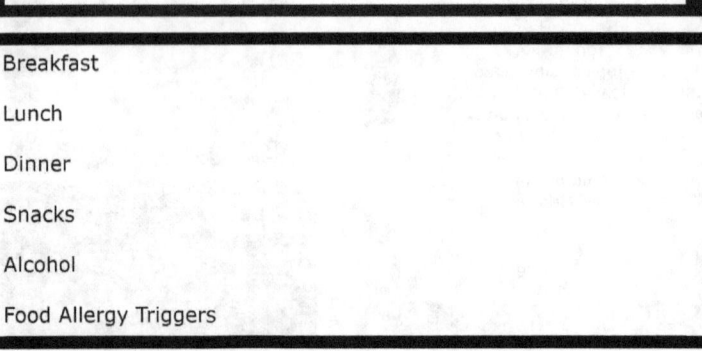

Breakfast

Lunch

Dinner

Snacks

Alcohol

Food Allergy Triggers

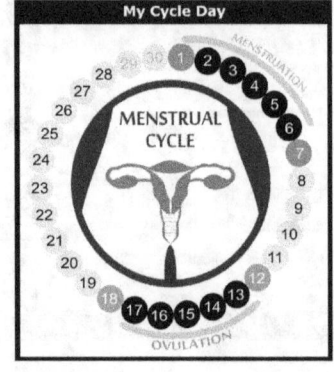

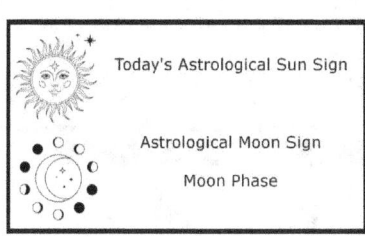

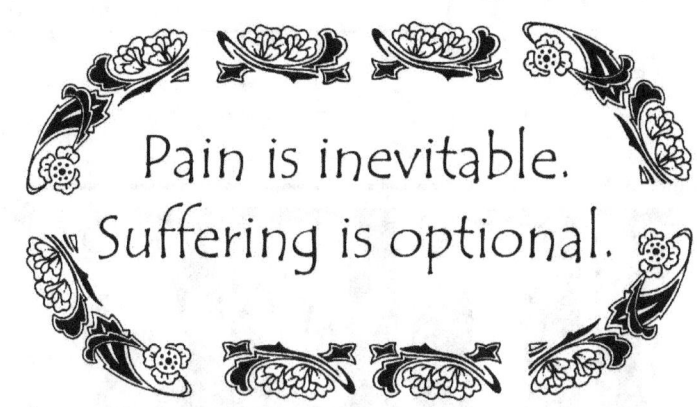

Notes

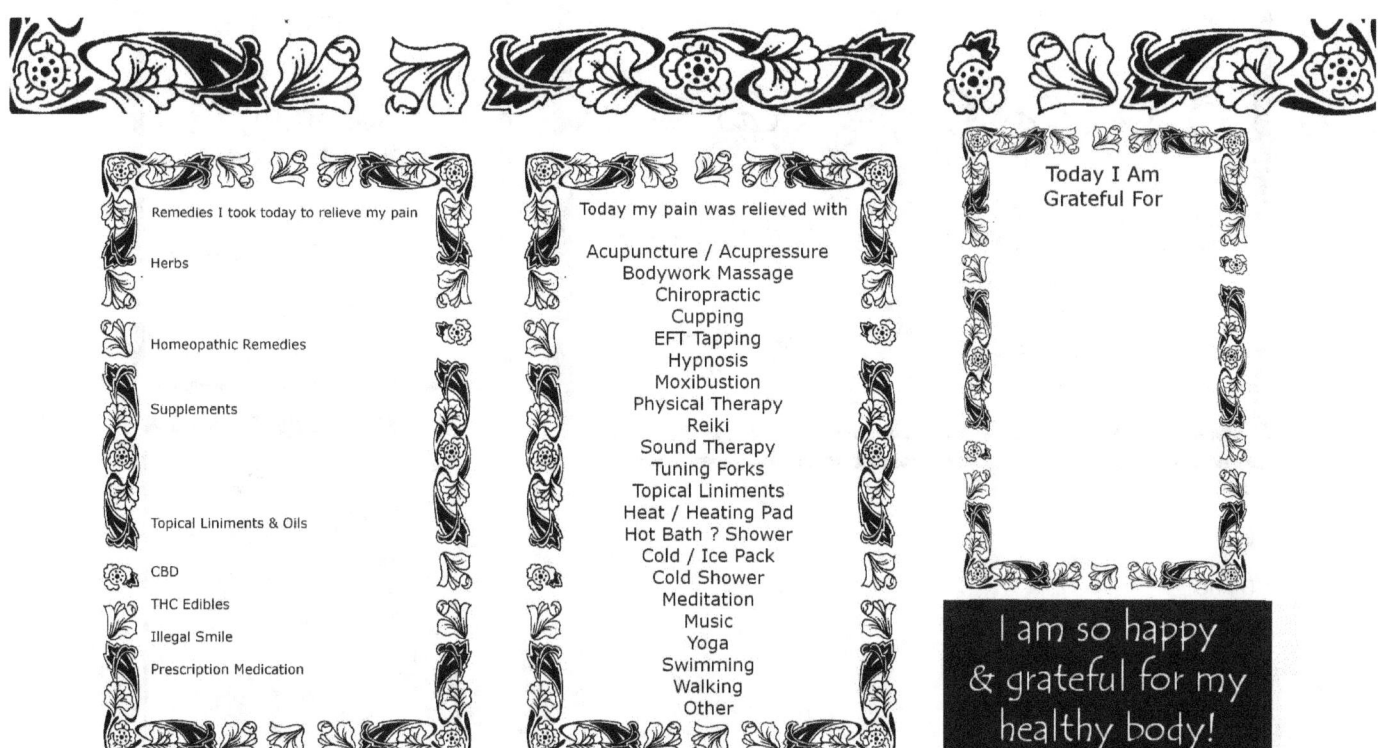

Today's Day & Date

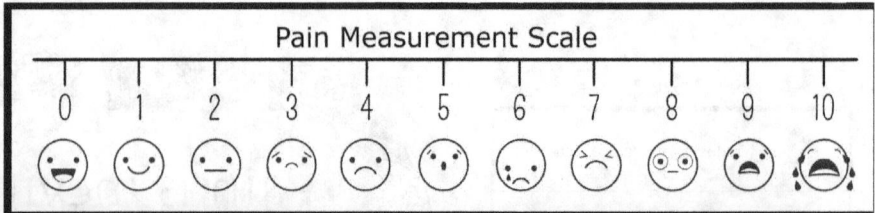

Highlight All Painful Areas

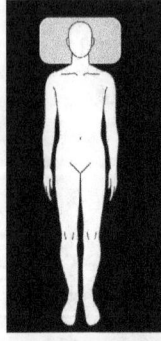 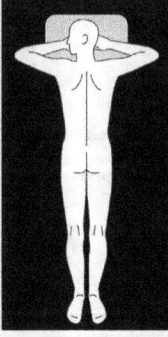 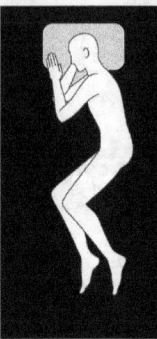 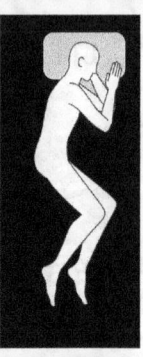

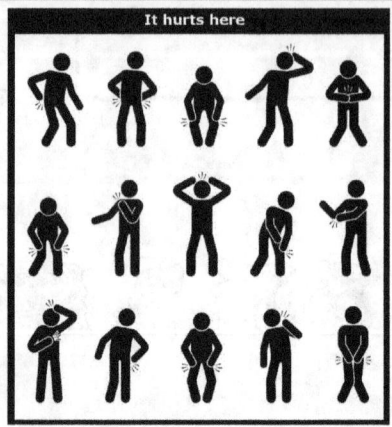
It hurts here

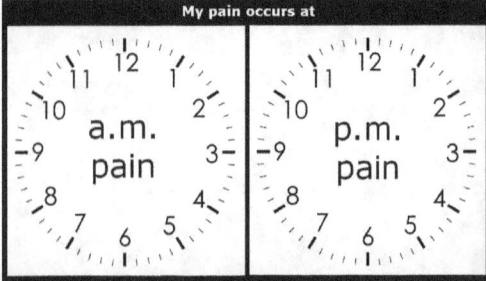

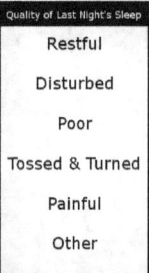
Quality of Last Night's Sleep
- Restful
- Disturbed
- Poor
- Tossed & Turned
- Painful
- Other

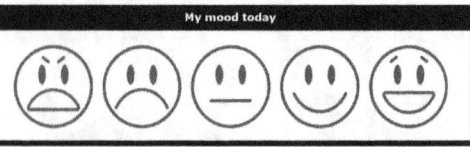
My mood today

My pain is

Hot
Burning
Cold
Stabbing
Throbbing
Fixed
Moving Traveling
Constant
On & Off

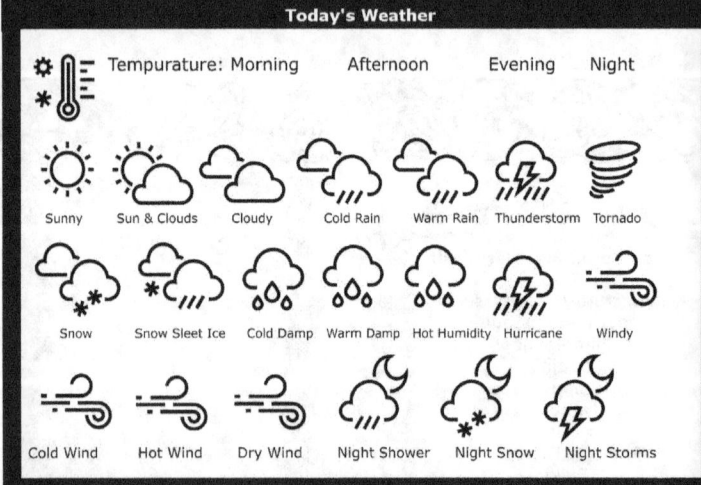

Breakfast

Lunch

Dinner

Snacks

Alcohol

Food Allergy Triggers

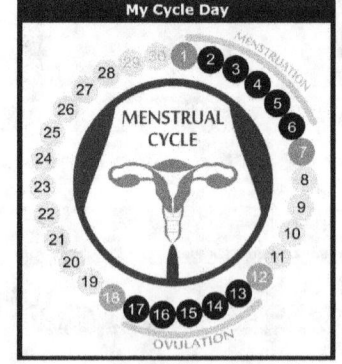

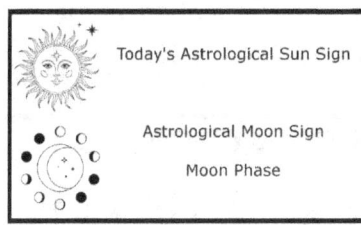

Today's Astrological Sun Sign

Astrological Moon Sign

Moon Phase

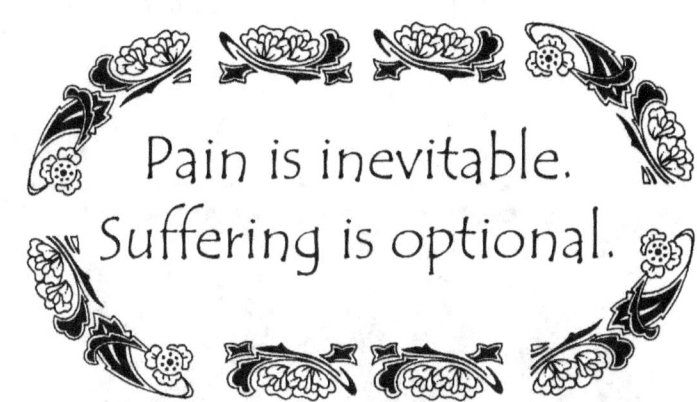

Pain is inevitable.
Suffering is optional.

Notes

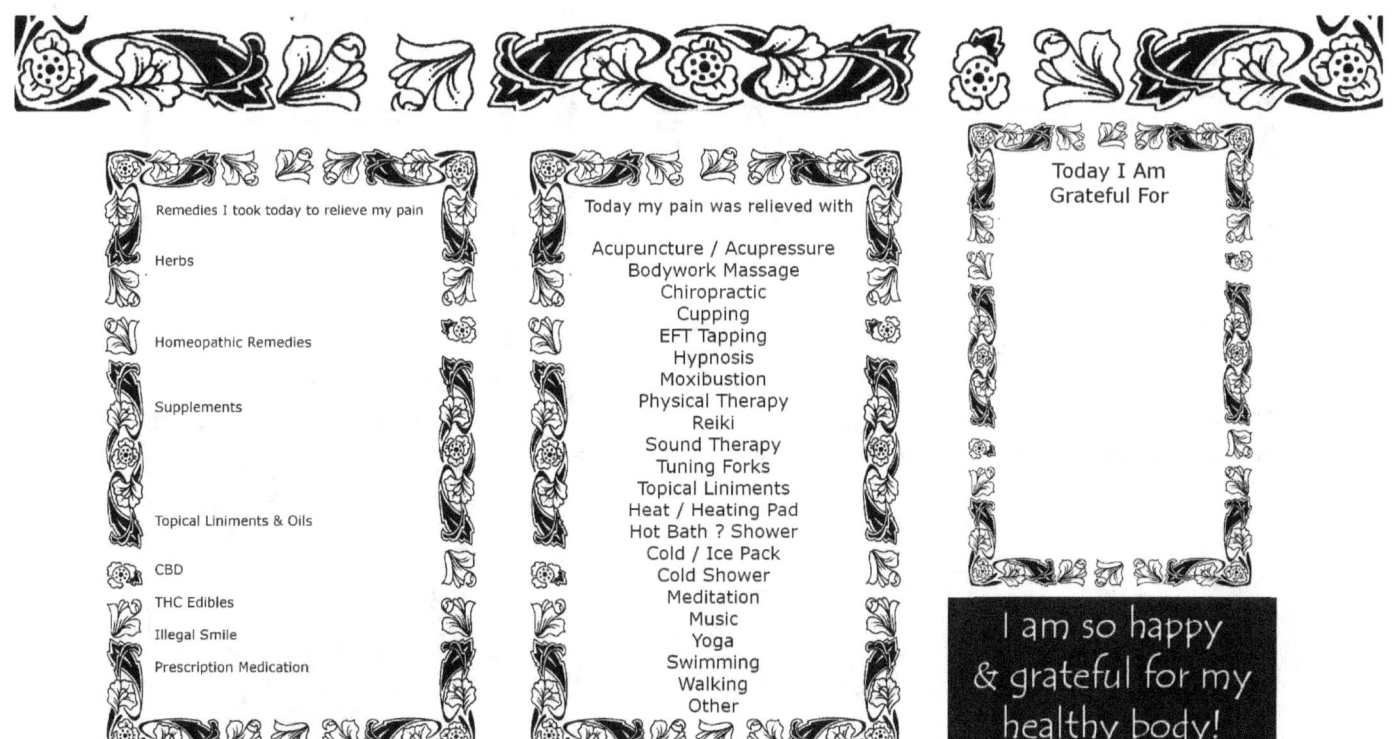

Remedies I took today to relieve my pain

Herbs

Homeopathic Remedies

Supplements

Topical Liniments & Oils

CBD

THC Edibles

Illegal Smile

Prescription Medication

Today my pain was relieved with

Acupuncture / Acupressure
Bodywork Massage
Chiropractic
Cupping
EFT Tapping
Hypnosis
Moxibustion
Physical Therapy
Reiki
Sound Therapy
Tuning Forks
Topical Liniments
Heat / Heating Pad
Hot Bath ? Shower
Cold / Ice Pack
Cold Shower
Meditation
Music
Yoga
Swimming
Walking
Other

Today I Am Grateful For

I am so happy & grateful for my healthy body!

Today's Day & Date

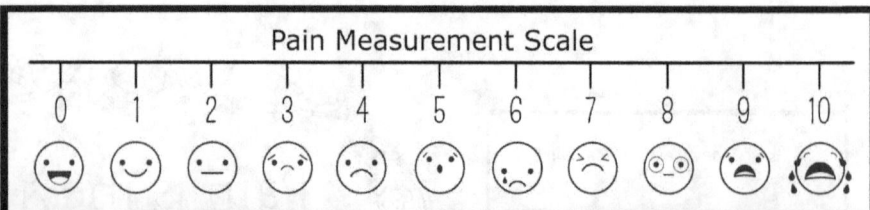

Pain Measurement Scale
0 1 2 3 4 5 6 7 8 9 10

Highlight All Painful Areas

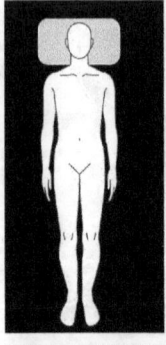 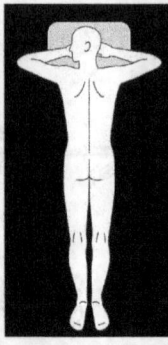 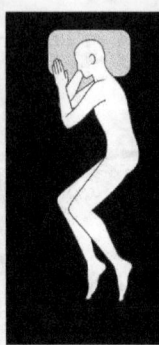 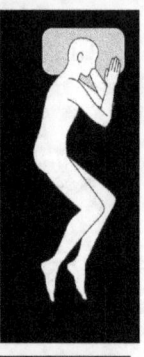

It hurts here

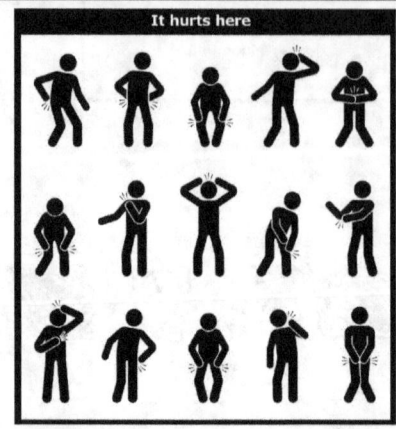

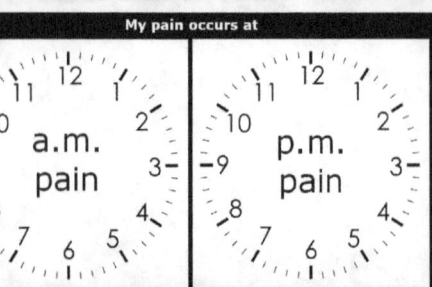

My pain occurs at — a.m. pain / p.m. pain

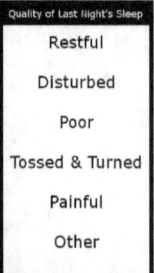

Quality of Last Night's Sleep
- Restful
- Disturbed
- Poor
- Tossed & Turned
- Painful
- Other

My mood today

Today's Weather

Tempurature: Morning Afternoon Evening Night

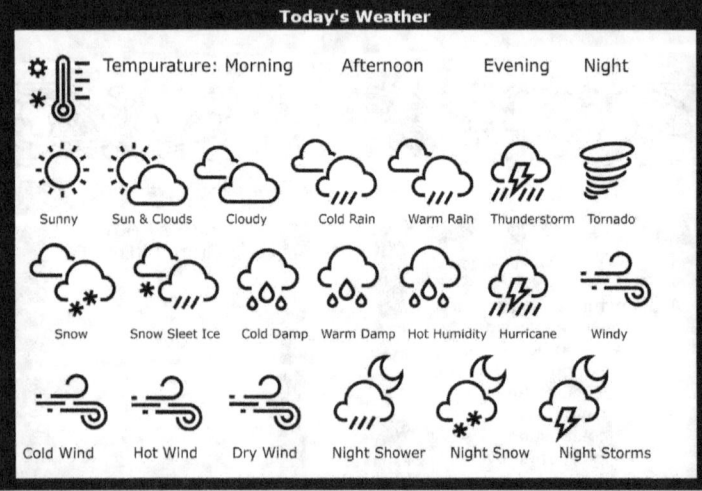

Sunny · Sun & Clouds · Cloudy · Cold Rain · Warm Rain · Thunderstorm · Tornado
Snow · Snow Sleet Ice · Cold Damp · Warm Damp · Hot Humidity · Hurricane · Windy
Cold Wind · Hot Wind · Dry Wind · Night Shower · Night Snow · Night Storms

My pain is

Hot
Burning
Cold
Stabbing
Throbbing
Fixed
Moving Traveling
Constant
On & Off

Breakfast

Lunch

Dinner

Snacks

Alcohol

Food Allergy Triggers

My Cycle Day

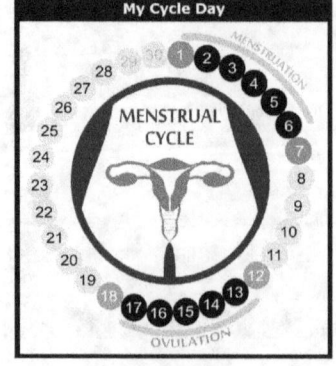

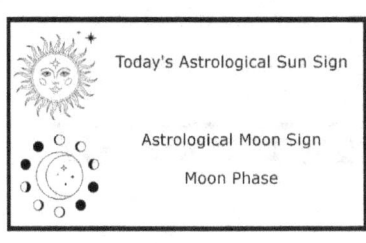

Today's Astrological Sun Sign

Astrological Moon Sign

Moon Phase

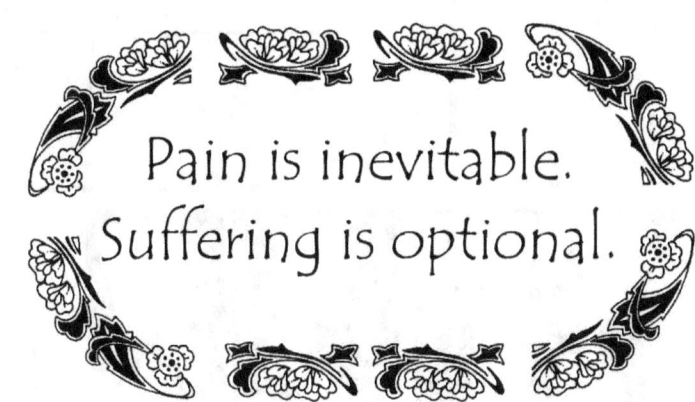

Pain is inevitable.
Suffering is optional.

Notes

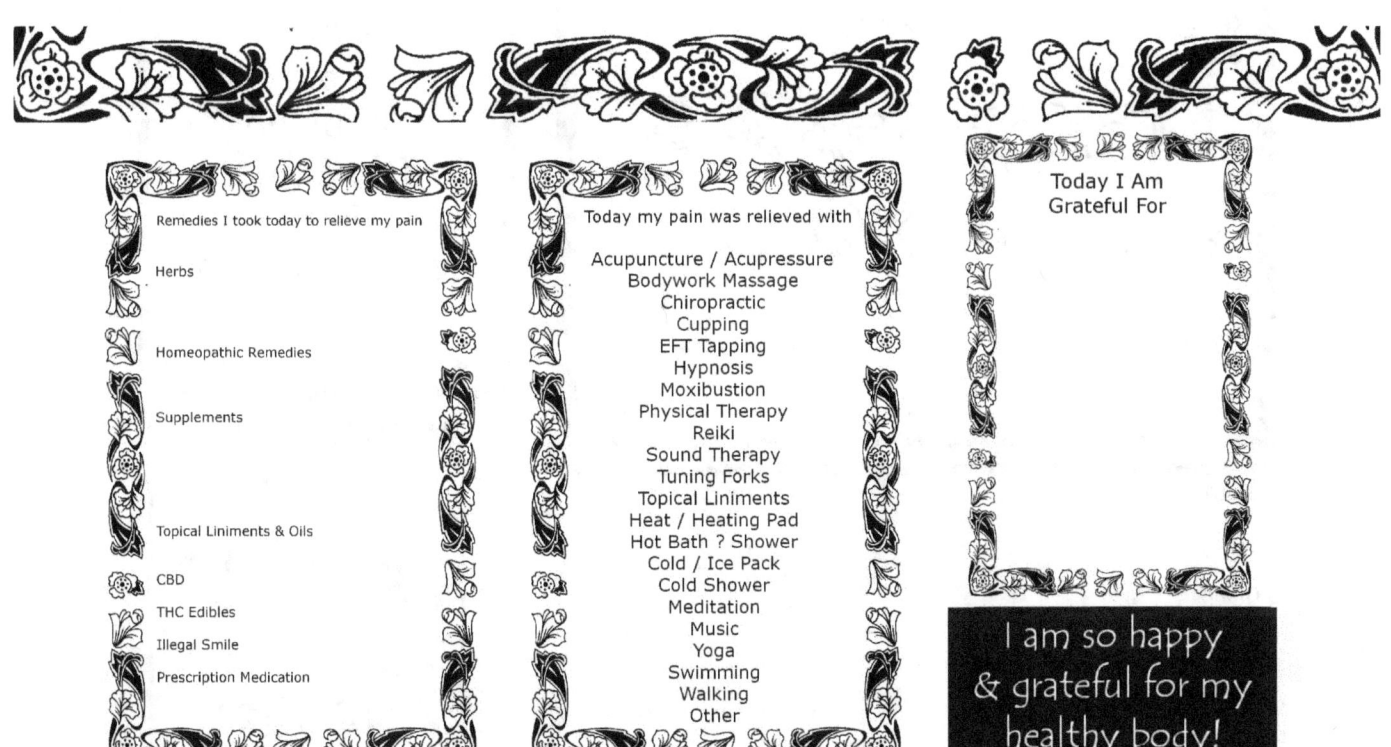

Remedies I took today to relieve my pain

Herbs

Homeopathic Remedies

Supplements

Topical Liniments & Oils

CBD

THC Edibles

Illegal Smile

Prescription Medication

Today my pain was relieved with

Acupuncture / Acupressure
Bodywork Massage
Chiropractic
Cupping
EFT Tapping
Hypnosis
Moxibustion
Physical Therapy
Reiki
Sound Therapy
Tuning Forks
Topical Liniments
Heat / Heating Pad
Hot Bath ? Shower
Cold / Ice Pack
Cold Shower
Meditation
Music
Yoga
Swimming
Walking
Other

Today I Am Grateful For

I am so happy & grateful for my healthy body!

Today's Day & Date

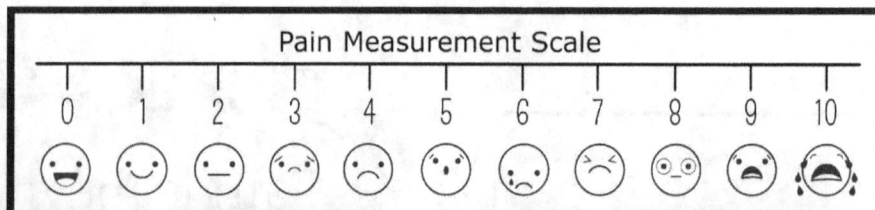

Highlight All Painful Areas

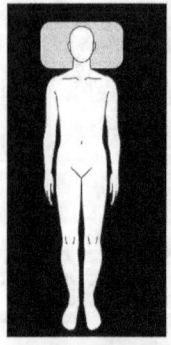 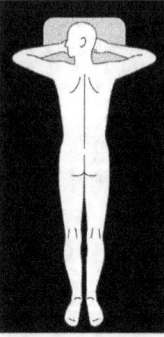 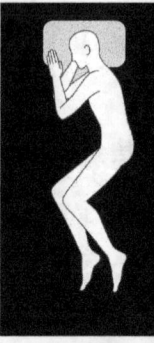 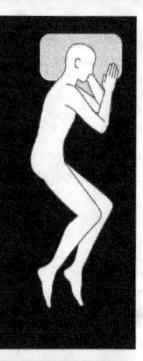

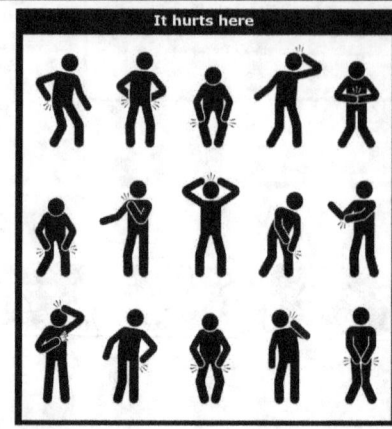
It hurts here

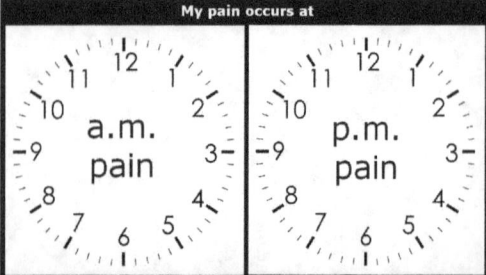
My pain occurs at

Quality of Last Night's Sleep
- Restful
- Disturbed
- Poor
- Tossed & Turned
- Painful
- Other

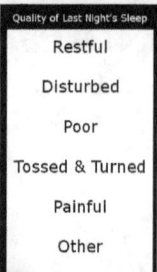

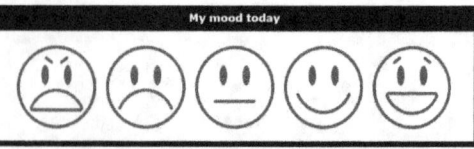
My mood today

My pain is
Hot
Burning
Cold
Stabbing
Throbbing
Fixed
Moving Traveling
Constant
On & Off

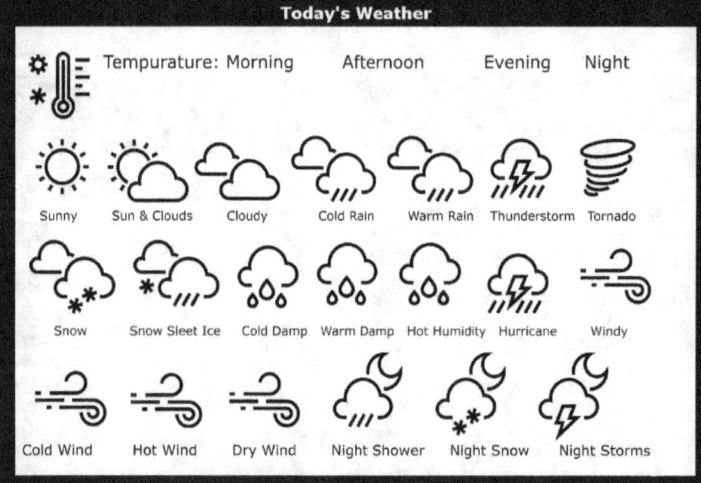
Today's Weather

Tempurature: Morning   Afternoon   Evening   Night

Breakfast

Lunch

Dinner

Snacks

Alcohol

Food Allergy Triggers

My Cycle Day

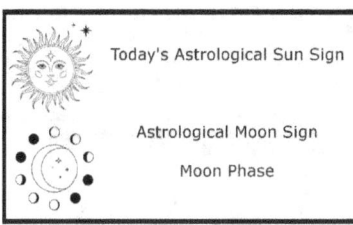

Today's Astrological Sun Sign

Astrological Moon Sign

Moon Phase

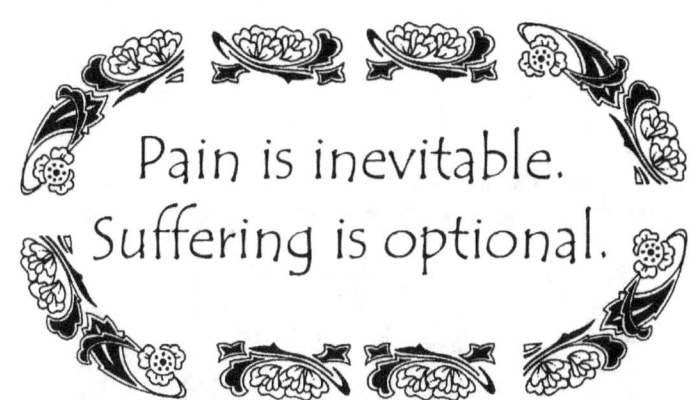

Pain is inevitable.
Suffering is optional.

Notes

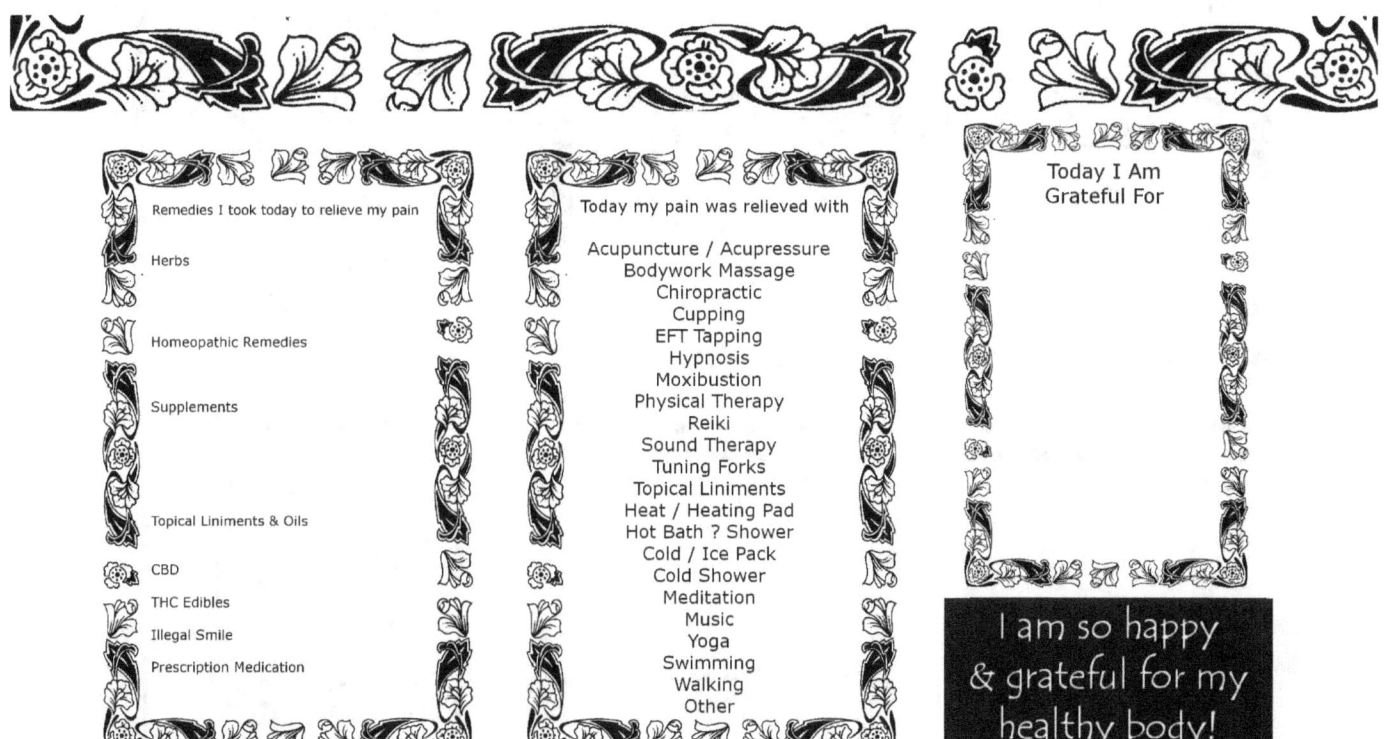

Remedies I took today to relieve my pain

Herbs

Homeopathic Remedies

Supplements

Topical Liniments & Oils

CBD

THC Edibles

Illegal Smile

Prescription Medication

Today my pain was relieved with

Acupuncture / Acupressure
Bodywork Massage
Chiropractic
Cupping
EFT Tapping
Hypnosis
Moxibustion
Physical Therapy
Reiki
Sound Therapy
Tuning Forks
Topical Liniments
Heat / Heating Pad
Hot Bath ? Shower
Cold / Ice Pack
Cold Shower
Meditation
Music
Yoga
Swimming
Walking
Other

Today I Am Grateful For

I am so happy & grateful for my healthy body!

Today's Day & Date

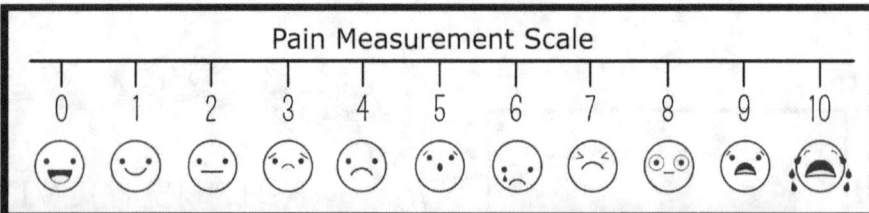

Highlight All Painful Areas

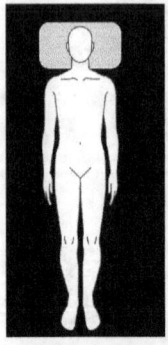 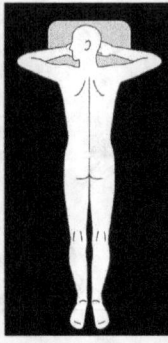 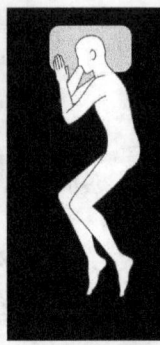 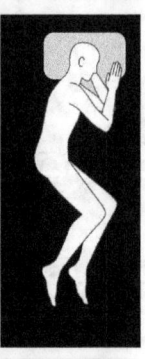

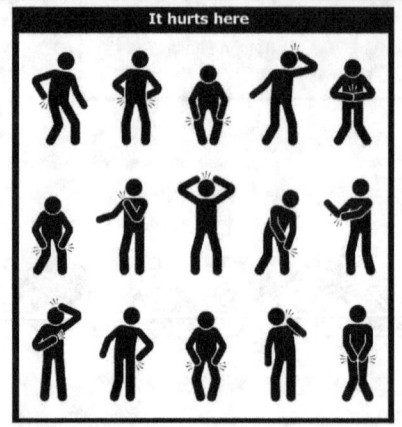
It hurts here

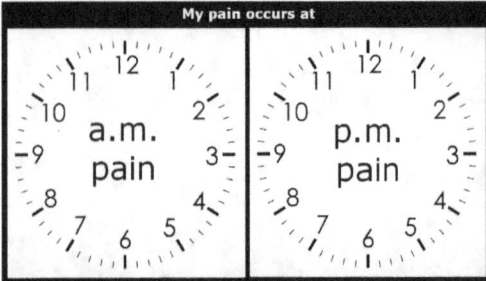
My pain occurs at — a.m. pain / p.m. pain

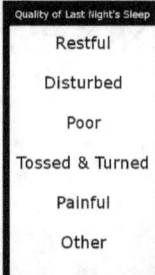
Quality of Last Night's Sleep
- Restful
- Disturbed
- Poor
- Tossed & Turned
- Painful
- Other

My mood today

My pain is
Hot
Burning
Cold
Stabbing
Throbbing
Fixed
Moving Traveling
Constant
On & Off

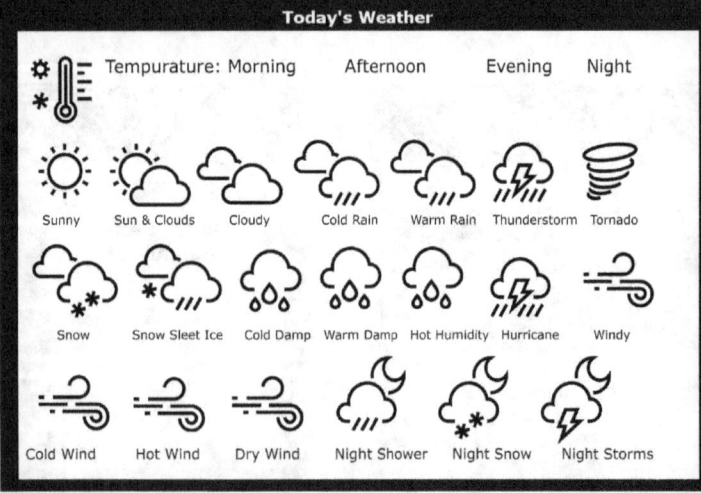
Today's Weather

Tempurature: Morning Afternoon Evening Night

Sunny, Sun & Clouds, Cloudy, Cold Rain, Warm Rain, Thunderstorm, Tornado
Snow, Snow Sleet Ice, Cold Damp, Warm Damp, Hot Humidity, Hurricane, Windy
Cold Wind, Hot Wind, Dry Wind, Night Shower, Night Snow, Night Storms

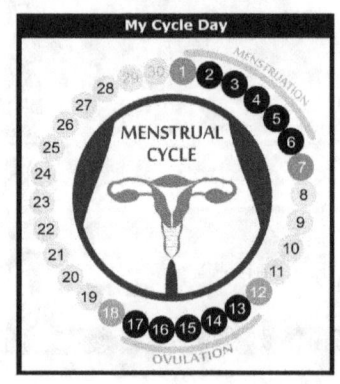
My Cycle Day

Breakfast

Lunch

Dinner

Snacks

Alcohol

Food Allergy Triggers

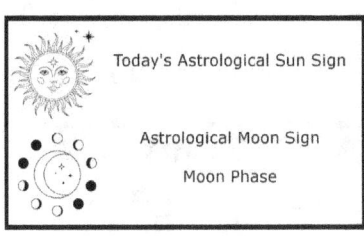

Today's Astrological Sun Sign

Astrological Moon Sign

Moon Phase

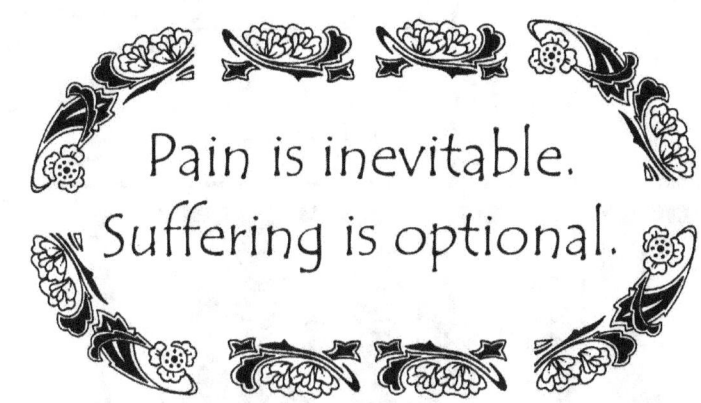

Pain is inevitable.
Suffering is optional.

Notes

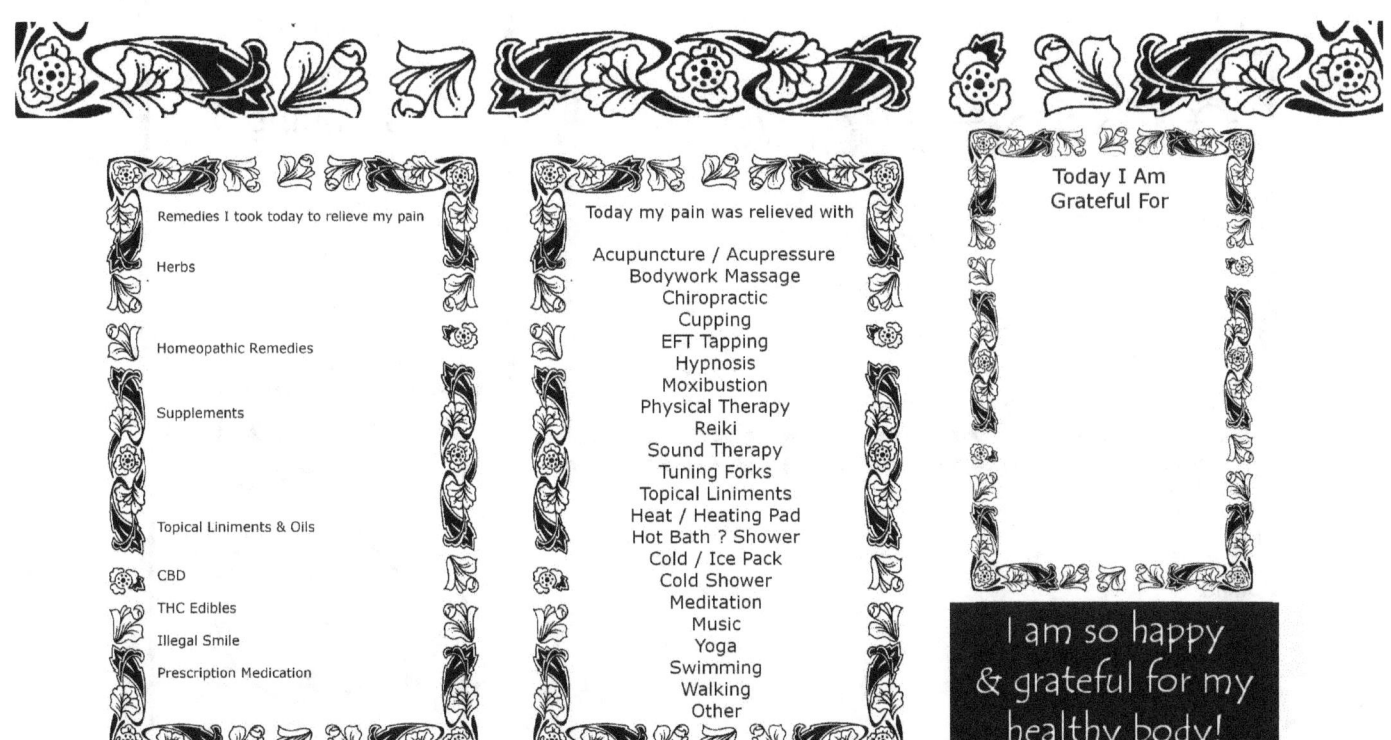

Remedies I took today to relieve my pain

Herbs

Homeopathic Remedies

Supplements

Topical Liniments & Oils

CBD

THC Edibles

Illegal Smile

Prescription Medication

Today my pain was relieved with

Acupuncture / Acupressure
Bodywork Massage
Chiropractic
Cupping
EFT Tapping
Hypnosis
Moxibustion
Physical Therapy
Reiki
Sound Therapy
Tuning Forks
Topical Liniments
Heat / Heating Pad
Hot Bath ? Shower
Cold / Ice Pack
Cold Shower
Meditation
Music
Yoga
Swimming
Walking
Other

Today I Am Grateful For

I am so happy & grateful for my healthy body!

Today's Day & Date

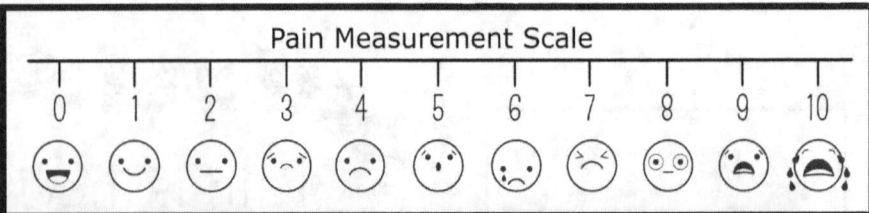

Highlight All Painful Areas

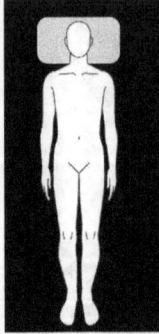 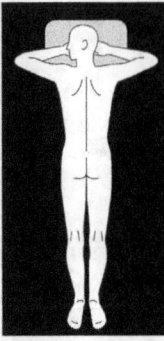 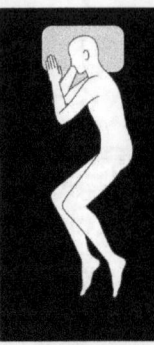 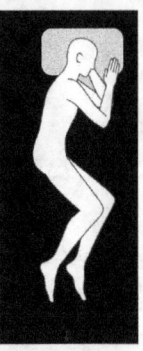

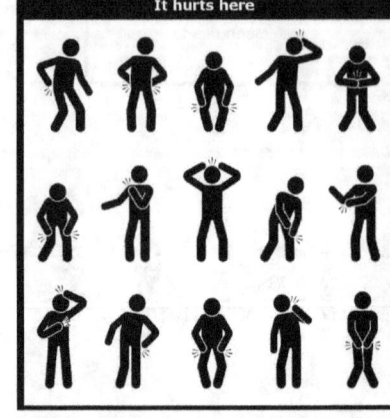

It hurts here

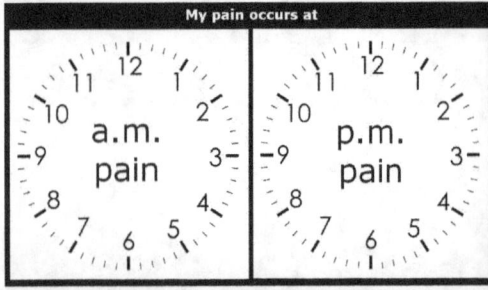
My pain occurs at — a.m. pain / p.m. pain

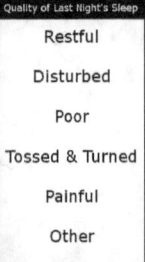

Quality of Last Night's Sleep
- Restful
- Disturbed
- Poor
- Tossed & Turned
- Painful
- Other

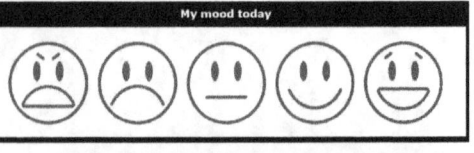

My mood today

My pain is
Hot
Burning
Cold
Stabbing
Throbbing
Fixed
Moving Traveling
Constant
On & Off

Today's Weather

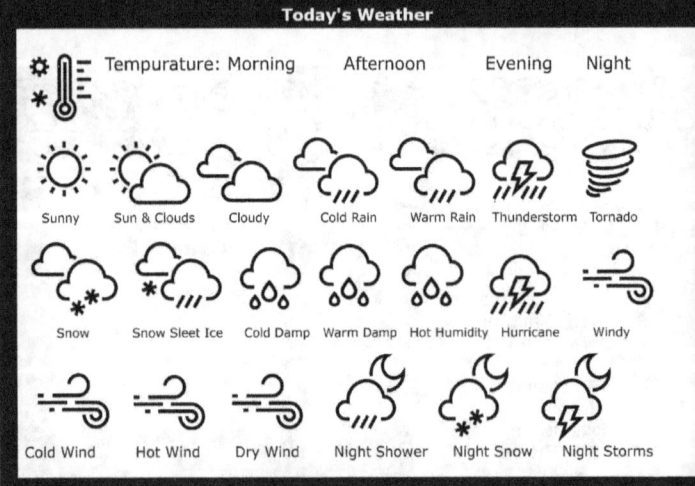

Temperature: Morning Afternoon Evening Night

Sunny, Sun & Clouds, Cloudy, Cold Rain, Warm Rain, Thunderstorm, Tornado
Snow, Snow Sleet Ice, Cold Damp, Warm Damp, Hot Humidity, Hurricane, Windy
Cold Wind, Hot Wind, Dry Wind, Night Shower, Night Snow, Night Storms

Breakfast

Lunch

Dinner

Snacks

Alcohol

Food Allergy Triggers

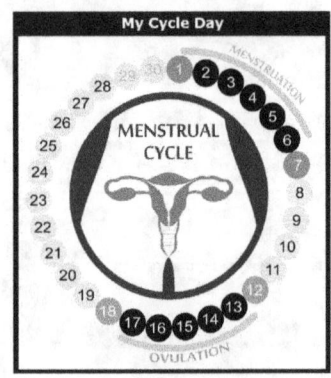

My Cycle Day

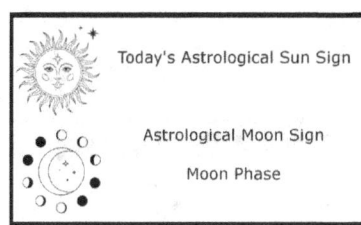

Today's Astrological Sun Sign

Astrological Moon Sign
Moon Phase

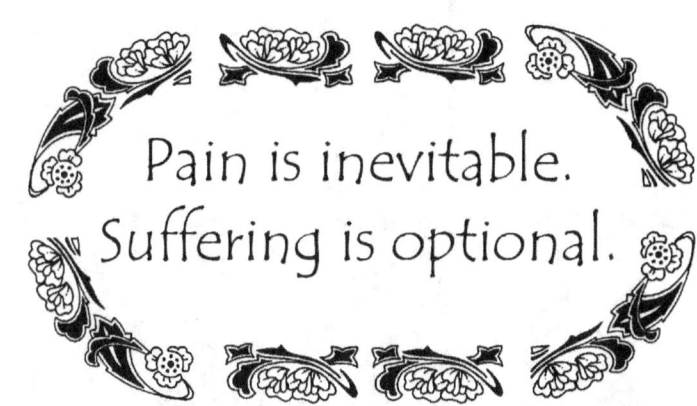

Pain is inevitable.
Suffering is optional.

Notes

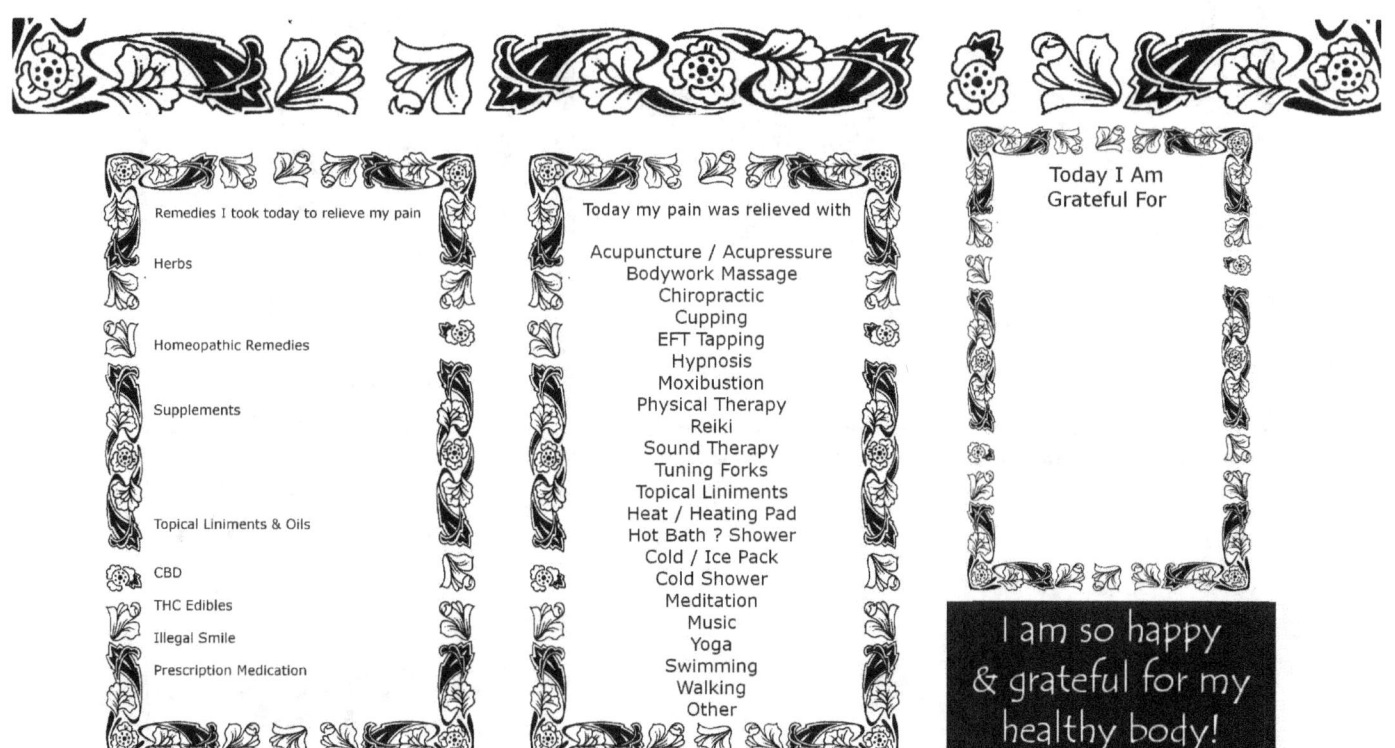

Remedies I took today to relieve my pain

Herbs

Homeopathic Remedies

Supplements

Topical Liniments & Oils

CBD
THC Edibles
Illegal Smile
Prescription Medication

Today my pain was relieved with

Acupuncture / Acupressure
Bodywork Massage
Chiropractic
Cupping
EFT Tapping
Hypnosis
Moxibustion
Physical Therapy
Reiki
Sound Therapy
Tuning Forks
Topical Liniments
Heat / Heating Pad
Hot Bath ? Shower
Cold / Ice Pack
Cold Shower
Meditation
Music
Yoga
Swimming
Walking
Other

Today I Am Grateful For

I am so happy & grateful for my healthy body!

Today's Day & Date

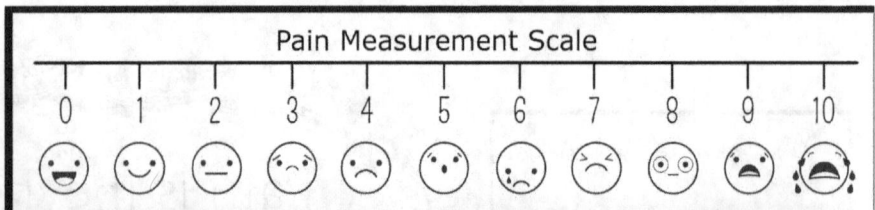

Highlight All Painful Areas

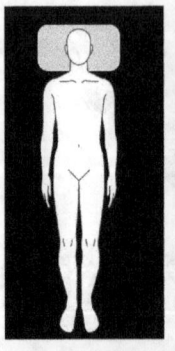 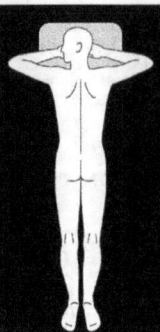 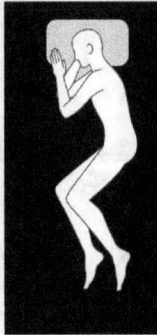 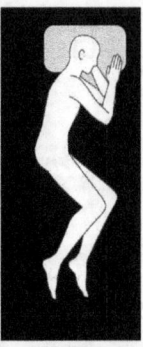

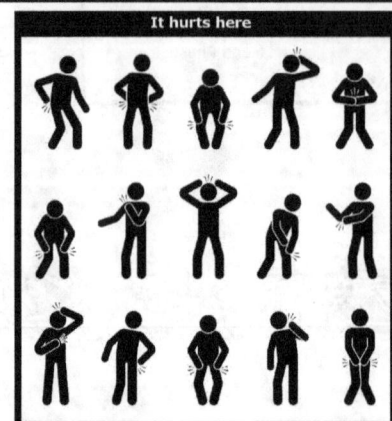
It hurts here

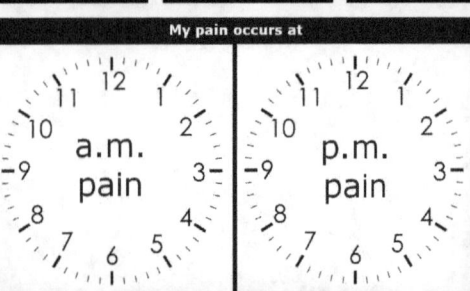
My pain occurs at — a.m. pain / p.m. pain

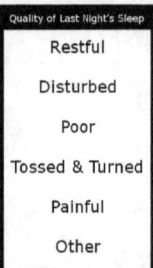

Quality of Last Night's Sleep
- Restful
- Disturbed
- Poor
- Tossed & Turned
- Painful
- Other

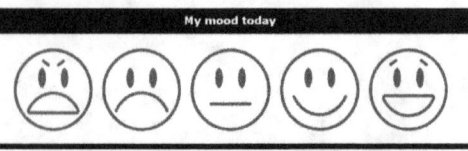
My mood today

My pain is
Hot
Burning
Cold
Stabbing
Throbbing
Fixed
Moving Traveling
Constant
On & Off

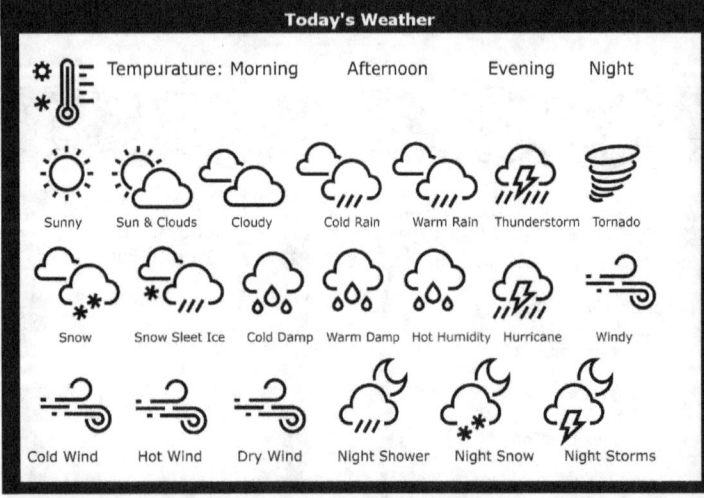
Today's Weather

Tempurature: Morning Afternoon Evening Night

Sunny, Sun & Clouds, Cloudy, Cold Rain, Warm Rain, Thunderstorm, Tornado
Snow, Snow Sleet Ice, Cold Damp, Warm Damp, Hot Humidity, Hurricane, Windy
Cold Wind, Hot Wind, Dry Wind, Night Shower, Night Snow, Night Storms

Breakfast

Lunch

Dinner

Snacks

Alcohol

Food Allergy Triggers

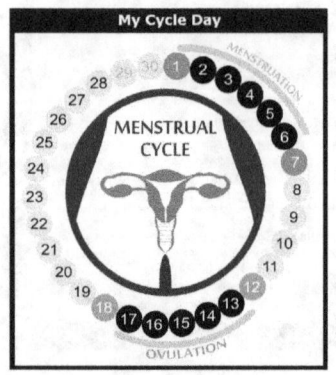
My Cycle Day

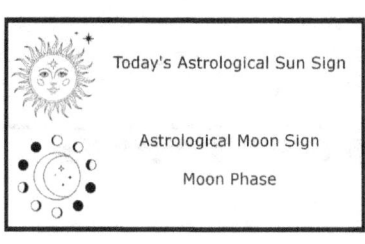

Today's Astrological Sun Sign

Astrological Moon Sign

Moon Phase

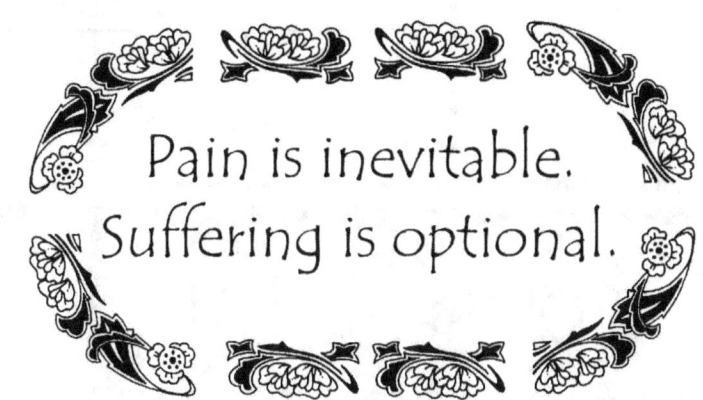

Pain is inevitable.
Suffering is optional.

Notes

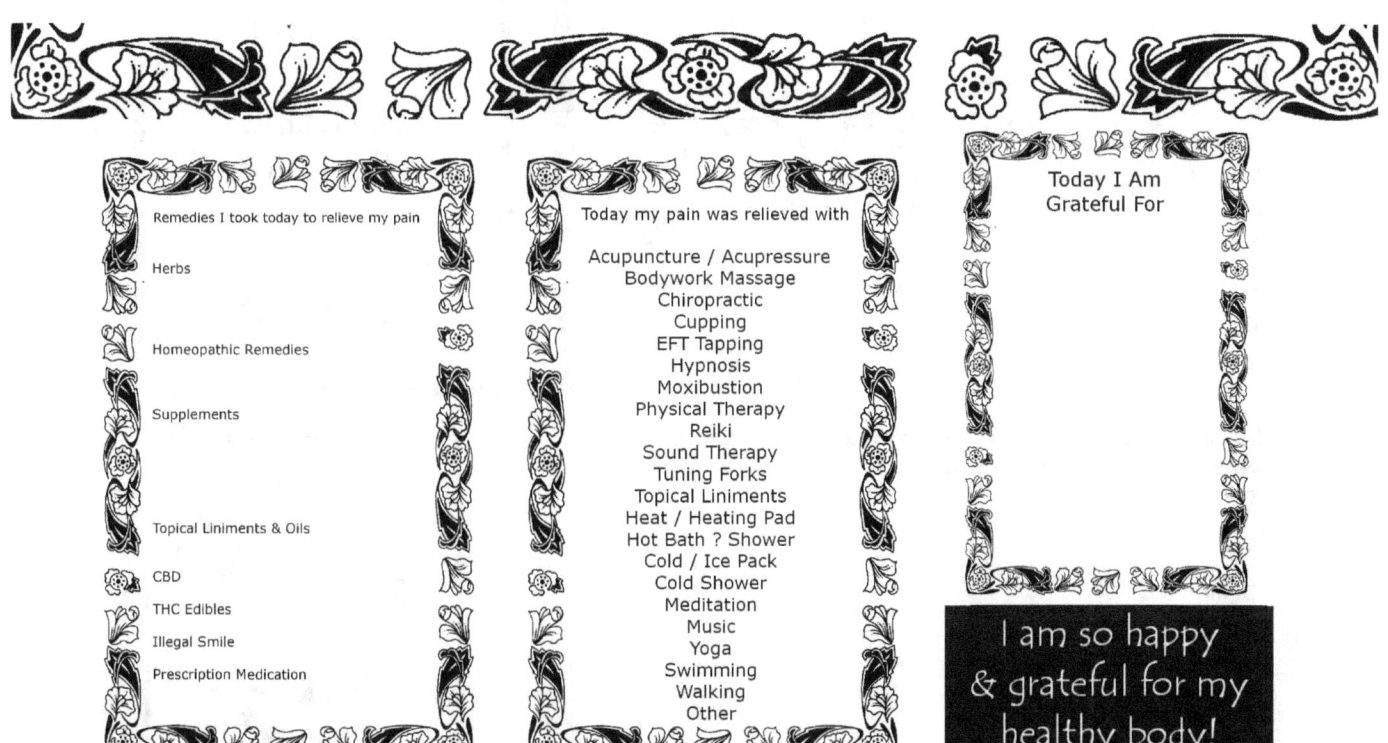

Remedies I took today to relieve my pain

Herbs

Homeopathic Remedies

Supplements

Topical Liniments & Oils

CBD

THC Edibles

Illegal Smile

Prescription Medication

Today my pain was relieved with

Acupuncture / Acupressure
Bodywork Massage
Chiropractic
Cupping
EFT Tapping
Hypnosis
Moxibustion
Physical Therapy
Reiki
Sound Therapy
Tuning Forks
Topical Liniments
Heat / Heating Pad
Hot Bath ? Shower
Cold / Ice Pack
Cold Shower
Meditation
Music
Yoga
Swimming
Walking
Other

Today I Am
Grateful For

I am so happy
& grateful for my
healthy body!

Today's Day & Date

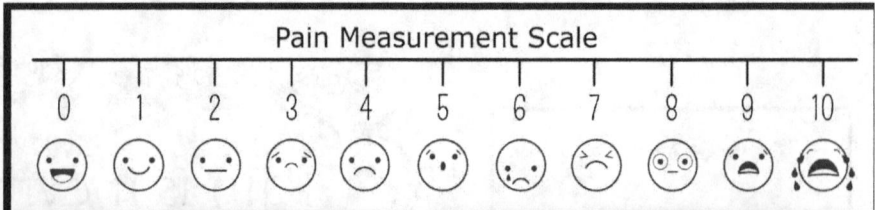

Pain Measurement Scale
0 1 2 3 4 5 6 7 8 9 10

Highlight All Painful Areas

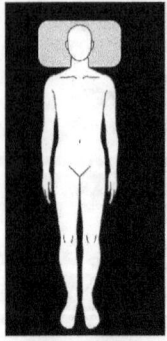 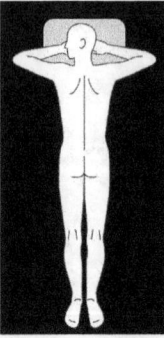 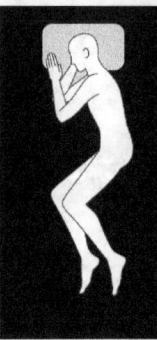 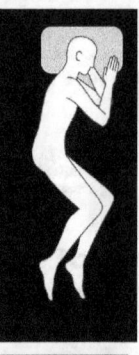

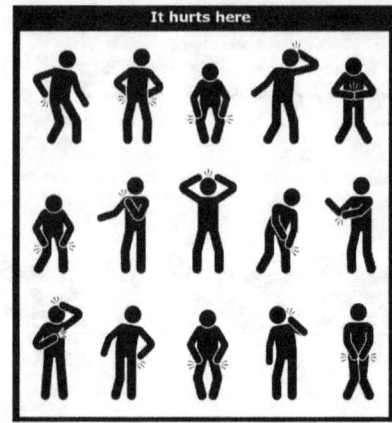
It hurts here

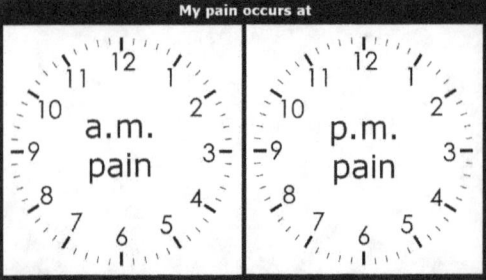
My pain occurs at — a.m. pain / p.m. pain

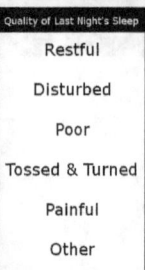

Quality of Last Night's Sleep
- Restful
- Disturbed
- Poor
- Tossed & Turned
- Painful
- Other

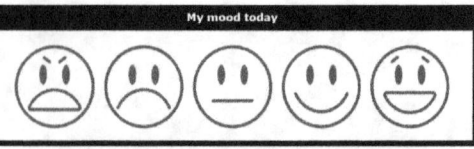
My mood today

My pain is
Hot
Burning
Cold
Stabbing
Throbbing
Fixed
Moving Traveling
Constant
On & Off

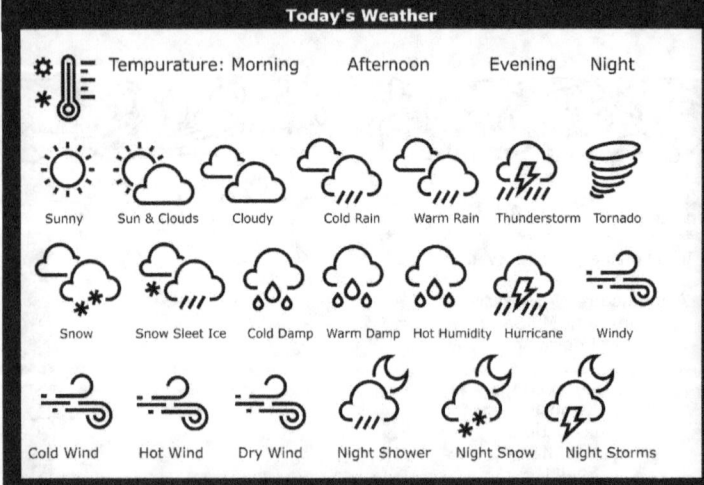
Today's Weather

Tempurature: Morning   Afternoon   Evening   Night

Sunny, Sun & Clouds, Cloudy, Cold Rain, Warm Rain, Thunderstorm, Tornado
Snow, Snow Sleet Ice, Cold Damp, Warm Damp, Hot Humidity, Hurricane, Windy
Cold Wind, Hot Wind, Dry Wind, Night Shower, Night Snow, Night Storms

Breakfast

Lunch

Dinner

Snacks

Alcohol

Food Allergy Triggers

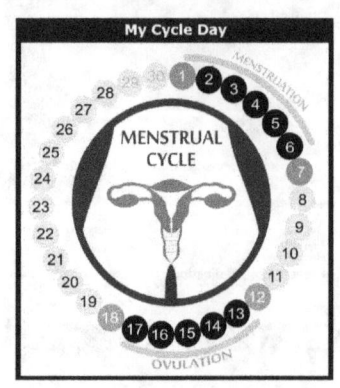
My Cycle Day

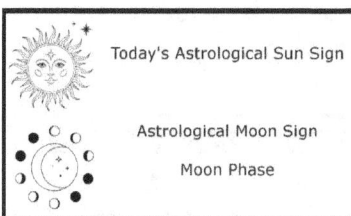

Today's Astrological Sun Sign

Astrological Moon Sign

Moon Phase

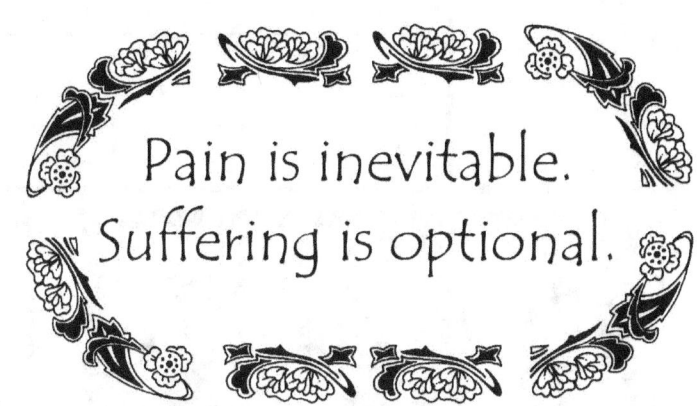

Pain is inevitable.
Suffering is optional.

Notes

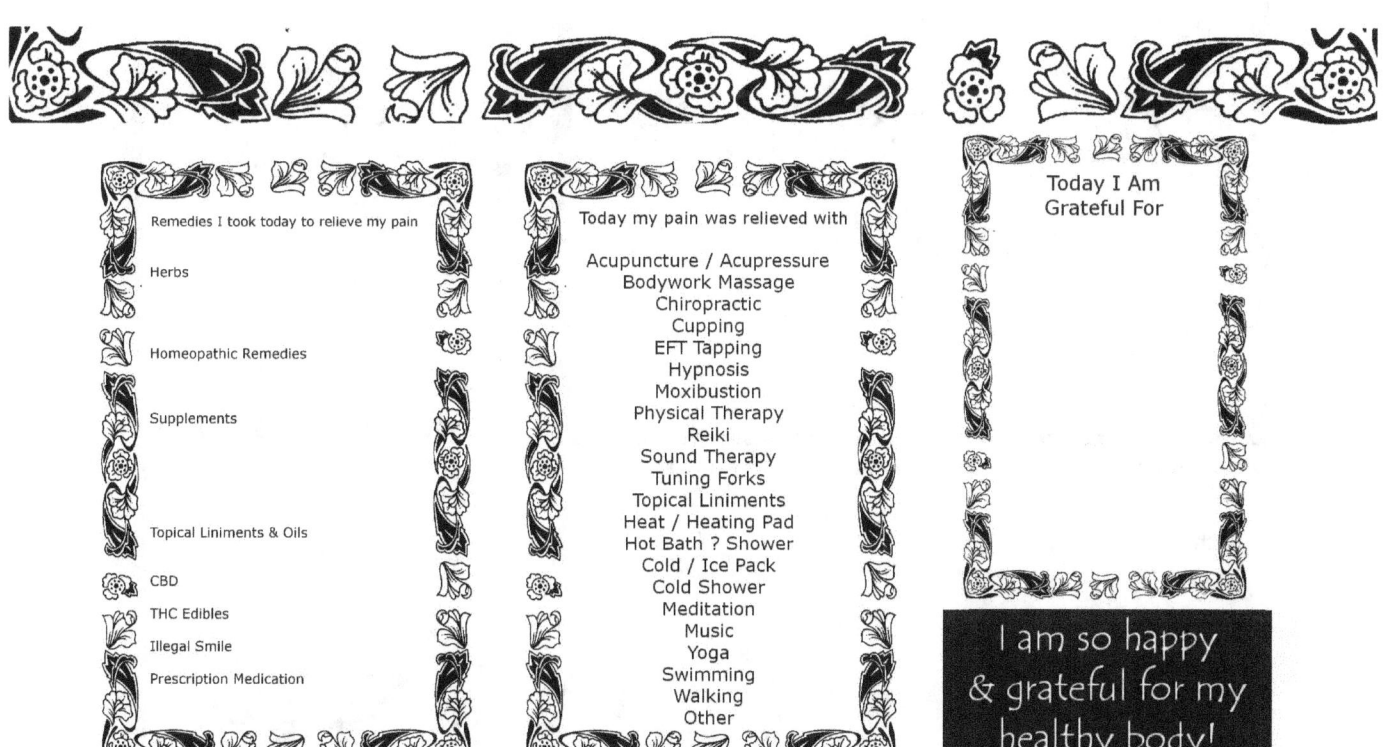

Remedies I took today to relieve my pain

Herbs

Homeopathic Remedies

Supplements

Topical Liniments & Oils

CBD

THC Edibles

Illegal Smile

Prescription Medication

Today my pain was relieved with

Acupuncture / Acupressure
Bodywork Massage
Chiropractic
Cupping
EFT Tapping
Hypnosis
Moxibustion
Physical Therapy
Reiki
Sound Therapy
Tuning Forks
Topical Liniments
Heat / Heating Pad
Hot Bath ? Shower
Cold / Ice Pack
Cold Shower
Meditation
Music
Yoga
Swimming
Walking
Other

Today I Am Grateful For

I am so happy & grateful for my healthy body!

Today's Day & Date

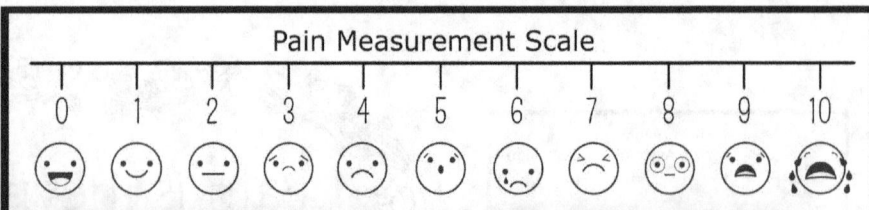

Highlight All Painful Areas

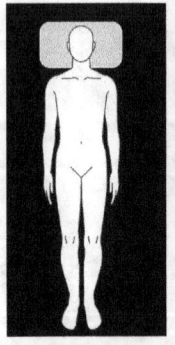 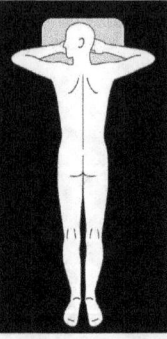 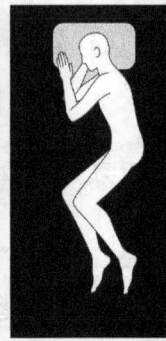 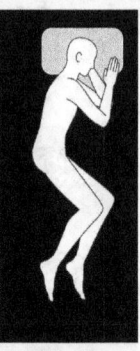

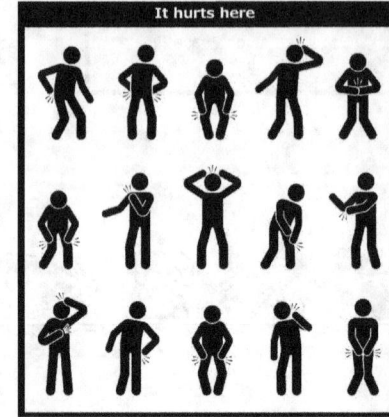

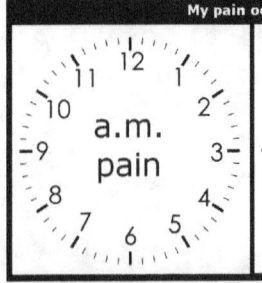 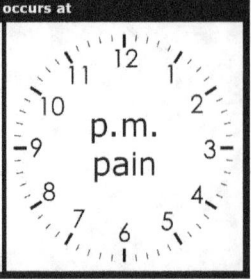 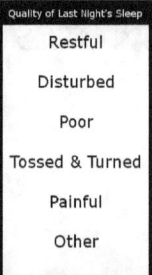

Quality of Last Night's Sleep
- Restful
- Disturbed
- Poor
- Tossed & Turned
- Painful
- Other

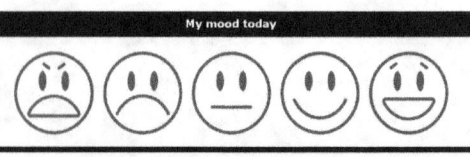

My pain is
Hot
Burning
Cold
Stabbing
Throbbing
Fixed
Moving Traveling
Constant
On & Off

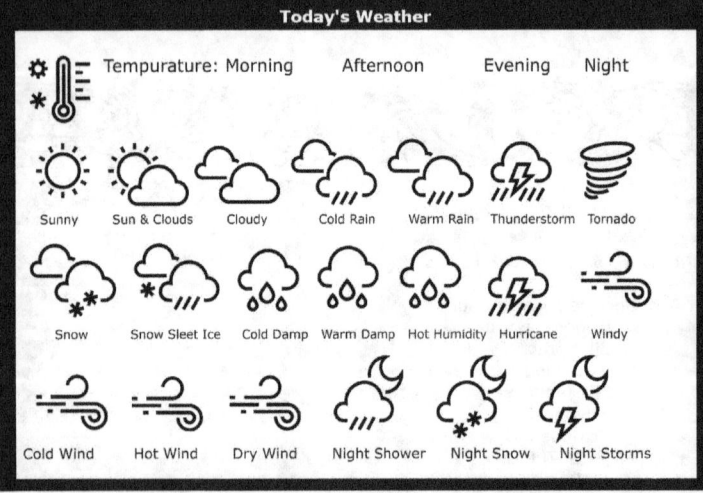

Breakfast

Lunch

Dinner

Snacks

Alcohol

Food Allergy Triggers

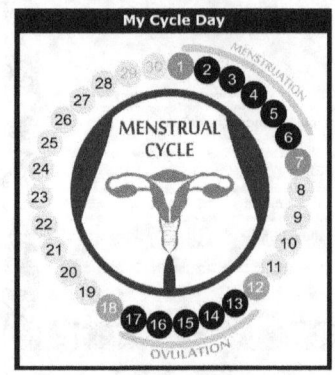

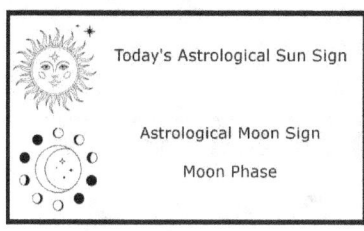

Today's Astrological Sun Sign

Astrological Moon Sign

Moon Phase

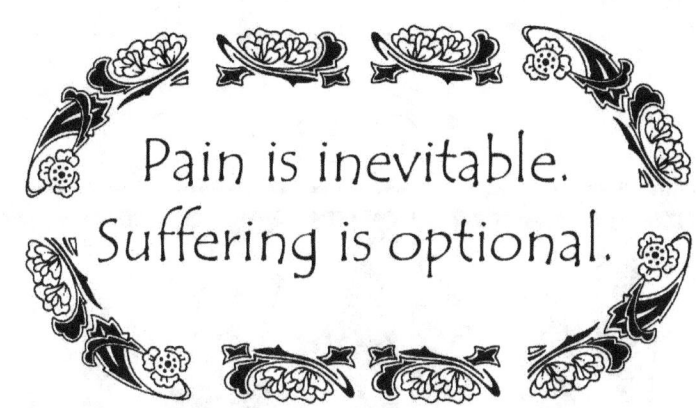

Pain is inevitable.
Suffering is optional.

Notes

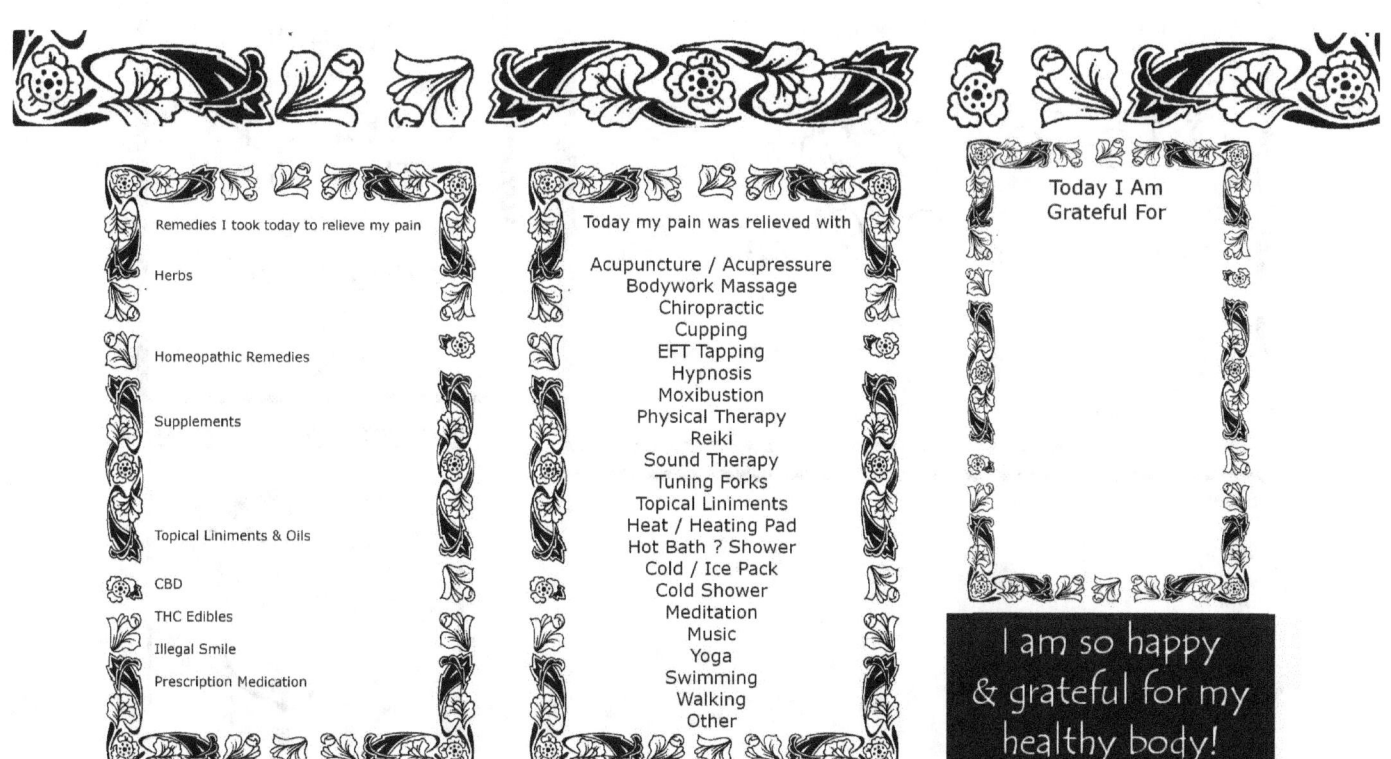

Remedies I took today to relieve my pain

Herbs

Homeopathic Remedies

Supplements

Topical Liniments & Oils

CBD

THC Edibles

Illegal Smile

Prescription Medication

Today my pain was relieved with

Acupuncture / Acupressure
Bodywork Massage
Chiropractic
Cupping
EFT Tapping
Hypnosis
Moxibustion
Physical Therapy
Reiki
Sound Therapy
Tuning Forks
Topical Liniments
Heat / Heating Pad
Hot Bath ? Shower
Cold / Ice Pack
Cold Shower
Meditation
Music
Yoga
Swimming
Walking
Other

Today I Am Grateful For

I am so happy & grateful for my healthy body!

Today's Day & Date

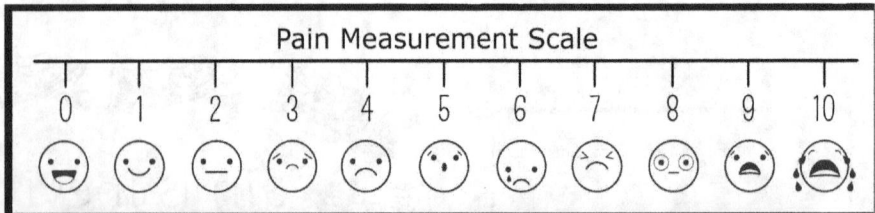

Highlight All Painful Areas

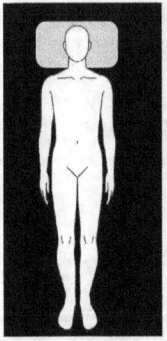 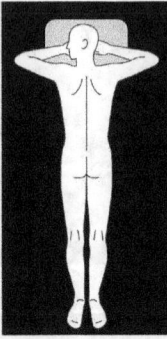 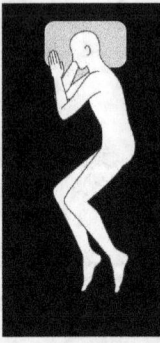 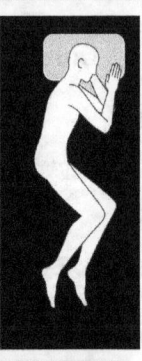

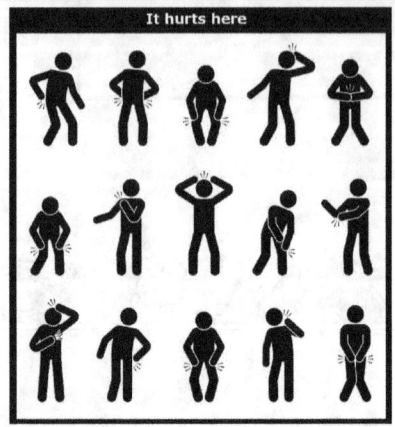
It hurts here

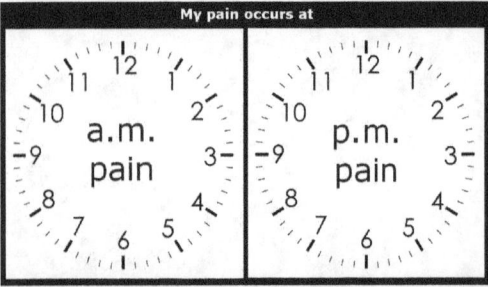
My pain occurs at — a.m. pain / p.m. pain

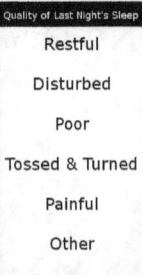
Quality of Last Night's Sleep
- Restful
- Disturbed
- Poor
- Tossed & Turned
- Painful
- Other

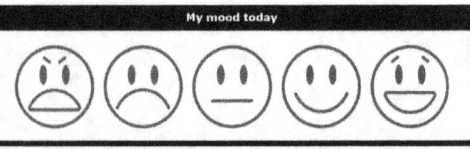
My mood today

My pain is
Hot
Burning
Cold
Stabbing
Throbbing
Fixed
Moving Traveling
Constant
On & Off

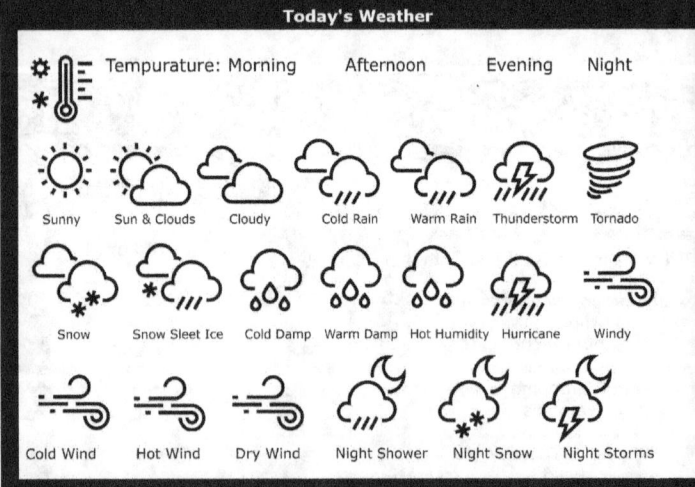
Today's Weather — Temperature: Morning, Afternoon, Evening, Night

Breakfast

Lunch

Dinner

Snacks

Alcohol

Food Allergy Triggers

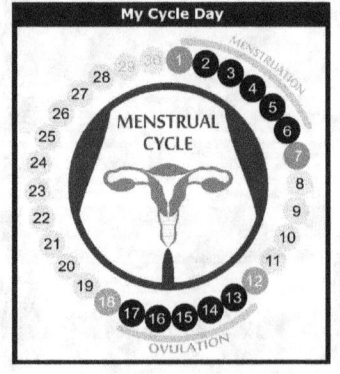
My Cycle Day

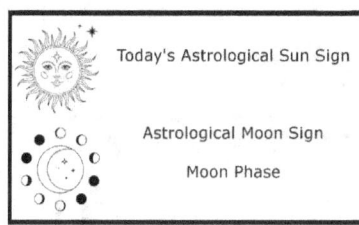

Today's Astrological Sun Sign

Astrological Moon Sign

Moon Phase

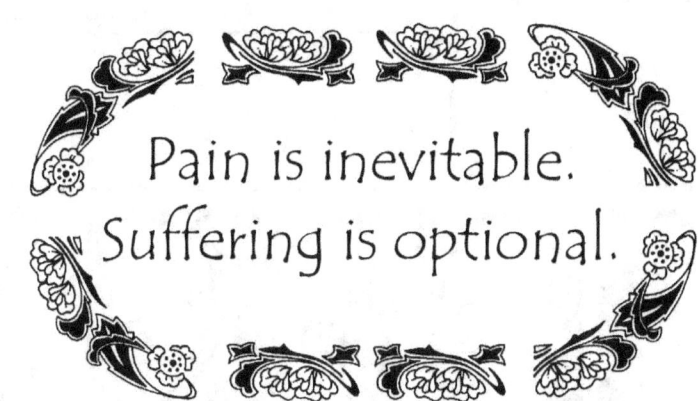

Pain is inevitable.
Suffering is optional.

Notes

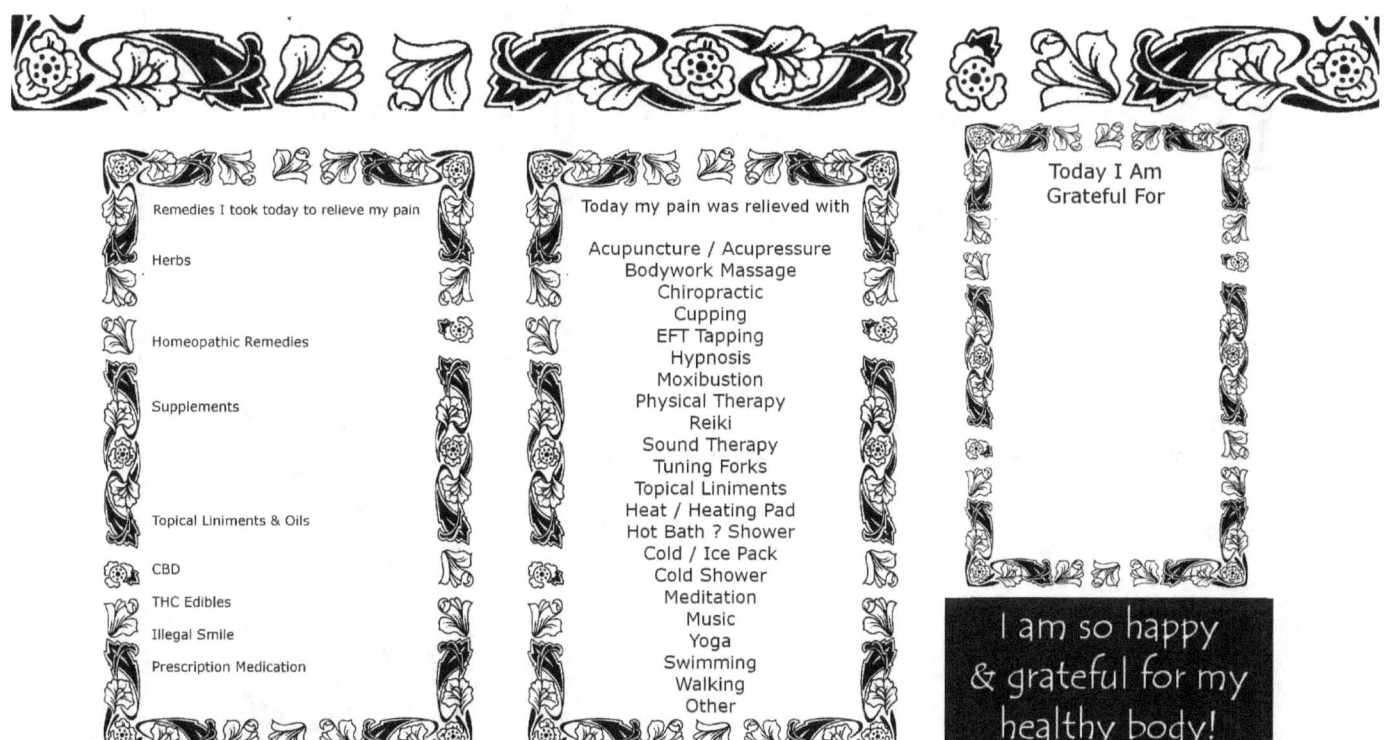

Remedies I took today to relieve my pain

Herbs

Homeopathic Remedies

Supplements

Topical Liniments & Oils

CBD
THC Edibles
Illegal Smile
Prescription Medication

Today my pain was relieved with

Acupuncture / Acupressure
Bodywork Massage
Chiropractic
Cupping
EFT Tapping
Hypnosis
Moxibustion
Physical Therapy
Reiki
Sound Therapy
Tuning Forks
Topical Liniments
Heat / Heating Pad
Hot Bath ? Shower
Cold / Ice Pack
Cold Shower
Meditation
Music
Yoga
Swimming
Walking
Other

Today I Am Grateful For

I am so happy & grateful for my healthy body!

Today's Day & Date

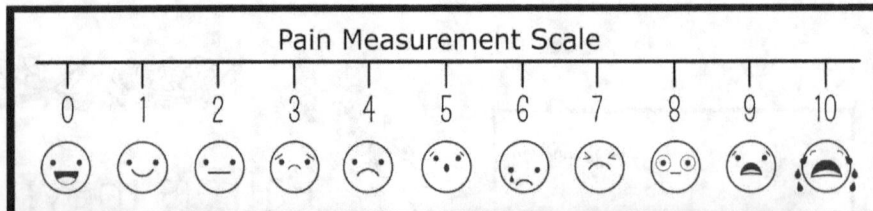

Highlight All Painful Areas

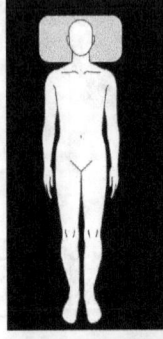 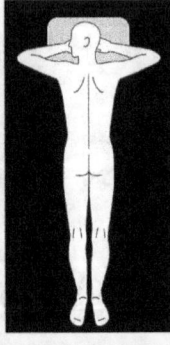 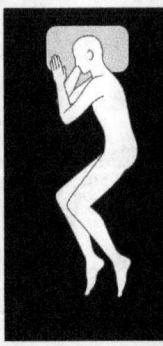 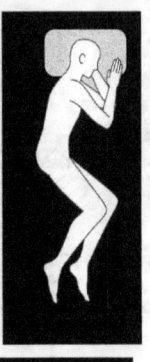

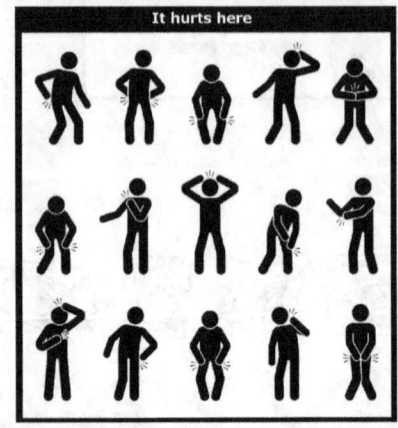

It hurts here

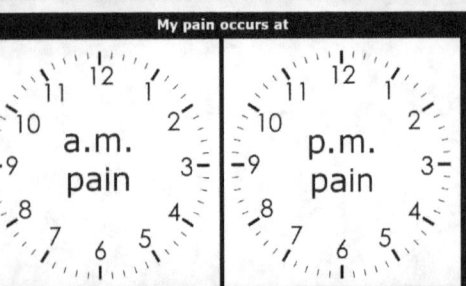

My pain occurs at — a.m. pain / p.m. pain

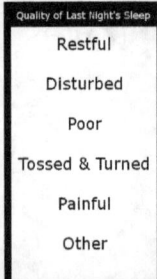

Quality of Last Night's Sleep
- Restful
- Disturbed
- Poor
- Tossed & Turned
- Painful
- Other

My mood today

My pain is
Hot
Burning
Cold
Stabbing
Throbbing
Fixed
Moving Traveling
Constant
On & Off

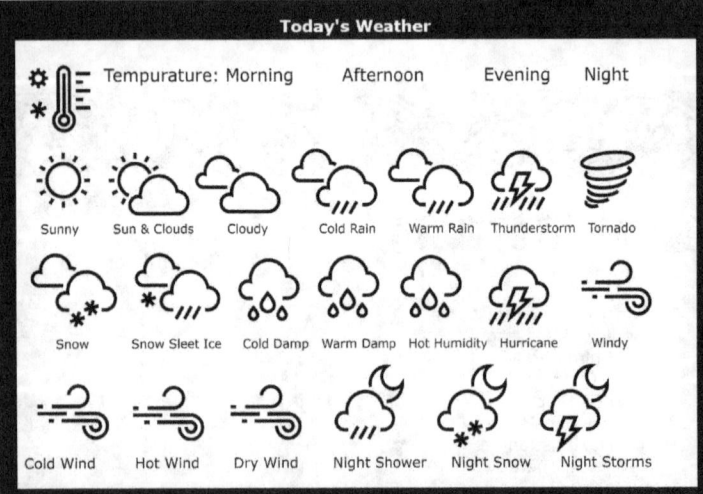

Today's Weather — Temperature: Morning, Afternoon, Evening, Night

Sunny, Sun & Clouds, Cloudy, Cold Rain, Warm Rain, Thunderstorm, Tornado, Snow, Snow Sleet Ice, Cold Damp, Warm Damp, Hot Humidity, Hurricane, Windy, Cold Wind, Hot Wind, Dry Wind, Night Shower, Night Snow, Night Storms

Breakfast

Lunch

Dinner

Snacks

Alcohol

Food Allergy Triggers

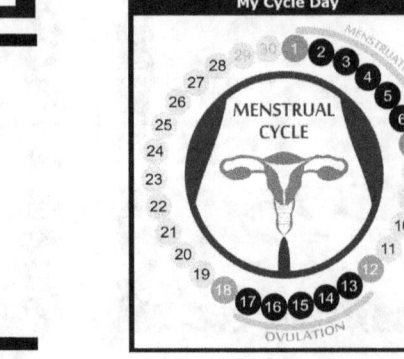

My Cycle Day

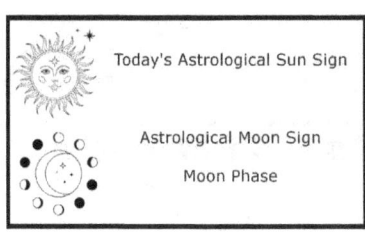

Today's Astrological Sun Sign

Astrological Moon Sign

Moon Phase

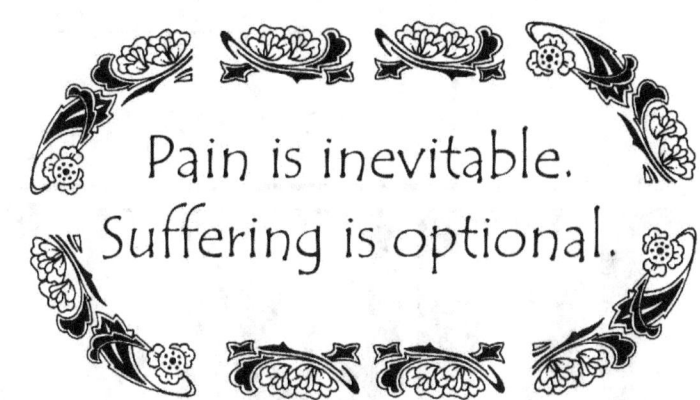

Pain is inevitable.
Suffering is optional.

Notes

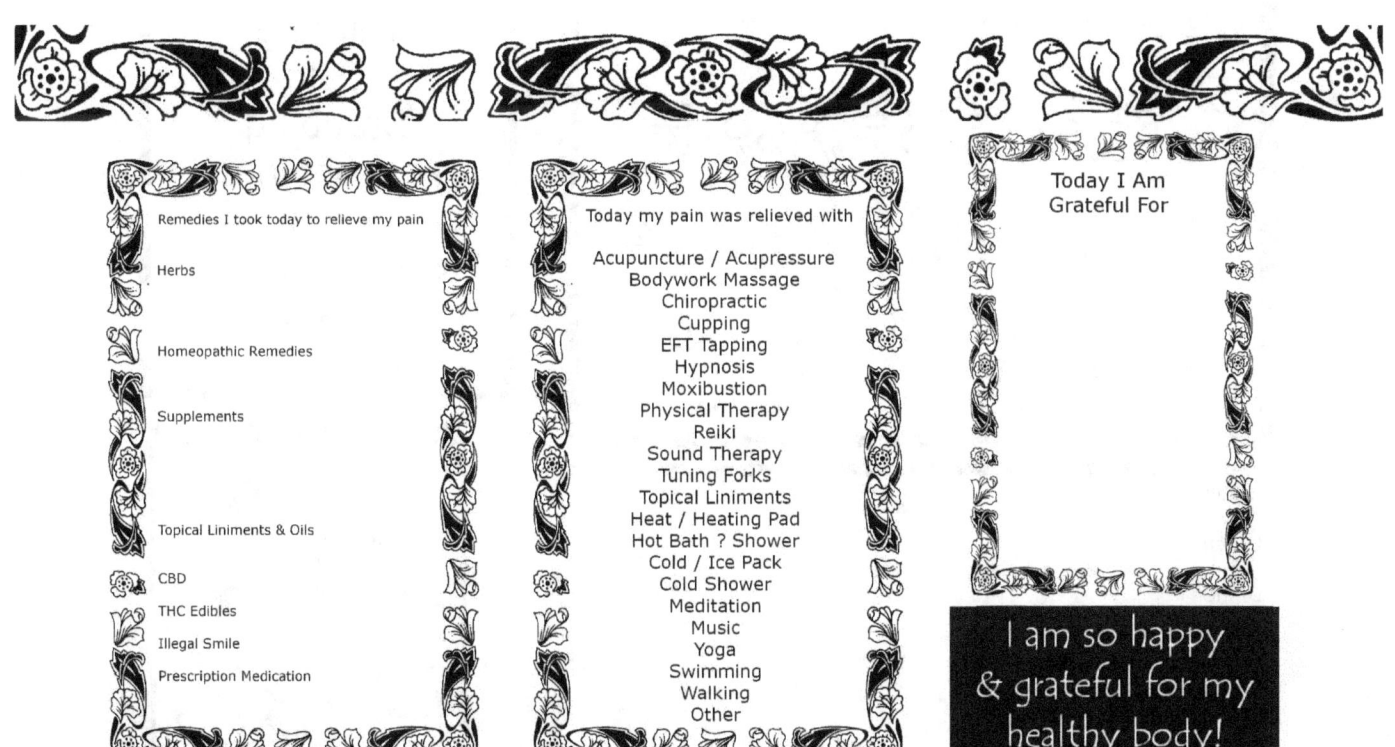

Remedies I took today to relieve my pain

Herbs

Homeopathic Remedies

Supplements

Topical Liniments & Oils

CBD

THC Edibles

Illegal Smile

Prescription Medication

Today my pain was relieved with

Acupuncture / Acupressure
Bodywork Massage
Chiropractic
Cupping
EFT Tapping
Hypnosis
Moxibustion
Physical Therapy
Reiki
Sound Therapy
Tuning Forks
Topical Liniments
Heat / Heating Pad
Hot Bath ? Shower
Cold / Ice Pack
Cold Shower
Meditation
Music
Yoga
Swimming
Walking
Other

Today I Am
Grateful For

I am so happy
& grateful for my
healthy body!

Today's Day & Date

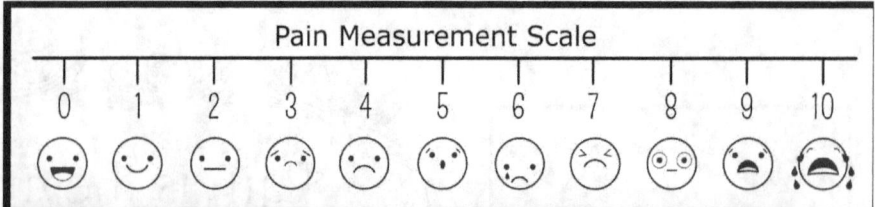

Highlight All Painful Areas

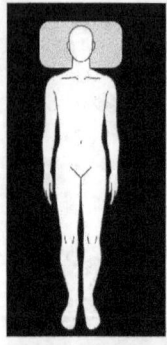 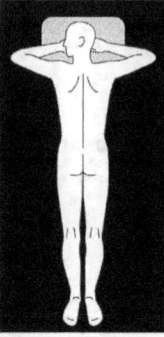 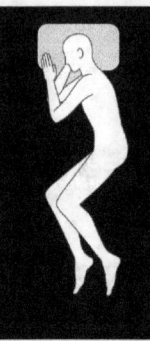 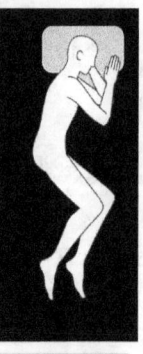

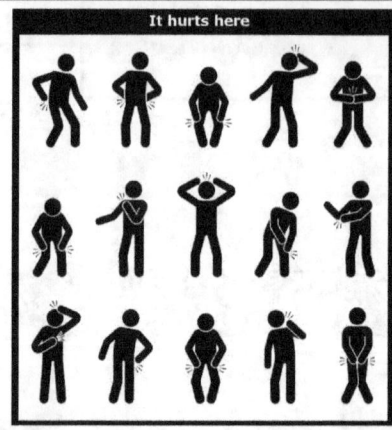
It hurts here

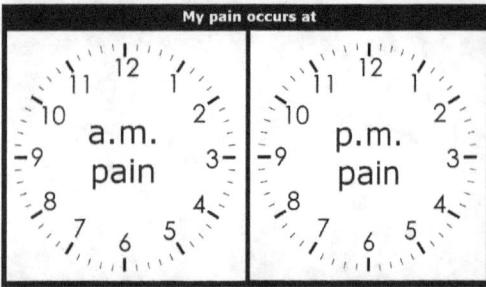
My pain occurs at — a.m. pain / p.m. pain

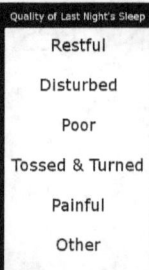
Quality of Last Night's Sleep
- Restful
- Disturbed
- Poor
- Tossed & Turned
- Painful
- Other

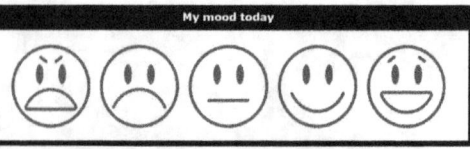
My mood today

My pain is
Hot
Burning
Cold
Stabbing
Throbbing
Fixed
Moving Traveling
Constant
On & Off

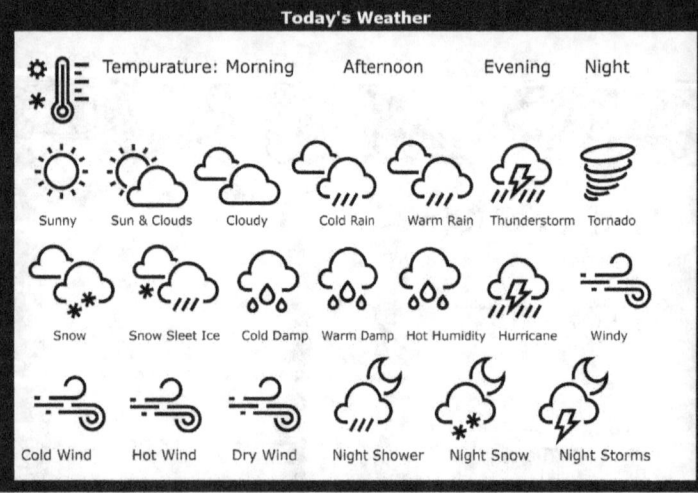
Today's Weather — Temperature: Morning, Afternoon, Evening, Night
Sunny, Sun & Clouds, Cloudy, Cold Rain, Warm Rain, Thunderstorm, Tornado
Snow, Snow Sleet Ice, Cold Damp, Warm Damp, Hot Humidity, Hurricane, Windy
Cold Wind, Hot Wind, Dry Wind, Night Shower, Night Snow, Night Storms

Breakfast

Lunch

Dinner

Snacks

Alcohol

Food Allergy Triggers

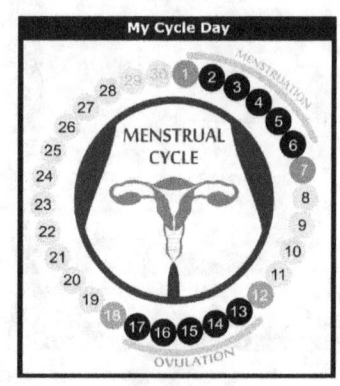
My Cycle Day

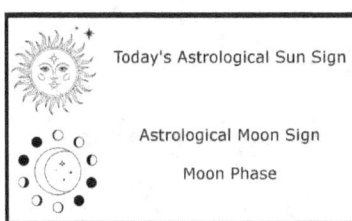

Today's Astrological Sun Sign

Astrological Moon Sign
Moon Phase

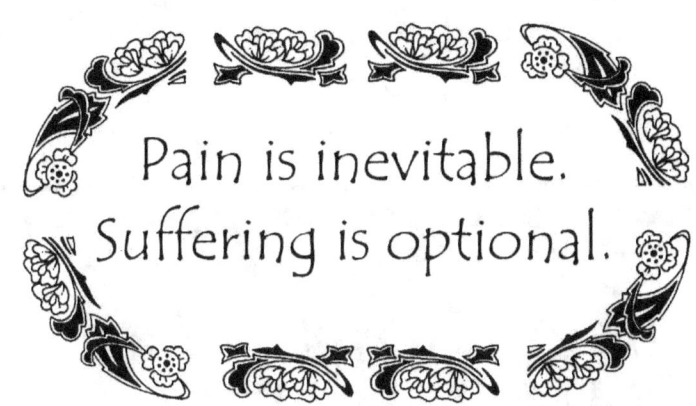

Pain is inevitable.
Suffering is optional.

Notes

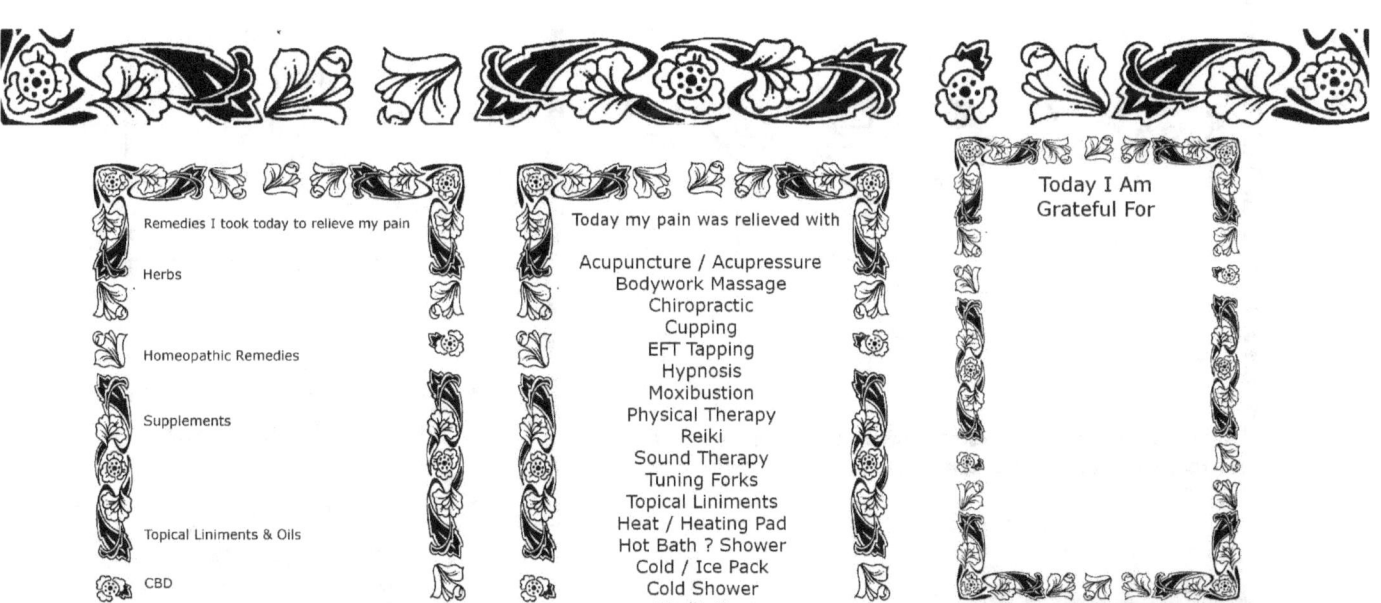

Remedies I took today to relieve my pain

Herbs

Homeopathic Remedies

Supplements

Topical Liniments & Oils

CBD
THC Edibles
Illegal Smile
Prescription Medication

Today my pain was relieved with

Acupuncture / Acupressure
Bodywork Massage
Chiropractic
Cupping
EFT Tapping
Hypnosis
Moxibustion
Physical Therapy
Reiki
Sound Therapy
Tuning Forks
Topical Liniments
Heat / Heating Pad
Hot Bath ? Shower
Cold / Ice Pack
Cold Shower
Meditation
Music
Yoga
Swimming
Walking
Other

Today I Am
Grateful For

I am so happy
& grateful for my
healthy body!

Today's Day & Date

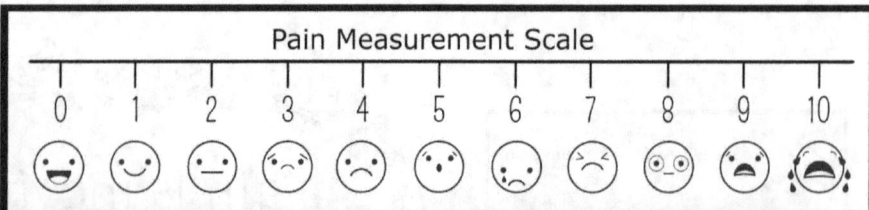

Highlight All Painful Areas

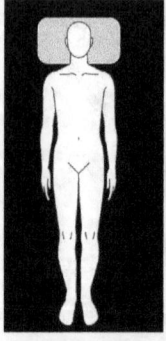 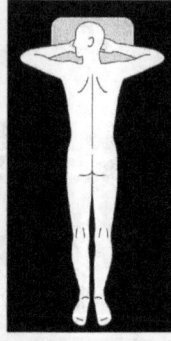 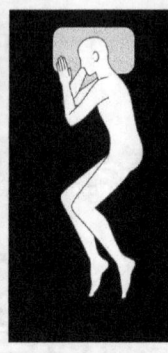 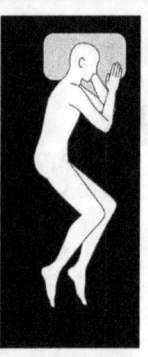

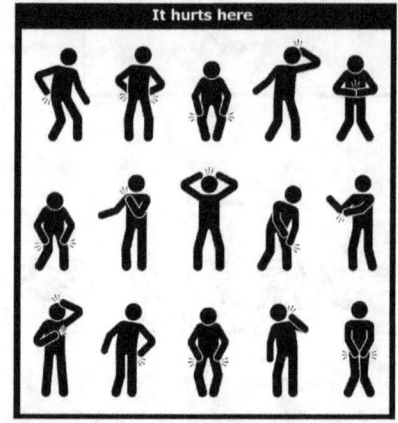

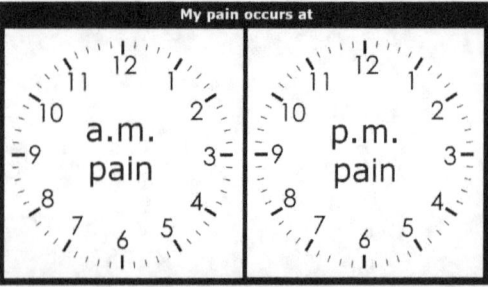

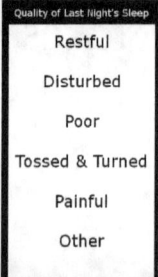

Quality of Last Night's Sleep
- Restful
- Disturbed
- Poor
- Tossed & Turned
- Painful
- Other

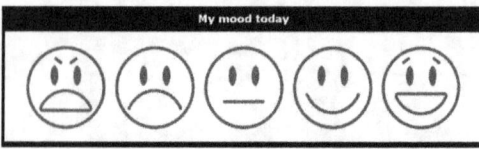

Today's Weather

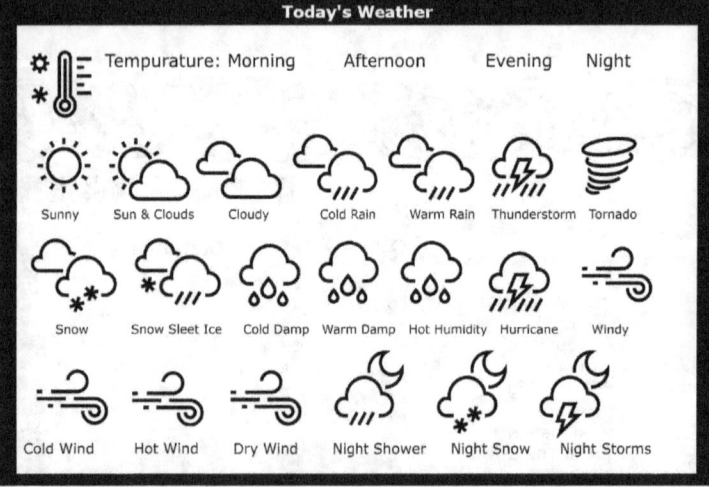

My pain is

Hot
Burning
Cold
Stabbing
Throbbing
Fixed
Moving Traveling
Constant
On & Off

Breakfast

Lunch

Dinner

Snacks

Alcohol

Food Allergy Triggers

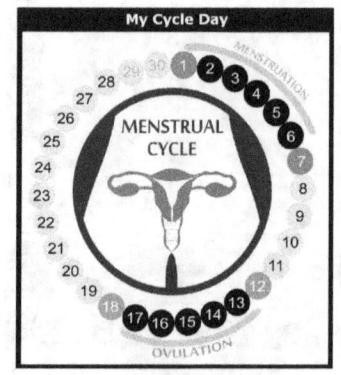

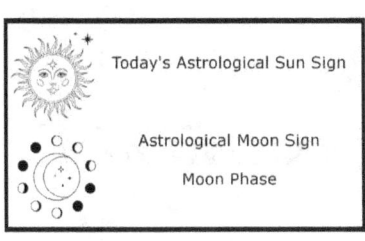

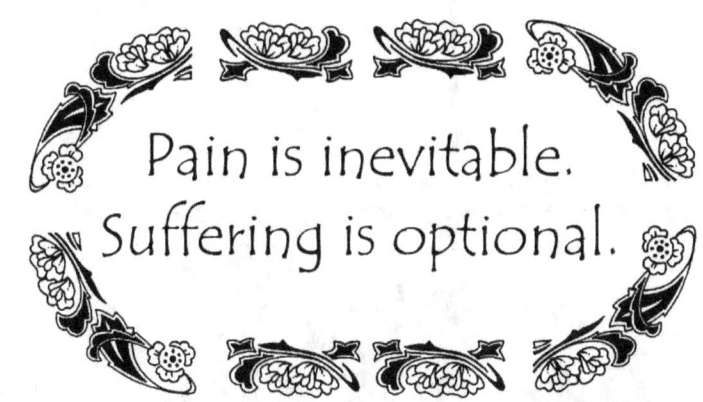

Pain is inevitable. Suffering is optional.

Notes

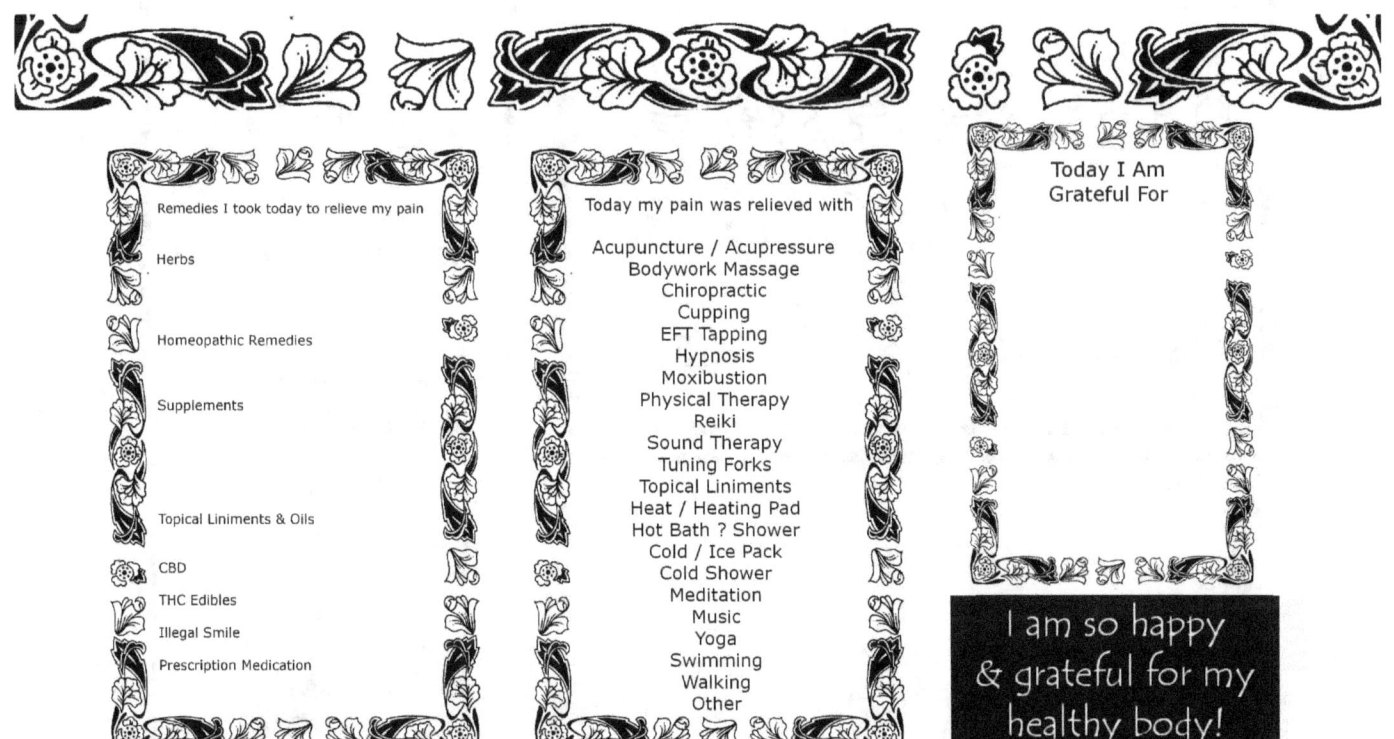

Remedies I took today to relieve my pain

Herbs

Homeopathic Remedies

Supplements

Topical Liniments & Oils

CBD
THC Edibles
Illegal Smile
Prescription Medication

Today my pain was relieved with

Acupuncture / Acupressure
Bodywork Massage
Chiropractic
Cupping
EFT Tapping
Hypnosis
Moxibustion
Physical Therapy
Reiki
Sound Therapy
Tuning Forks
Topical Liniments
Heat / Heating Pad
Hot Bath ? Shower
Cold / Ice Pack
Cold Shower
Meditation
Music
Yoga
Swimming
Walking
Other

Today I Am Grateful For

I am so happy & grateful for my healthy body!

Today's Day & Date

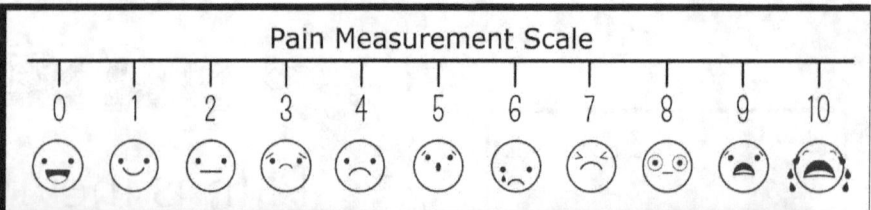

Highlight All Painful Areas

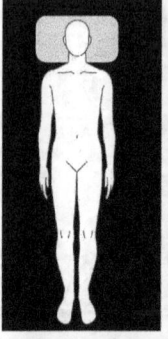
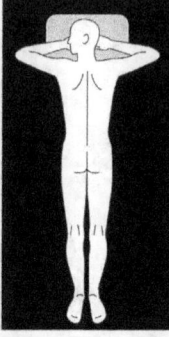
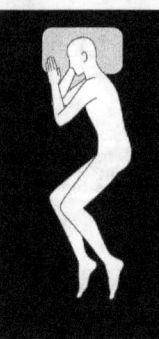
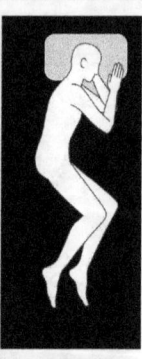

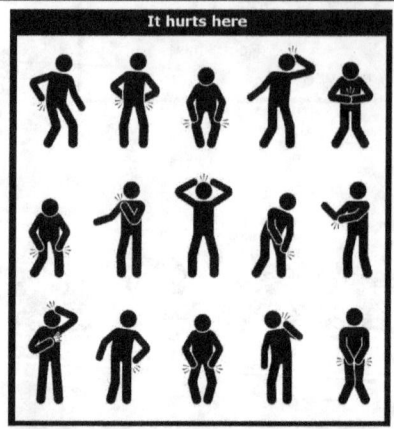

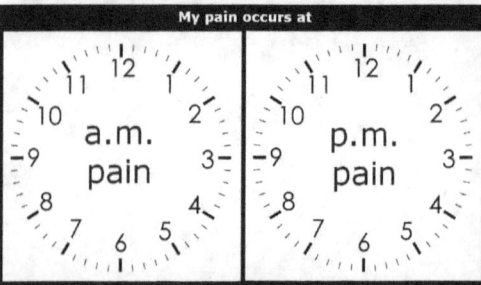

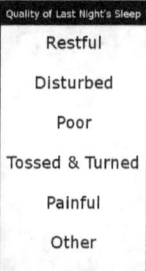

Quality of Last Night's Sleep
- Restful
- Disturbed
- Poor
- Tossed & Turned
- Painful
- Other

My pain is

Hot
Burning
Cold
Stabbing
Throbbing
Fixed
Moving Traveling
Constant
On & Off

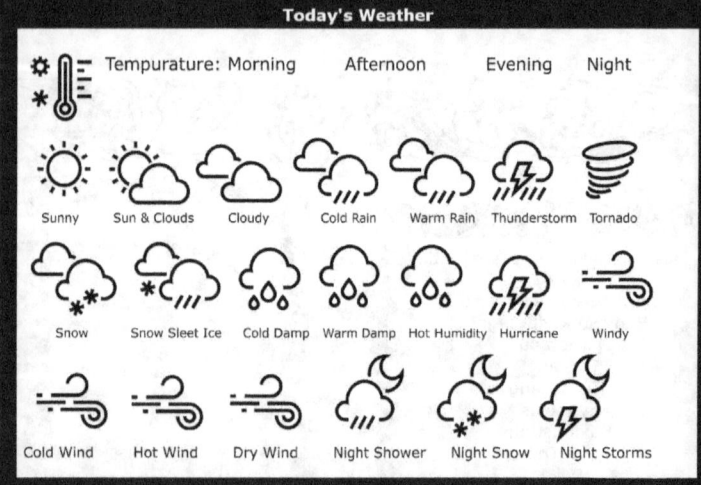

Breakfast

Lunch

Dinner

Snacks

Alcohol

Food Allergy Triggers

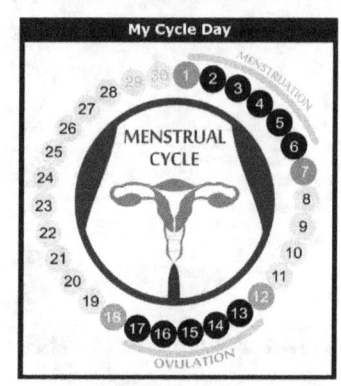

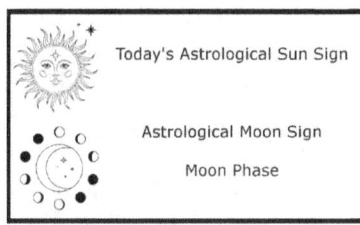

Today's Astrological Sun Sign

Astrological Moon Sign

Moon Phase

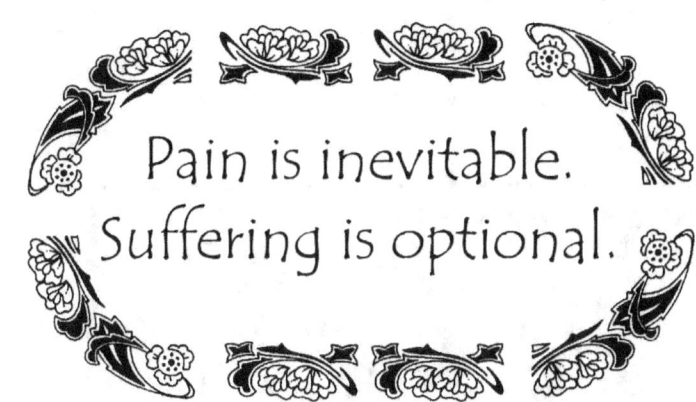

Pain is inevitable. Suffering is optional.

Notes

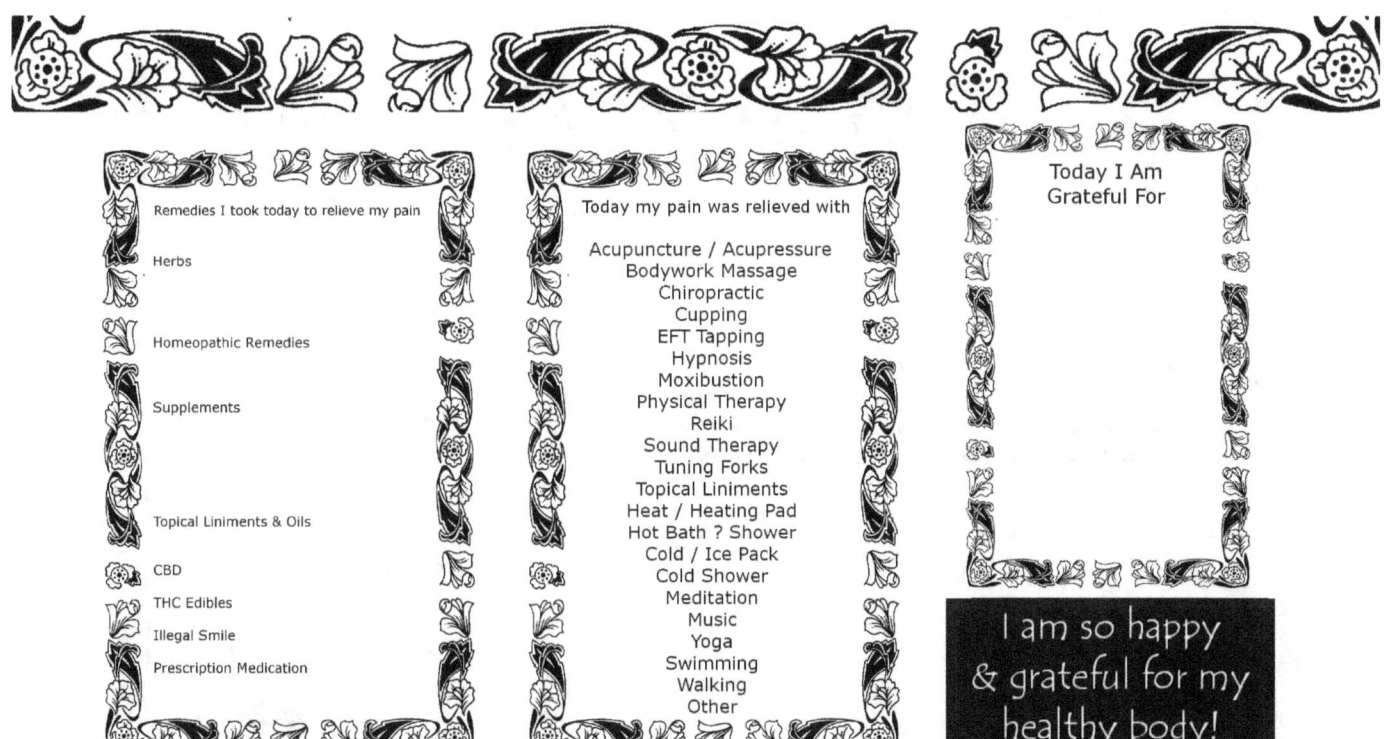

Remedies I took today to relieve my pain

Herbs

Homeopathic Remedies

Supplements

Topical Liniments & Oils

CBD

THC Edibles

Illegal Smile

Prescription Medication

Today my pain was relieved with

Acupuncture / Acupressure
Bodywork Massage
Chiropractic
Cupping
EFT Tapping
Hypnosis
Moxibustion
Physical Therapy
Reiki
Sound Therapy
Tuning Forks
Topical Liniments
Heat / Heating Pad
Hot Bath ? Shower
Cold / Ice Pack
Cold Shower
Meditation
Music
Yoga
Swimming
Walking
Other

Today I Am Grateful For

I am so happy & grateful for my healthy body!

Today's Day & Date

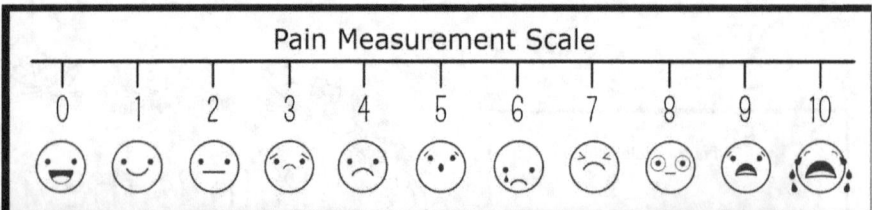

Highlight All Painful Areas

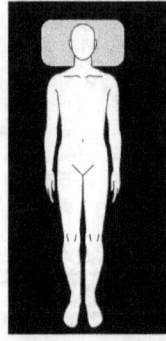 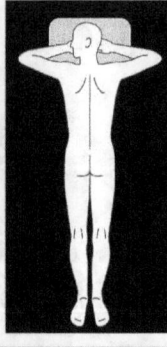 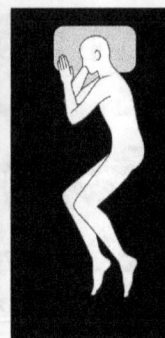 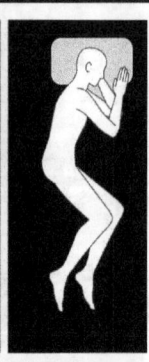

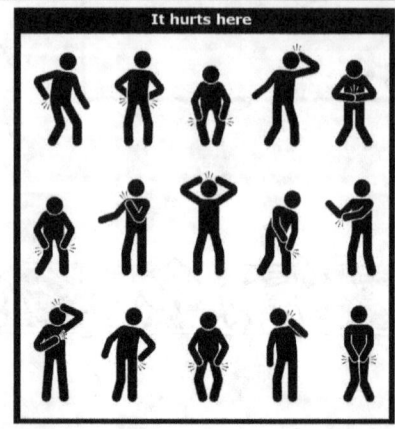

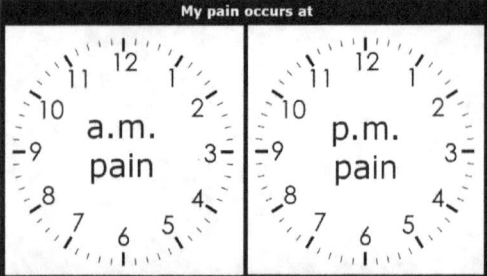

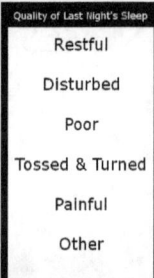

Quality of Last Night's Sleep
- Restful
- Disturbed
- Poor
- Tossed & Turned
- Painful
- Other

My pain is

Hot
Burning
Cold
Stabbing
Throbbing
Fixed
Moving Traveling
Constant
On & Off

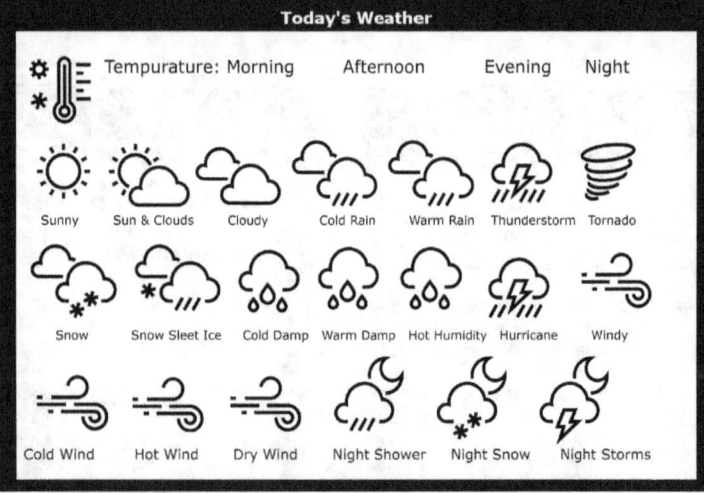

Breakfast

Lunch

Dinner

Snacks

Alcohol

Food Allergy Triggers

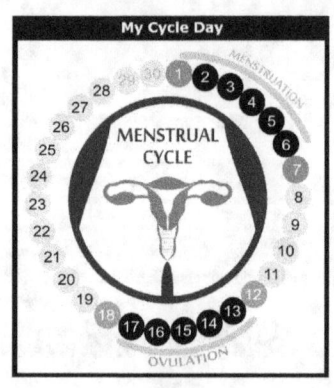

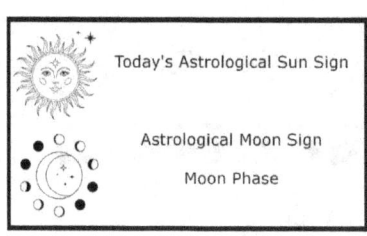

Today's Astrological Sun Sign

Astrological Moon Sign

Moon Phase

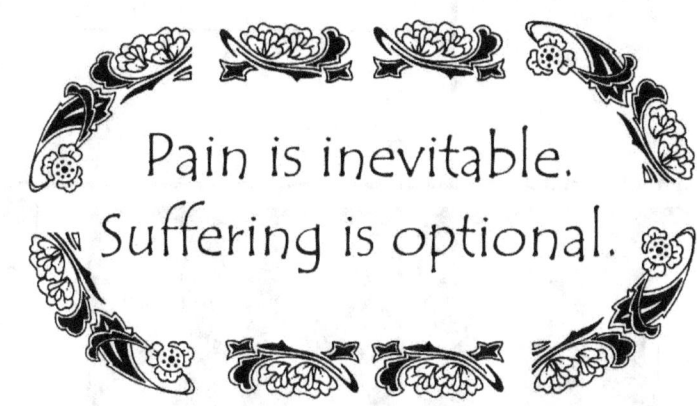

Pain is inevitable.
Suffering is optional.

Notes

Remedies I took today to relieve my pain

Herbs

Homeopathic Remedies

Supplements

Topical Liniments & Oils

CBD

THC Edibles

Illegal Smile

Prescription Medication

Today my pain was relieved with

Acupuncture / Acupressure
Bodywork Massage
Chiropractic
Cupping
EFT Tapping
Hypnosis
Moxibustion
Physical Therapy
Reiki
Sound Therapy
Tuning Forks
Topical Liniments
Heat / Heating Pad
Hot Bath ? Shower
Cold / Ice Pack
Cold Shower
Meditation
Music
Yoga
Swimming
Walking
Other

Today I Am Grateful For

I am so happy & grateful for my healthy body!

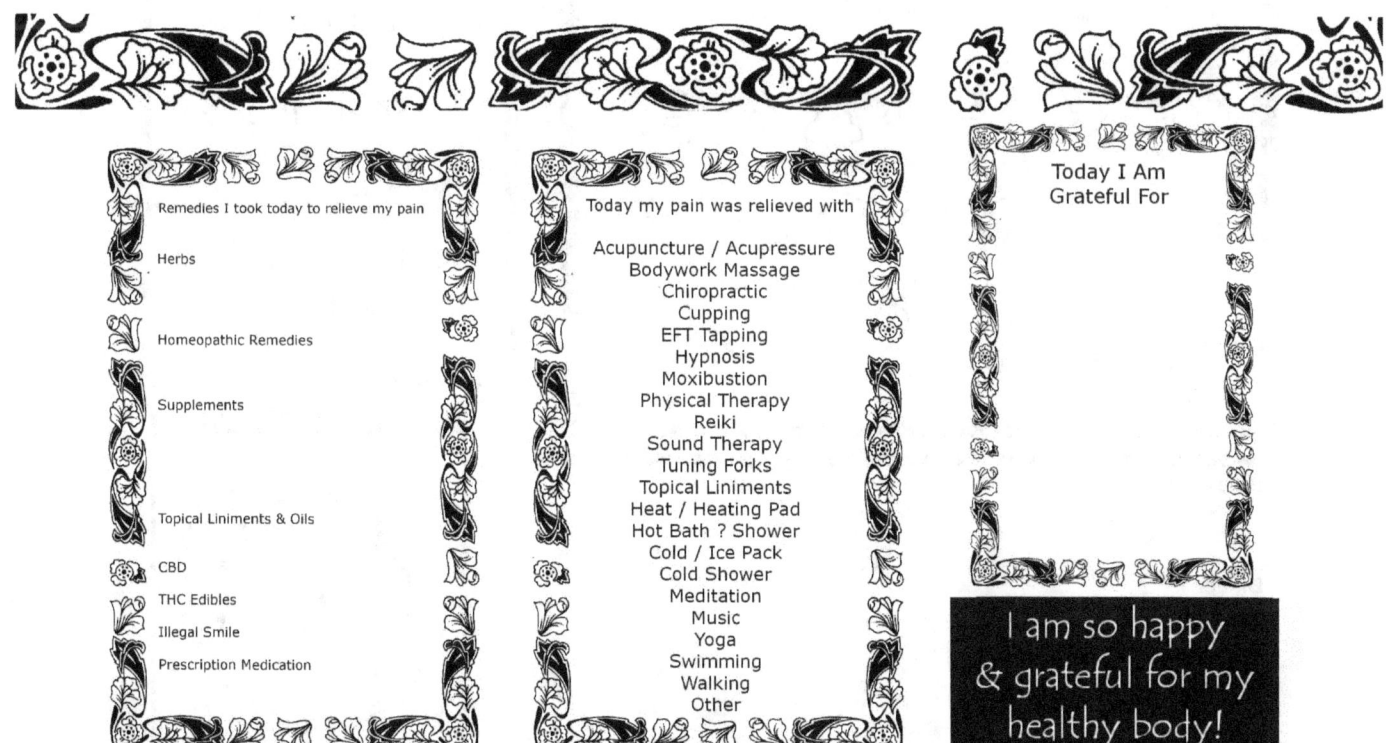

Today's Day & Date

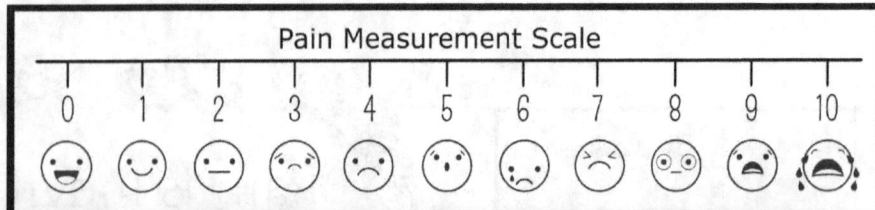

Highlight All Painful Areas

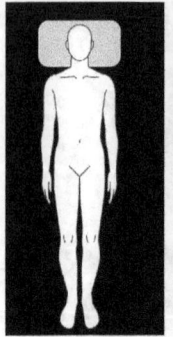 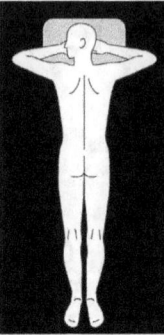 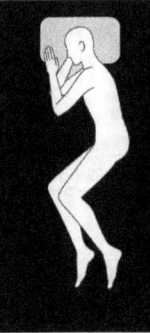 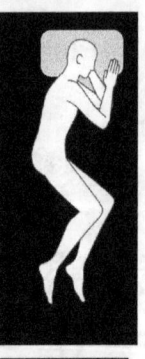

It hurts here

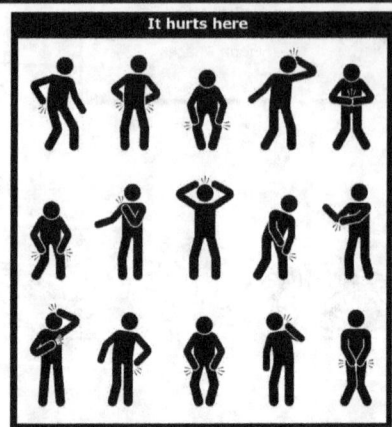

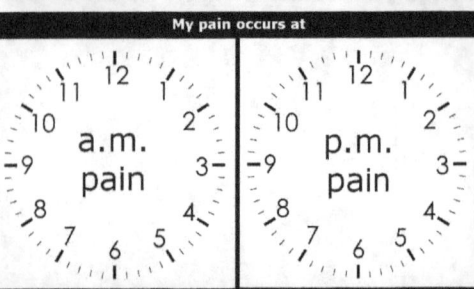

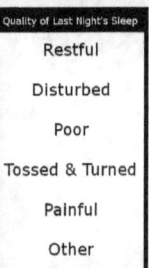

Quality of Last Night's Sleep
- Restful
- Disturbed
- Poor
- Tossed & Turned
- Painful
- Other

My mood today

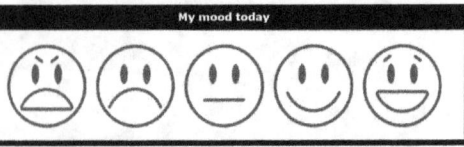

My pain is
Hot
Burning
Cold
Stabbing
Throbbing
Fixed
Moving Traveling
Constant
On & Off

Today's Weather

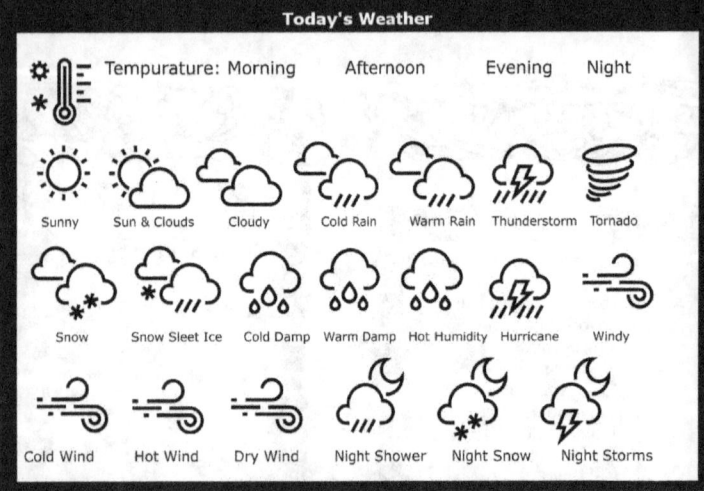

Tempurature: Morning   Afternoon   Evening   Night

My Cycle Day

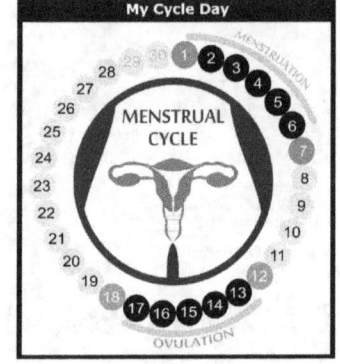

Breakfast

Lunch

Dinner

Snacks

Alcohol

Food Allergy Triggers

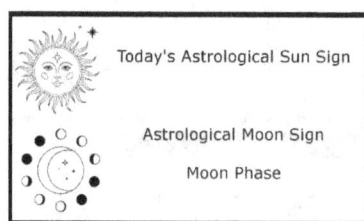

Today's Astrological Sun Sign

Astrological Moon Sign

Moon Phase

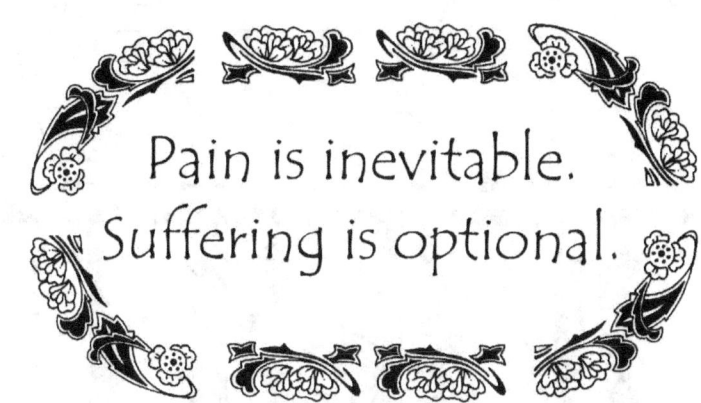

Pain is inevitable. Suffering is optional.

Notes

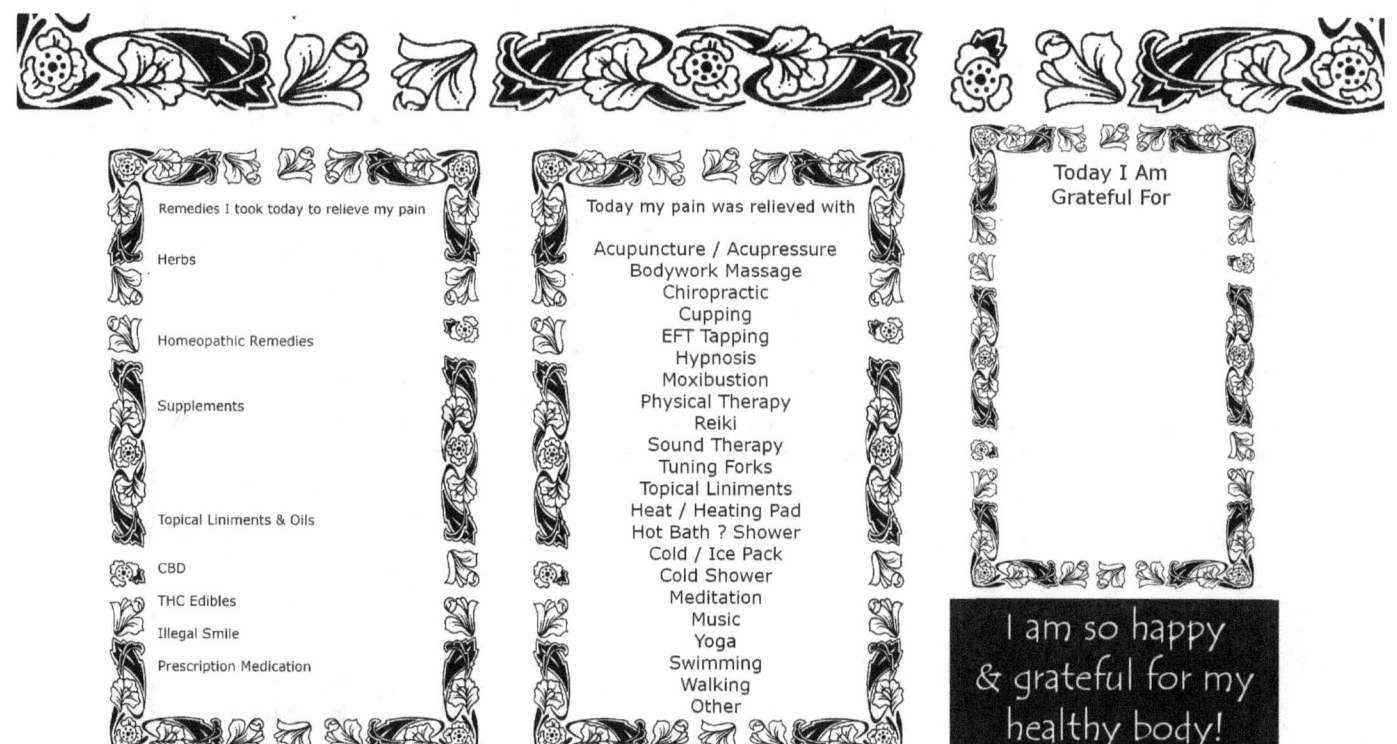

Remedies I took today to relieve my pain

Herbs

Homeopathic Remedies

Supplements

Topical Liniments & Oils

CBD
THC Edibles
Illegal Smile
Prescription Medication

Today my pain was relieved with

Acupuncture / Acupressure
Bodywork Massage
Chiropractic
Cupping
EFT Tapping
Hypnosis
Moxibustion
Physical Therapy
Reiki
Sound Therapy
Tuning Forks
Topical Liniments
Heat / Heating Pad
Hot Bath ? Shower
Cold / Ice Pack
Cold Shower
Meditation
Music
Yoga
Swimming
Walking
Other

Today I Am Grateful For

I am so happy & grateful for my healthy body!

Today's Day & Date

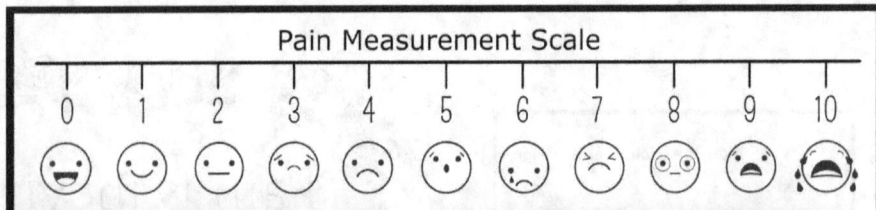

Highlight All Painful Areas

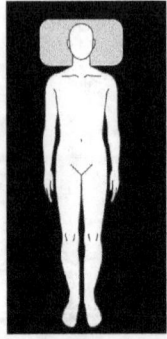 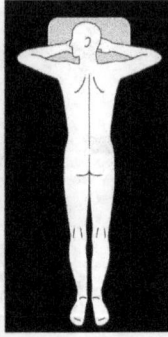 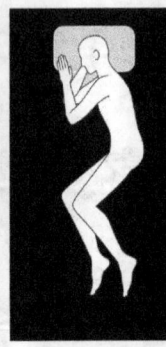 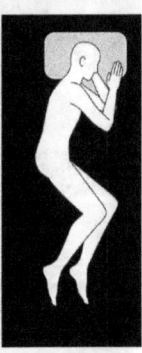

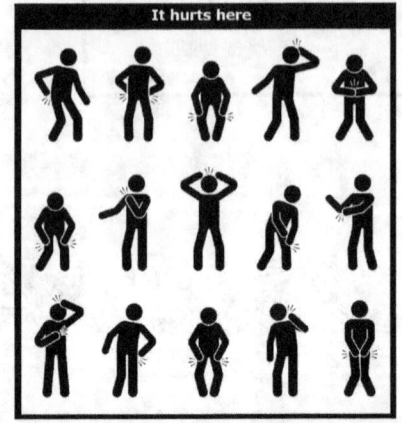
It hurts here

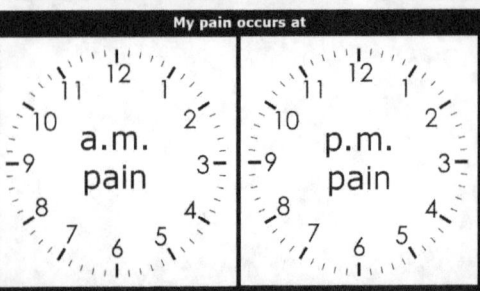
My pain occurs at — a.m. pain / p.m. pain

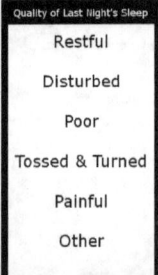
Quality of Last Night's Sleep
- Restful
- Disturbed
- Poor
- Tossed & Turned
- Painful
- Other

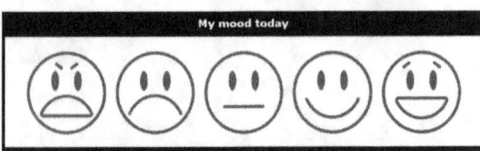
My mood today

My pain is
Hot
Burning
Cold
Stabbing
Throbbing
Fixed
Moving Traveling
Constant
On & Off

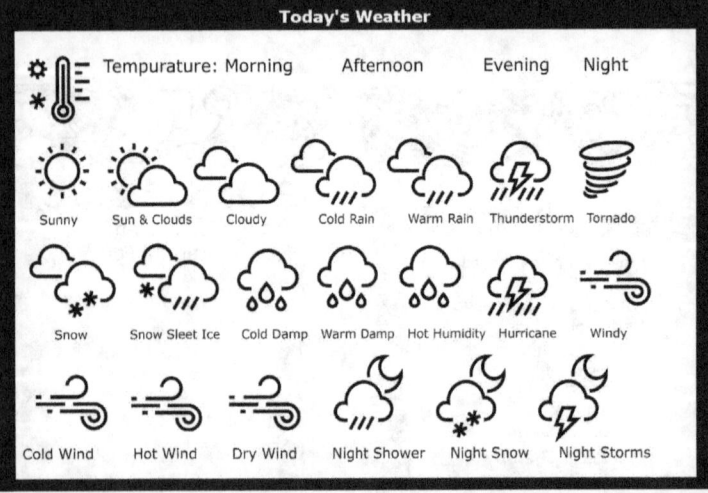
Today's Weather — Temperature: Morning, Afternoon, Evening, Night

Breakfast

Lunch

Dinner

Snacks

Alcohol

Food Allergy Triggers

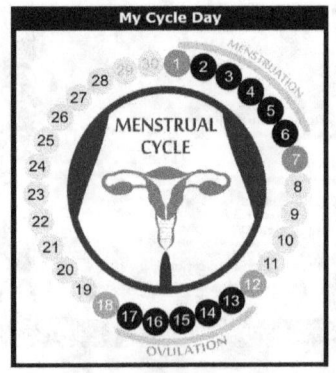
My Cycle Day

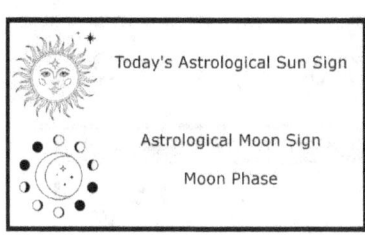

Today's Astrological Sun Sign

Astrological Moon Sign

Moon Phase

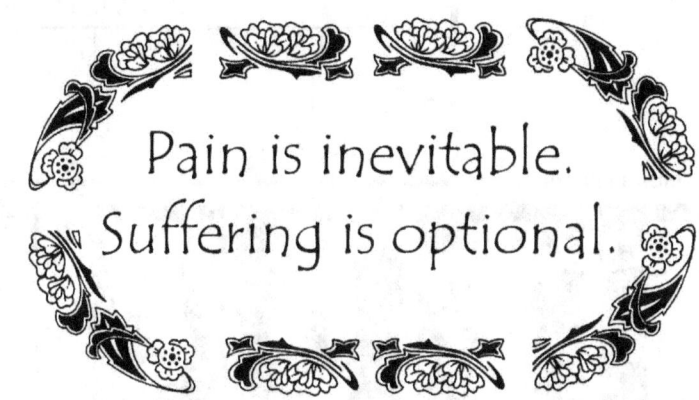

Pain is inevitable. Suffering is optional.

Notes

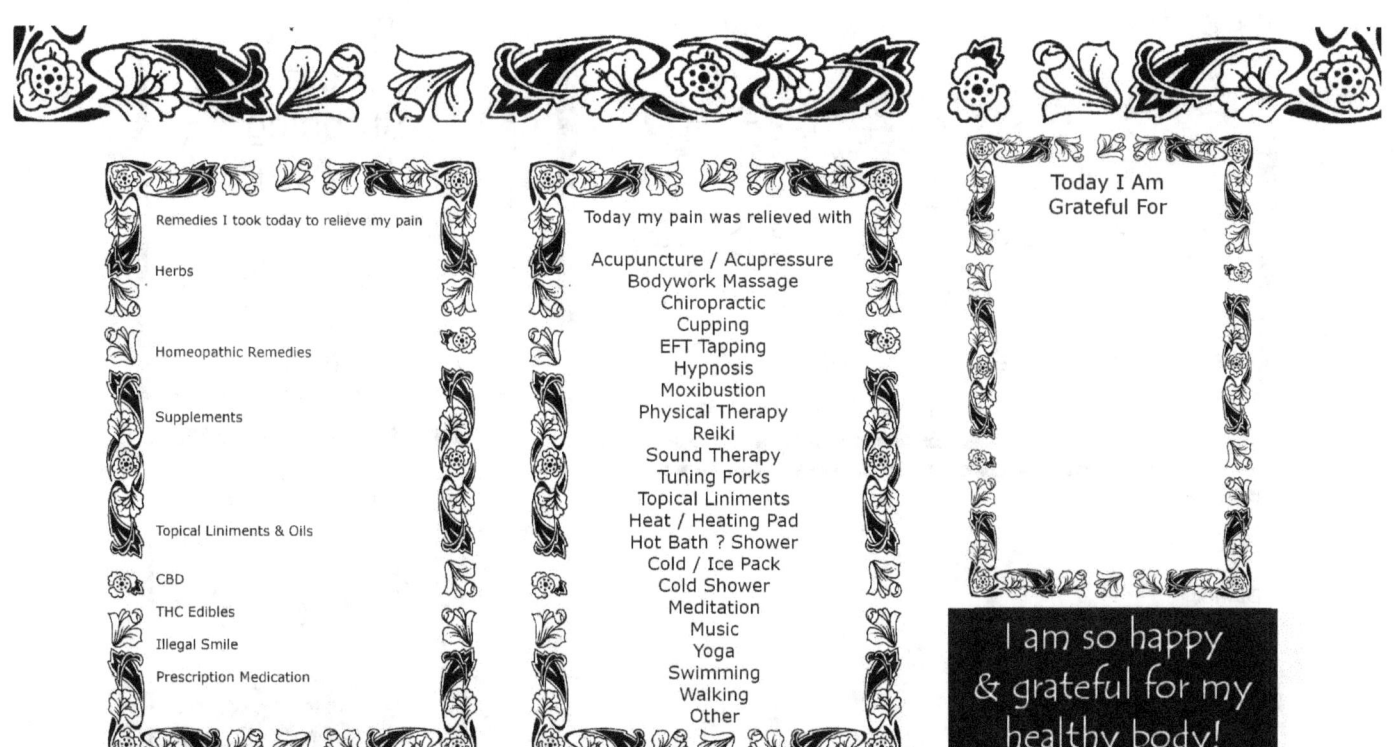

Remedies I took today to relieve my pain

Herbs

Homeopathic Remedies

Supplements

Topical Liniments & Oils

CBD

THC Edibles

Illegal Smile

Prescription Medication

Today my pain was relieved with

Acupuncture / Acupressure
Bodywork Massage
Chiropractic
Cupping
EFT Tapping
Hypnosis
Moxibustion
Physical Therapy
Reiki
Sound Therapy
Tuning Forks
Topical Liniments
Heat / Heating Pad
Hot Bath ? Shower
Cold / Ice Pack
Cold Shower
Meditation
Music
Yoga
Swimming
Walking
Other

Today I Am Grateful For

I am so happy & grateful for my healthy body!

Today's Day & Date

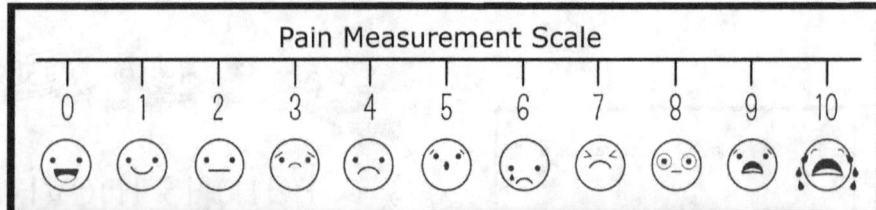

Highlight All Painful Areas

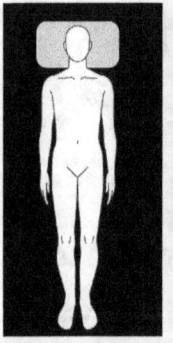 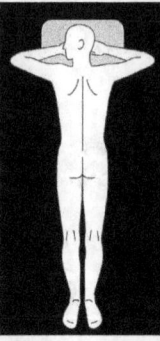 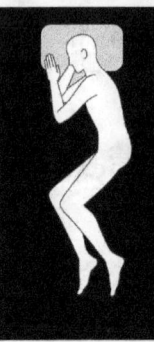 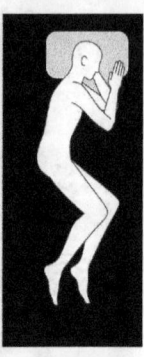

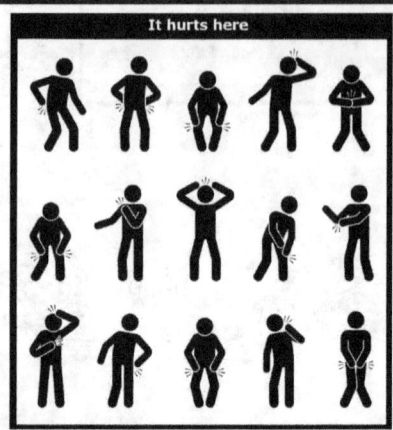

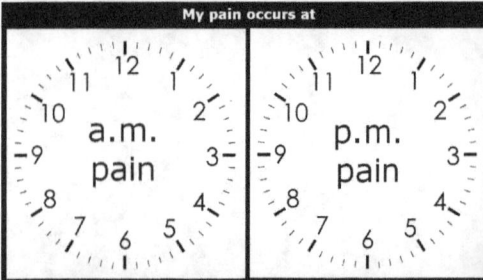

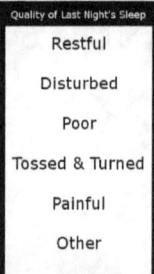
Quality of Last Night's Sleep
- Restful
- Disturbed
- Poor
- Tossed & Turned
- Painful
- Other

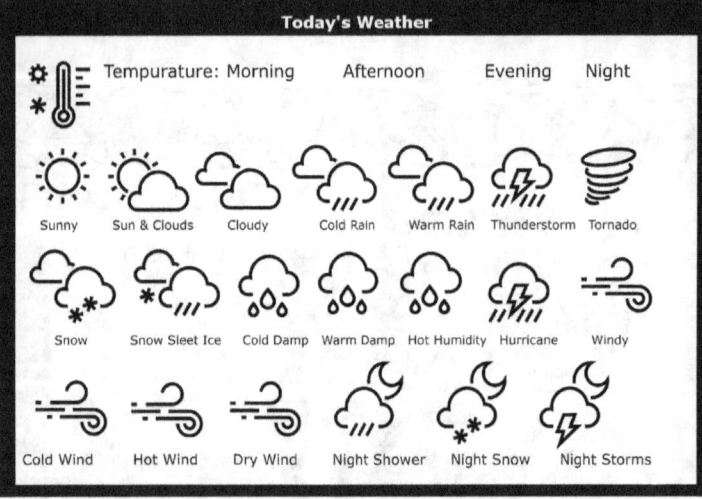

My pain is
Hot
Burning
Cold
Stabbing
Throbbing
Fixed
Moving Traveling
Constant
On & Off

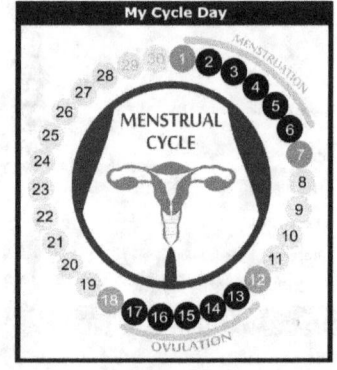

Breakfast

Lunch

Dinner

Snacks

Alcohol

Food Allergy Triggers

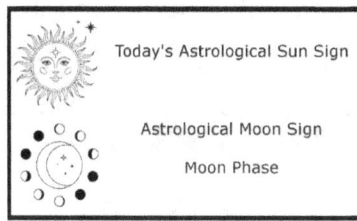

Today's Astrological Sun Sign

Astrological Moon Sign

Moon Phase

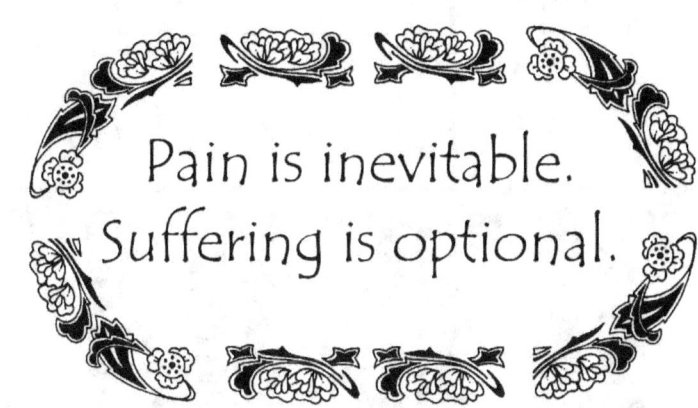

Pain is inevitable.
Suffering is optional.

Notes

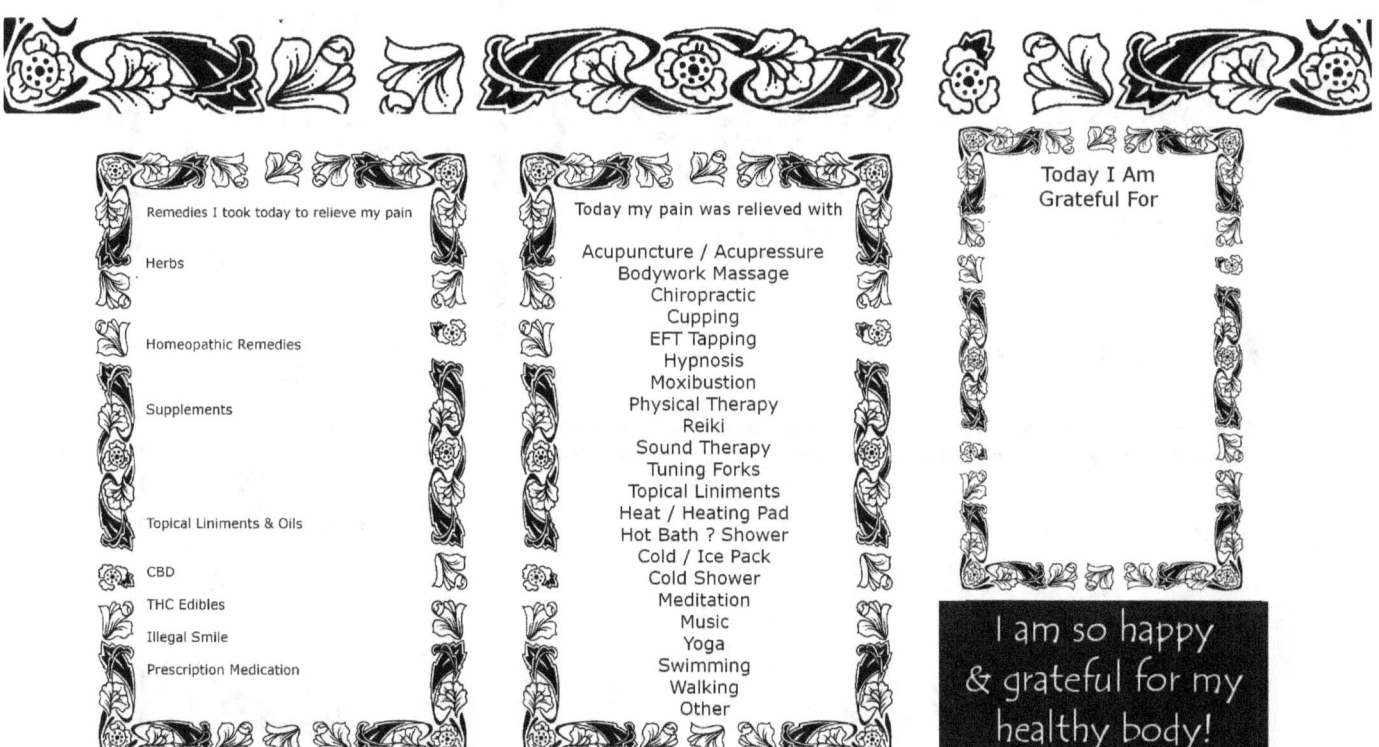

Remedies I took today to relieve my pain

Herbs

Homeopathic Remedies

Supplements

Topical Liniments & Oils

CBD

THC Edibles

Illegal Smile

Prescription Medication

Today my pain was relieved with

Acupuncture / Acupressure
Bodywork Massage
Chiropractic
Cupping
EFT Tapping
Hypnosis
Moxibustion
Physical Therapy
Reiki
Sound Therapy
Tuning Forks
Topical Liniments
Heat / Heating Pad
Hot Bath ? Shower
Cold / Ice Pack
Cold Shower
Meditation
Music
Yoga
Swimming
Walking
Other

Today I Am Grateful For

I am so happy & grateful for my healthy body!

Today's Day & Date

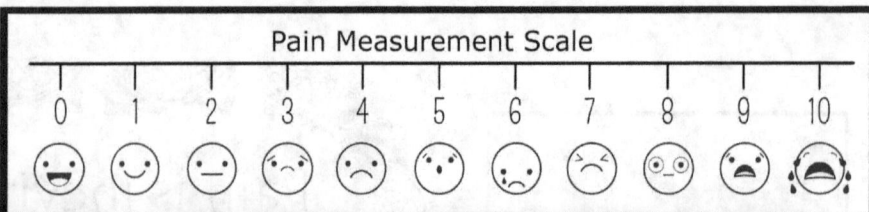

Pain Measurement Scale

Highlight All Painful Areas

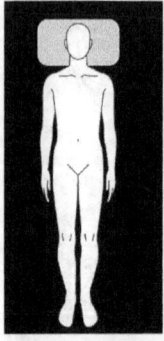 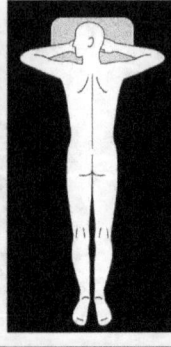 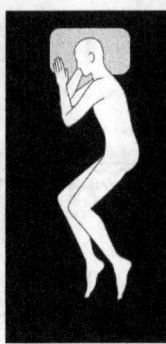 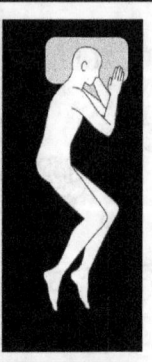

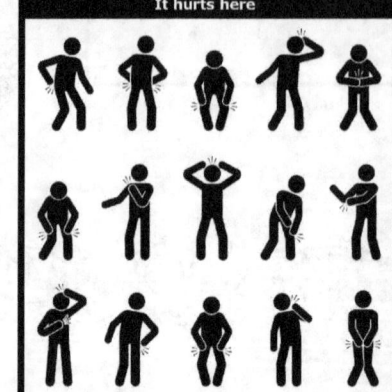
It hurts here

My pain occurs at

a.m. pain | p.m. pain

Quality of Last Night's Sleep
- Restful
- Disturbed
- Poor
- Tossed & Turned
- Painful
- Other

My mood today

My pain is
Hot
Burning
Cold
Stabbing
Throbbing
Fixed
Moving Traveling
Constant
On & Off

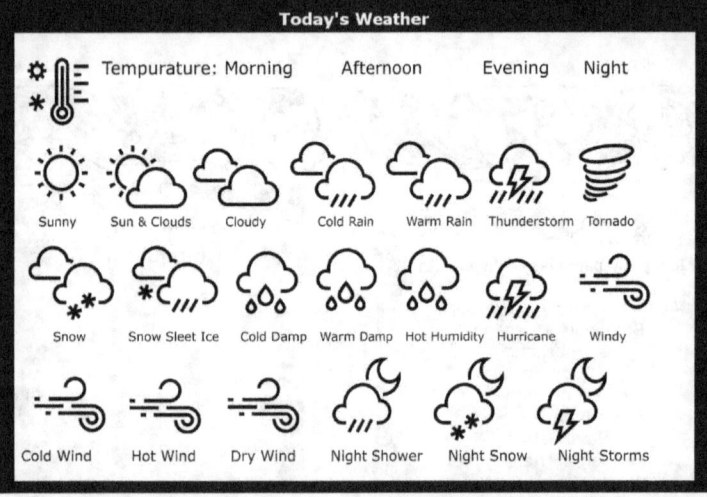
Today's Weather — Temperature: Morning, Afternoon, Evening, Night

Breakfast

Lunch

Dinner

Snacks

Alcohol

Food Allergy Triggers

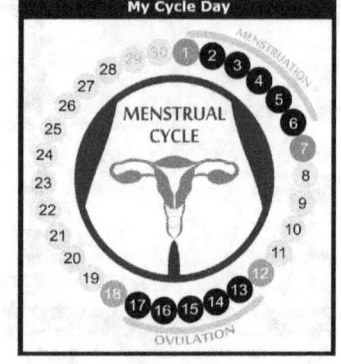
My Cycle Day

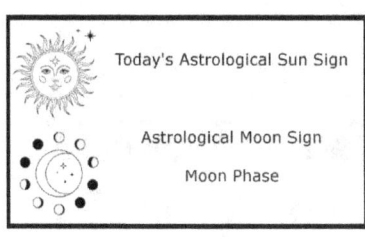

Today's Astrological Sun Sign

Astrological Moon Sign

Moon Phase

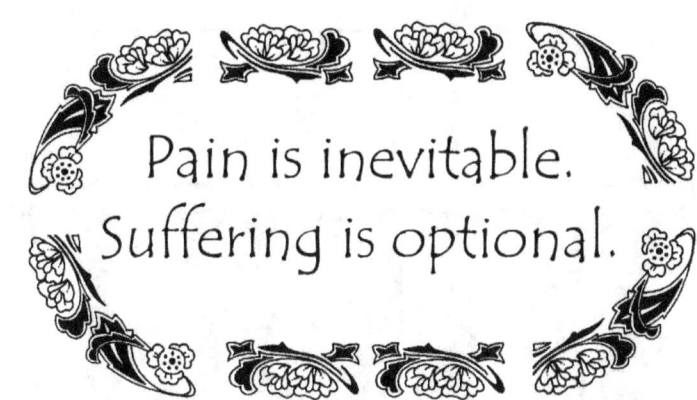

Pain is inevitable.
Suffering is optional.

Notes

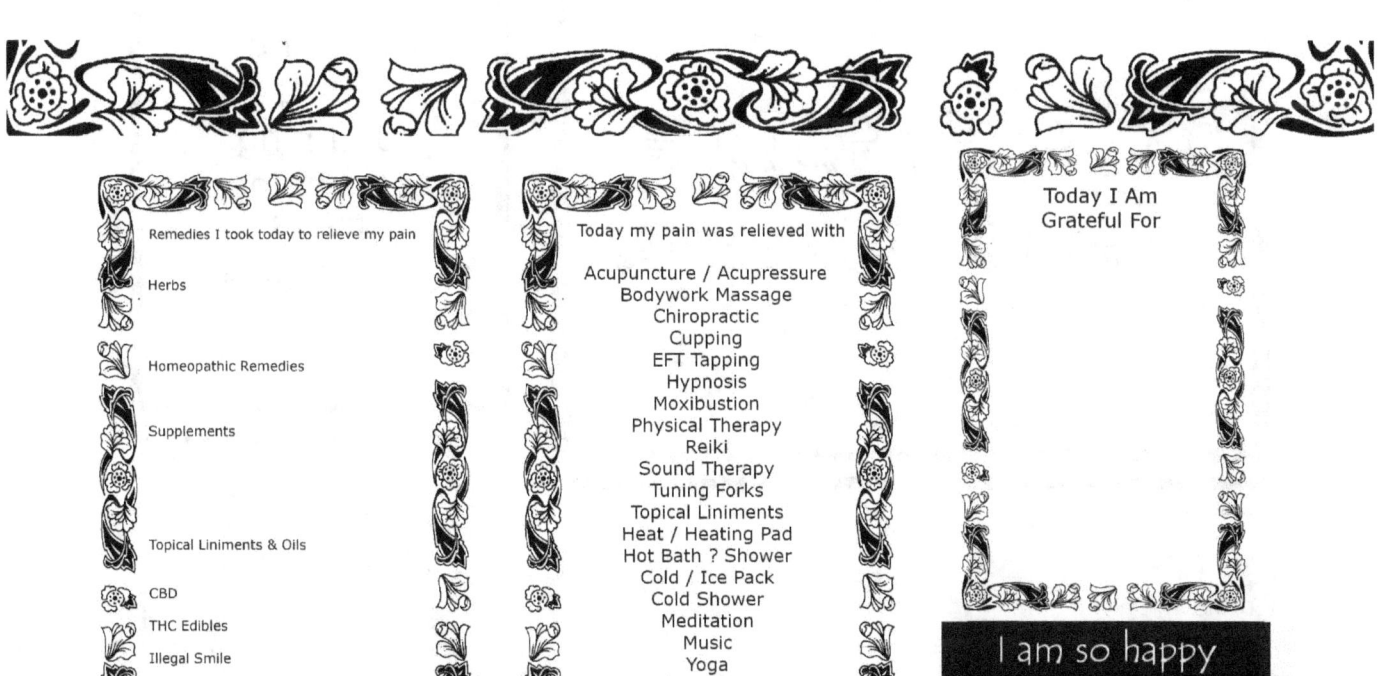

Remedies I took today to relieve my pain

Herbs

Homeopathic Remedies

Supplements

Topical Liniments & Oils

CBD

THC Edibles

Illegal Smile

Prescription Medication

Today my pain was relieved with

Acupuncture / Acupressure
Bodywork Massage
Chiropractic
Cupping
EFT Tapping
Hypnosis
Moxibustion
Physical Therapy
Reiki
Sound Therapy
Tuning Forks
Topical Liniments
Heat / Heating Pad
Hot Bath ? Shower
Cold / Ice Pack
Cold Shower
Meditation
Music
Yoga
Swimming
Walking
Other

Today I Am Grateful For

I am so happy & grateful for my healthy body!

Today's Day & Date

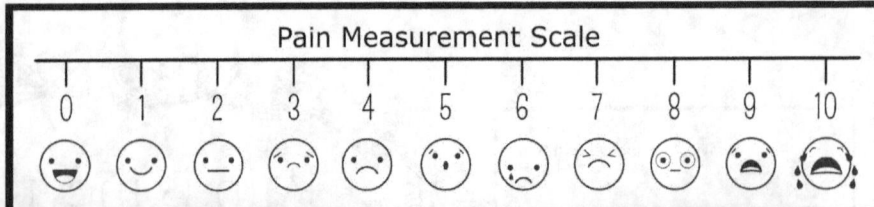

Highlight All Painful Areas

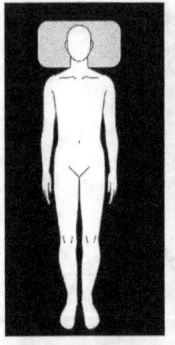 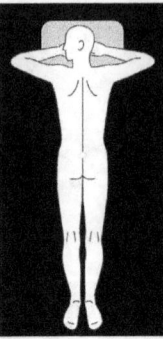 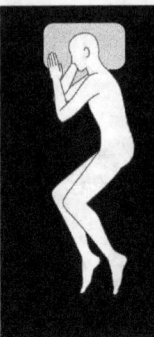 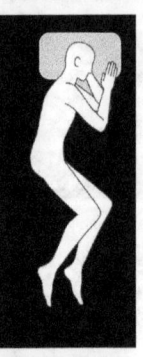

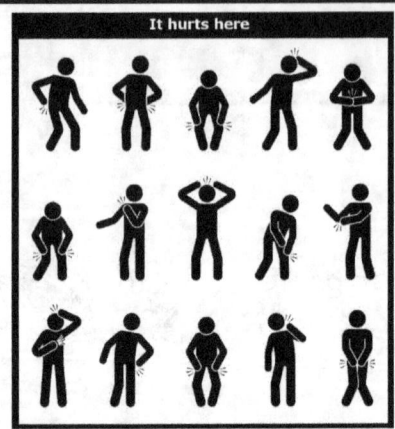
It hurts here

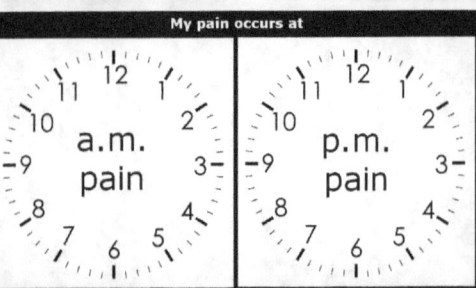
My pain occurs at — a.m. pain / p.m. pain

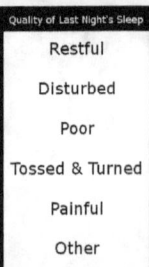

Quality of Last Night's Sleep
- Restful
- Disturbed
- Poor
- Tossed & Turned
- Painful
- Other

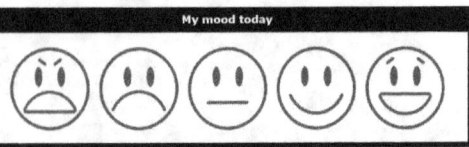
My mood today

My pain is
Hot
Burning
Cold
Stabbing
Throbbing
Fixed
Moving Traveling
Constant
On & Off

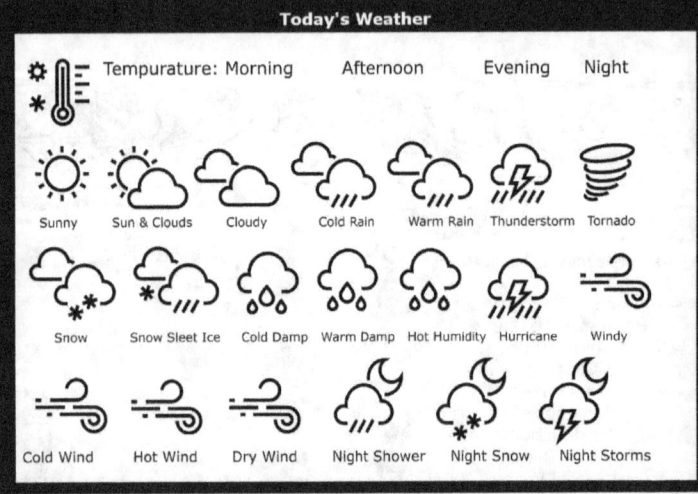
Today's Weather — Temperature: Morning, Afternoon, Evening, Night

Breakfast

Lunch

Dinner

Snacks

Alcohol

Food Allergy Triggers

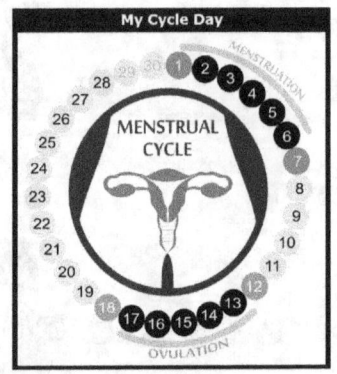
My Cycle Day

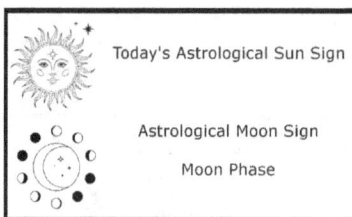

Today's Astrological Sun Sign

Astrological Moon Sign

Moon Phase

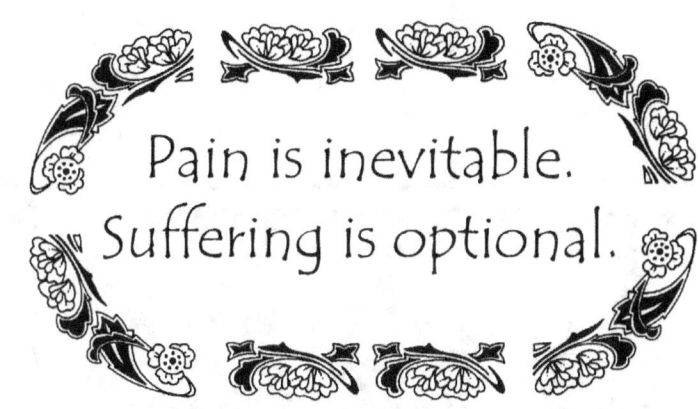

Pain is inevitable.
Suffering is optional.

Notes

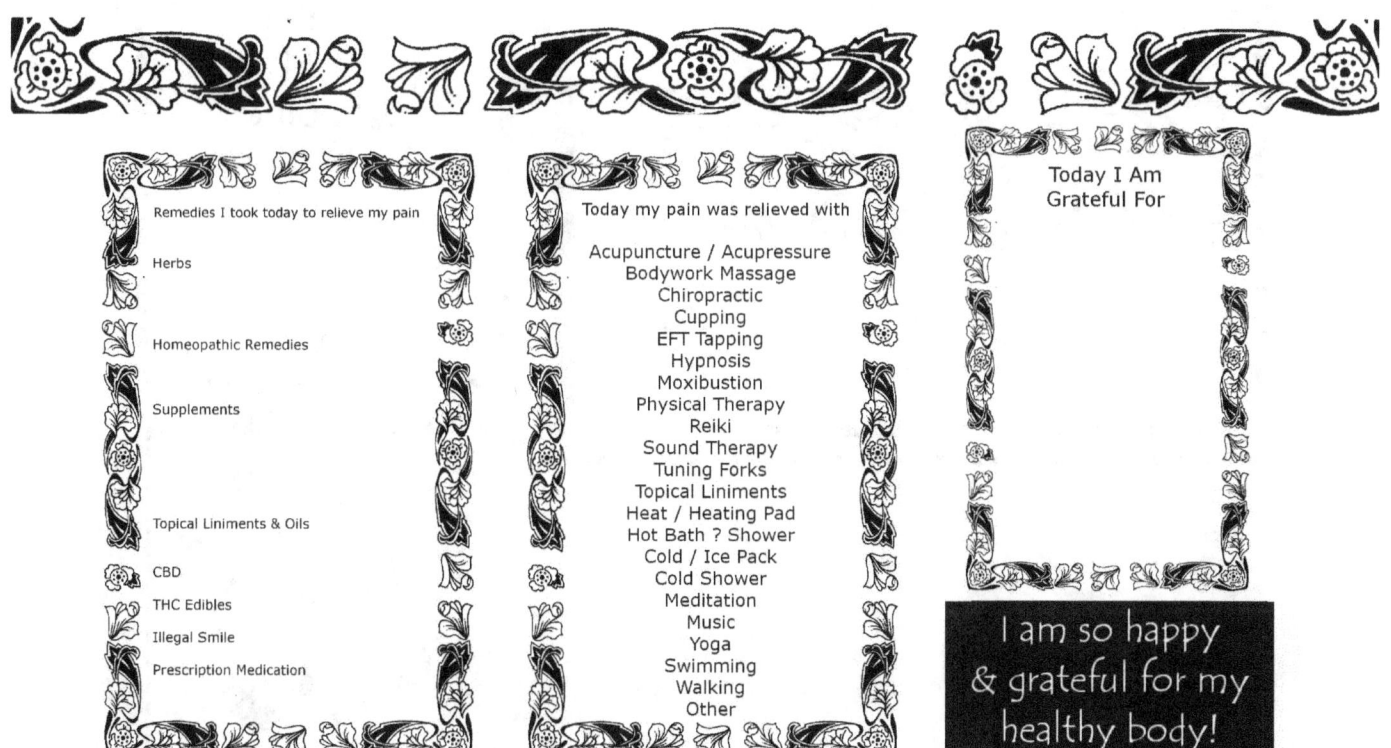

Remedies I took today to relieve my pain

Herbs

Homeopathic Remedies

Supplements

Topical Liniments & Oils

CBD

THC Edibles

Illegal Smile

Prescription Medication

Today my pain was relieved with

Acupuncture / Acupressure
Bodywork Massage
Chiropractic
Cupping
EFT Tapping
Hypnosis
Moxibustion
Physical Therapy
Reiki
Sound Therapy
Tuning Forks
Topical Liniments
Heat / Heating Pad
Hot Bath ? Shower
Cold / Ice Pack
Cold Shower
Meditation
Music
Yoga
Swimming
Walking
Other

Today I Am Grateful For

I am so happy & grateful for my healthy body!

Today's Day & Date

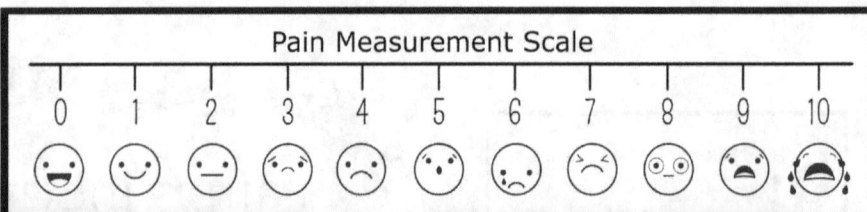

Highlight All Painful Areas

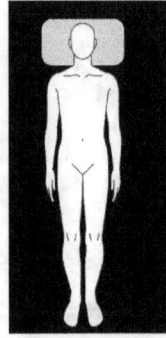 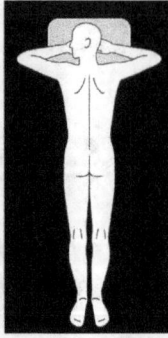 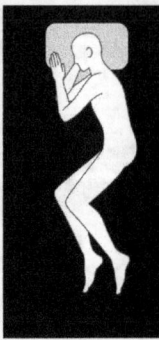 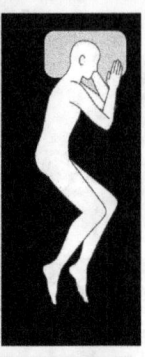

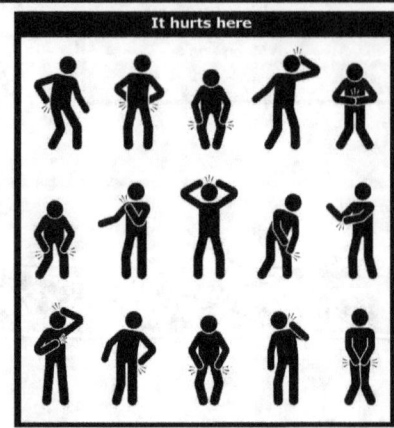

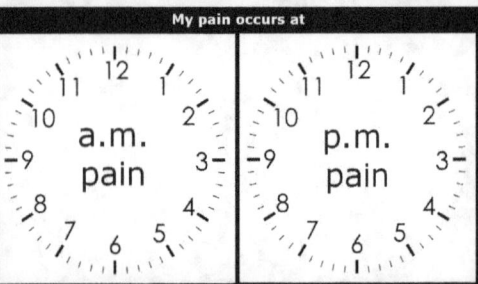

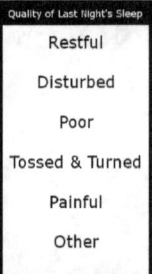

Quality of Last Night's Sleep
- Restful
- Disturbed
- Poor
- Tossed & Turned
- Painful
- Other

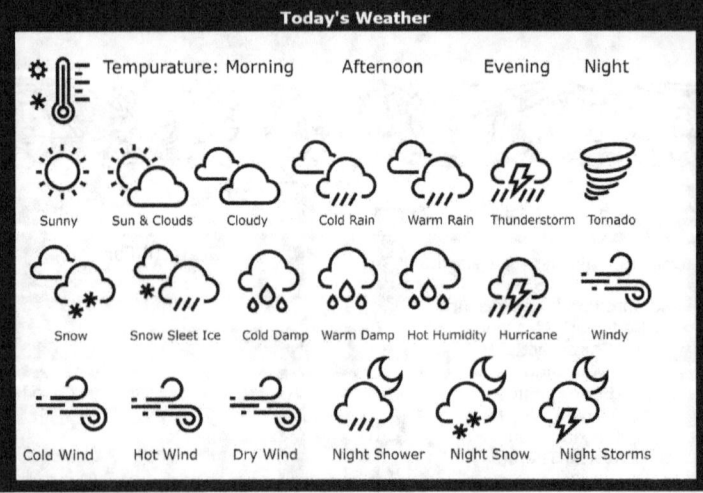

My pain is
Hot
Burning
Cold
Stabbing
Throbbing
Fixed
Moving Traveling
Constant
On & Off

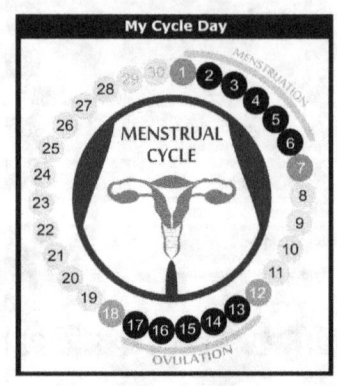

Breakfast

Lunch

Dinner

Snacks

Alcohol

Food Allergy Triggers

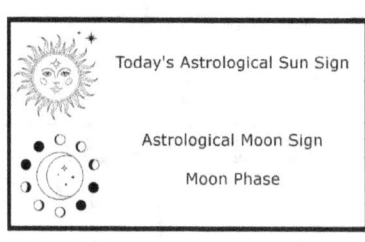

Today's Astrological Sun Sign

Astrological Moon Sign

Moon Phase

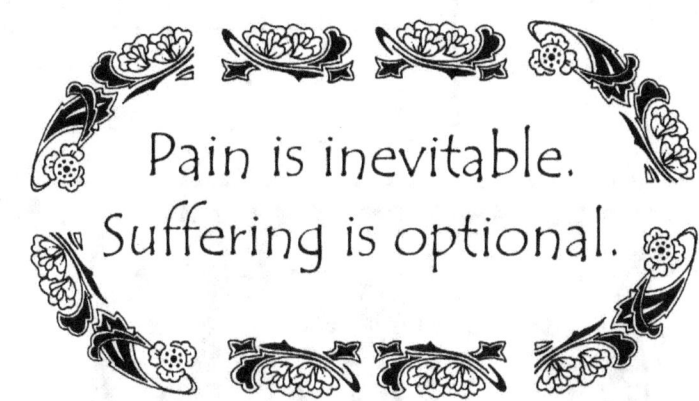

Pain is inevitable.
Suffering is optional.

Notes

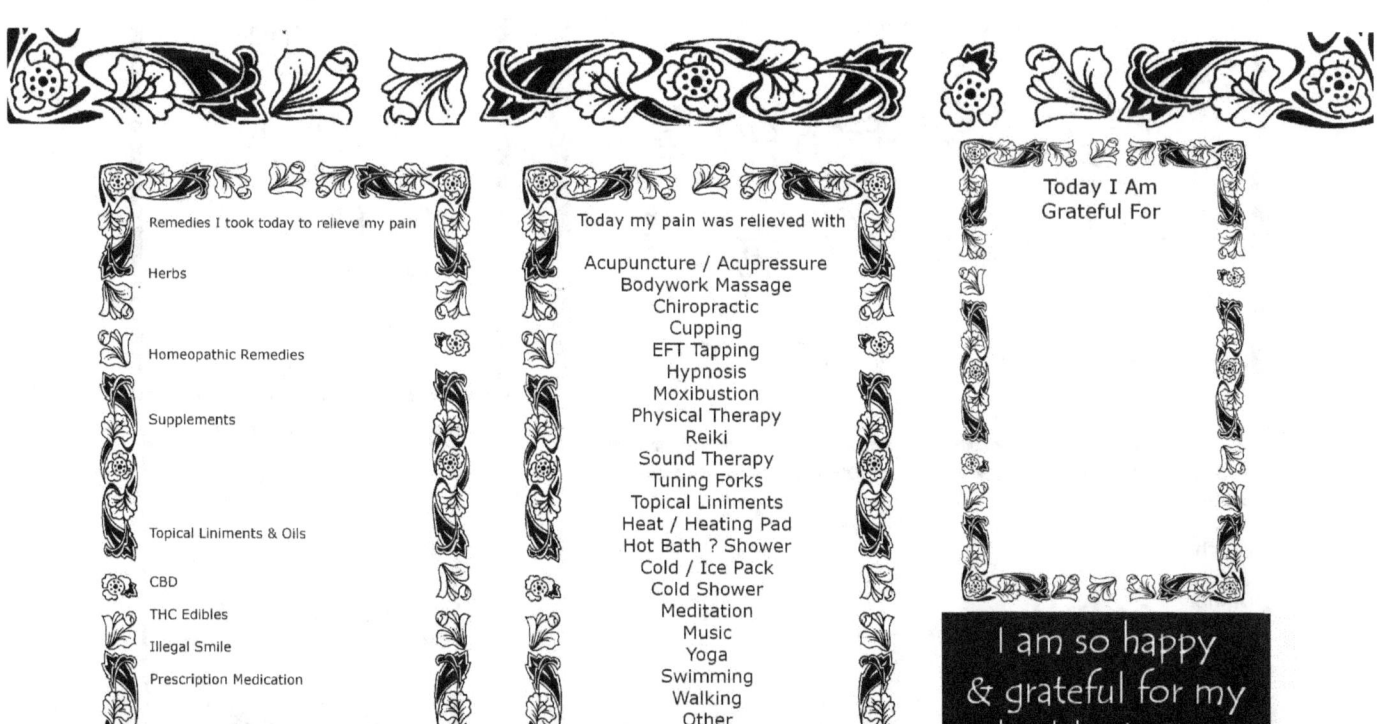

Remedies I took today to relieve my pain

Herbs

Homeopathic Remedies

Supplements

Topical Liniments & Oils

CBD
THC Edibles
Illegal Smile
Prescription Medication

Today my pain was relieved with

Acupuncture / Acupressure
Bodywork Massage
Chiropractic
Cupping
EFT Tapping
Hypnosis
Moxibustion
Physical Therapy
Reiki
Sound Therapy
Tuning Forks
Topical Liniments
Heat / Heating Pad
Hot Bath ? Shower
Cold / Ice Pack
Cold Shower
Meditation
Music
Yoga
Swimming
Walking
Other

Today I Am Grateful For

I am so happy & grateful for my healthy body!

Today's Day & Date

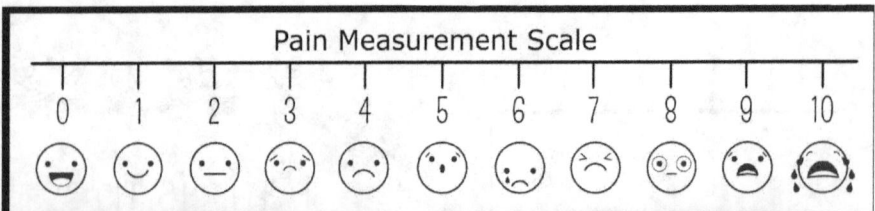

Highlight All Painful Areas

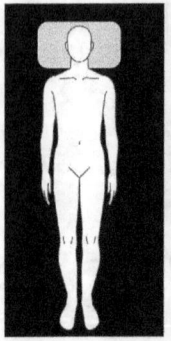 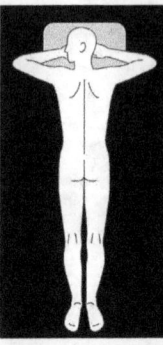 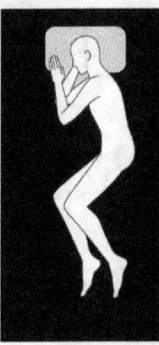 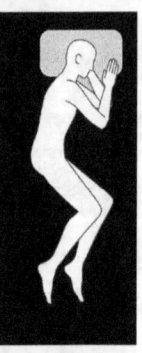

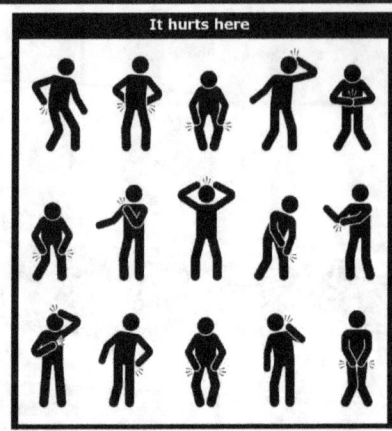
It hurts here

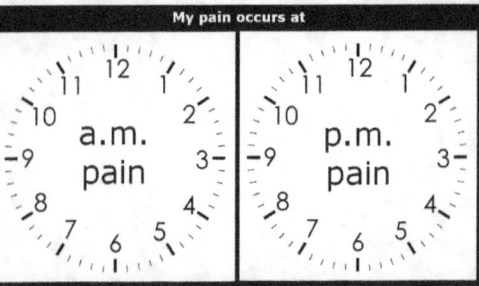
My pain occurs at — a.m. pain / p.m. pain

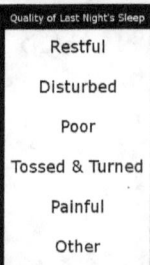

Quality of Last Night's Sleep
- Restful
- Disturbed
- Poor
- Tossed & Turned
- Painful
- Other

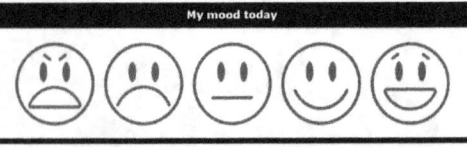
My mood today

My pain is
Hot
Burning
Cold
Stabbing
Throbbing
Fixed
Moving Traveling
Constant
On & Off

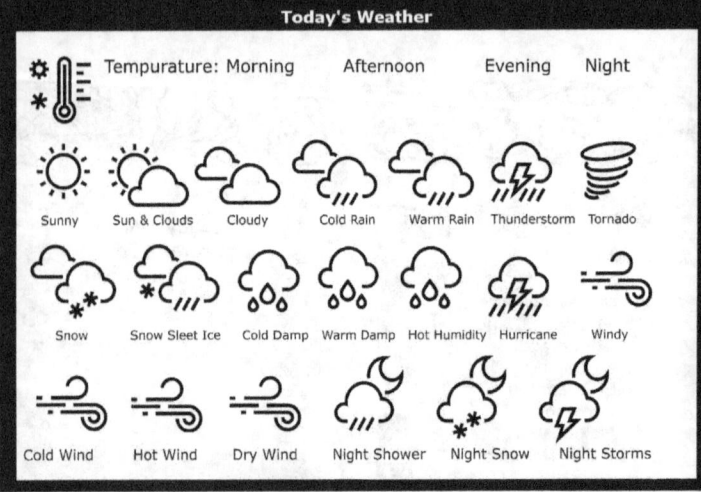
Today's Weather — Temperature: Morning, Afternoon, Evening, Night

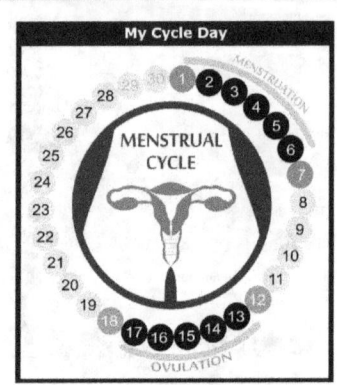
My Cycle Day

Breakfast

Lunch

Dinner

Snacks

Alcohol

Food Allergy Triggers

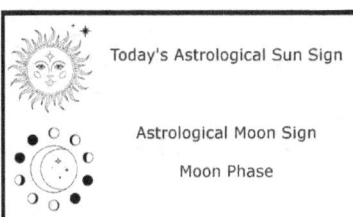

Today's Astrological Sun Sign

Astrological Moon Sign
Moon Phase

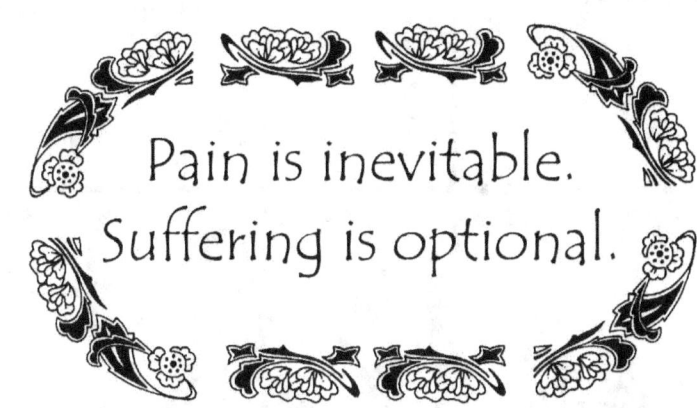

Pain is inevitable.
Suffering is optional.

Notes

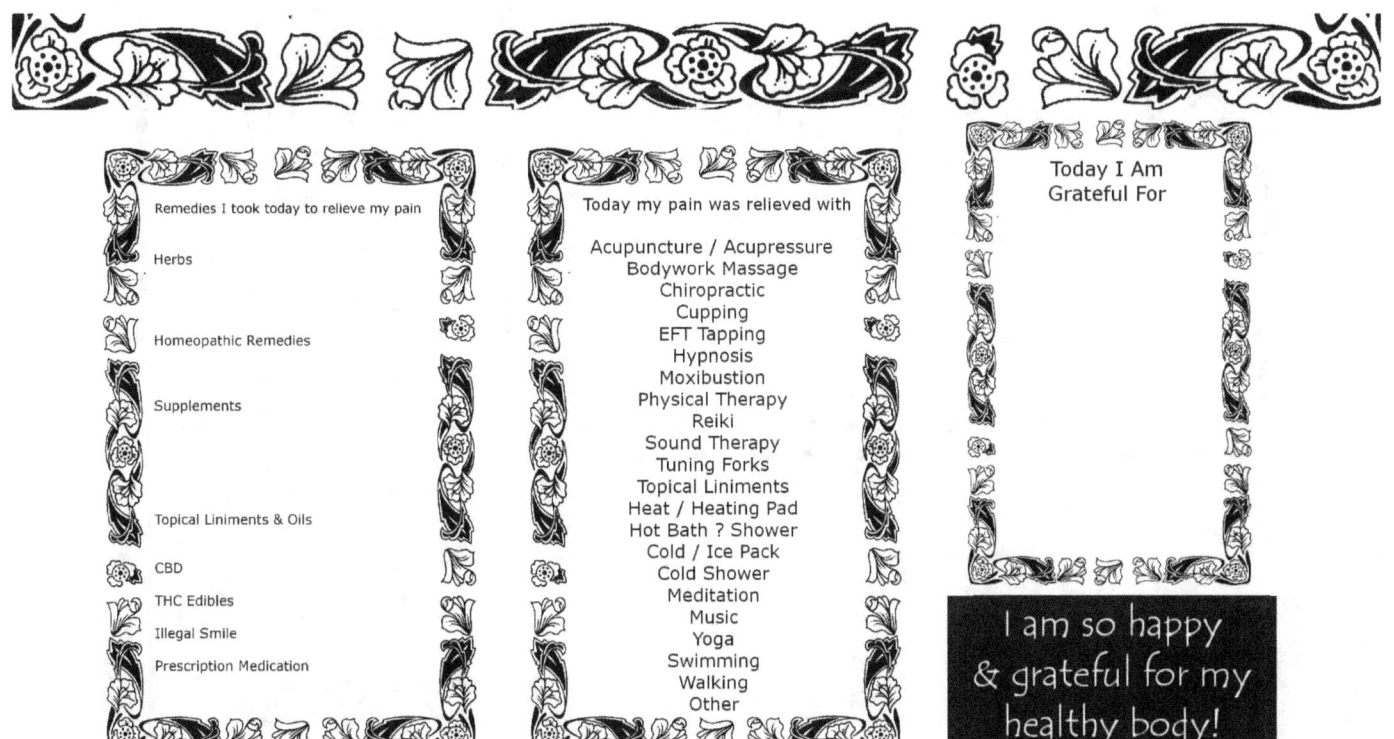

Remedies I took today to relieve my pain

Herbs

Homeopathic Remedies

Supplements

Topical Liniments & Oils

CBD
THC Edibles
Illegal Smile
Prescription Medication

Today my pain was relieved with

Acupuncture / Acupressure
Bodywork Massage
Chiropractic
Cupping
EFT Tapping
Hypnosis
Moxibustion
Physical Therapy
Reiki
Sound Therapy
Tuning Forks
Topical Liniments
Heat / Heating Pad
Hot Bath ? Shower
Cold / Ice Pack
Cold Shower
Meditation
Music
Yoga
Swimming
Walking
Other

Today I Am Grateful For

I am so happy & grateful for my healthy body!

Today's Day & Date

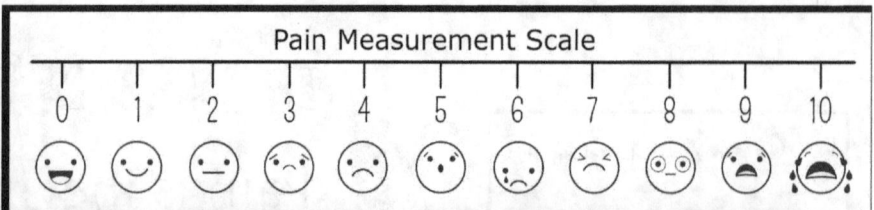

Highlight All Painful Areas

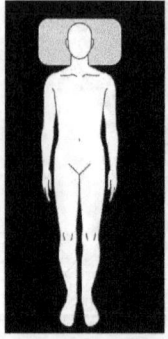 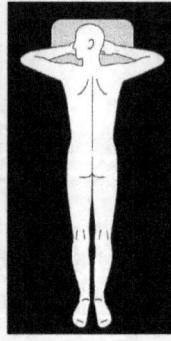 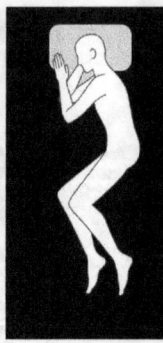 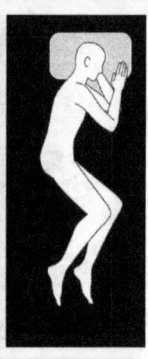

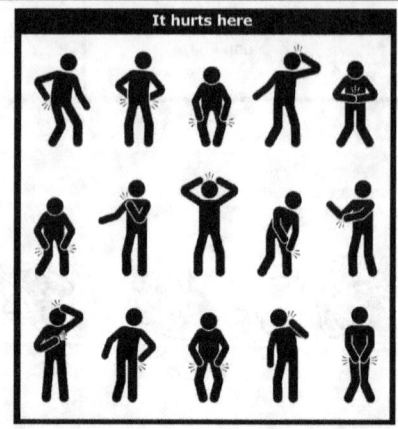

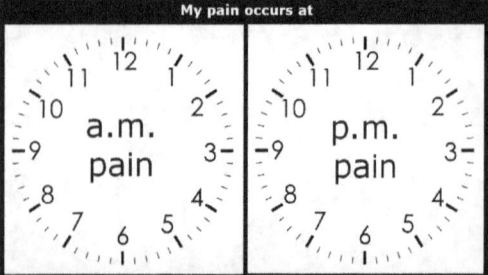

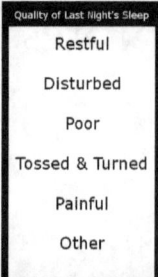

Quality of Last Night's Sleep
- Restful
- Disturbed
- Poor
- Tossed & Turned
- Painful
- Other

My pain is

Hot
Burning
Cold
Stabbing
Throbbing
Fixed
Moving Traveling
Constant
On & Off

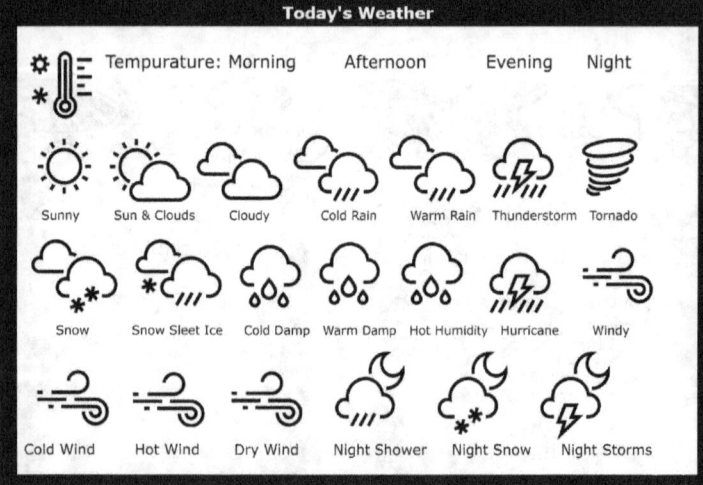

Breakfast

Lunch

Dinner

Snacks

Alcohol

Food Allergy Triggers

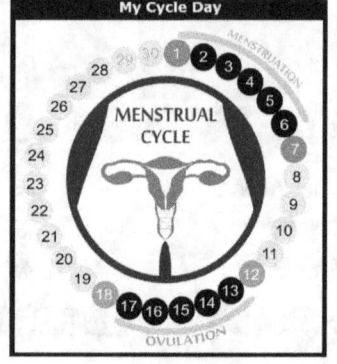

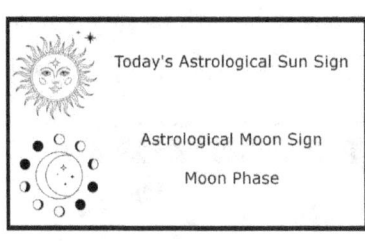

Today's Astrological Sun Sign

Astrological Moon Sign

Moon Phase

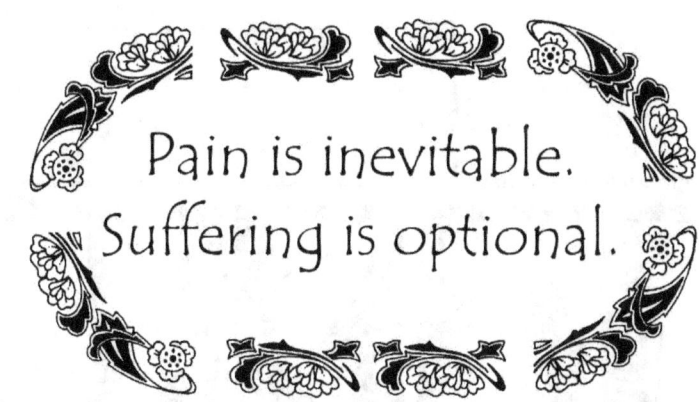

Pain is inevitable.
Suffering is optional.

Notes

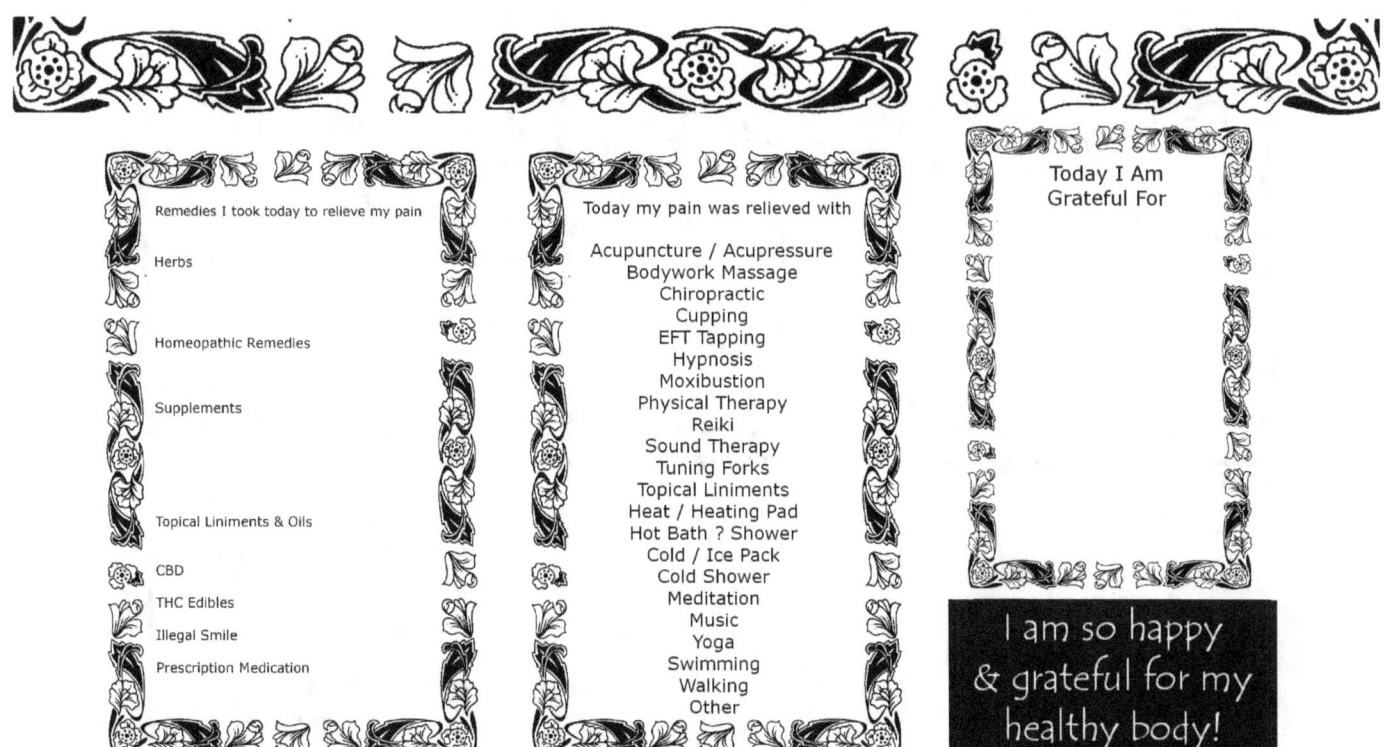

Remedies I took today to relieve my pain

Herbs

Homeopathic Remedies

Supplements

Topical Liniments & Oils

CBD

THC Edibles

Illegal Smile

Prescription Medication

Today my pain was relieved with

Acupuncture / Acupressure
Bodywork Massage
Chiropractic
Cupping
EFT Tapping
Hypnosis
Moxibustion
Physical Therapy
Reiki
Sound Therapy
Tuning Forks
Topical Liniments
Heat / Heating Pad
Hot Bath ? Shower
Cold / Ice Pack
Cold Shower
Meditation
Music
Yoga
Swimming
Walking
Other

Today I Am Grateful For

I am so happy & grateful for my healthy body!

Today's Day & Date

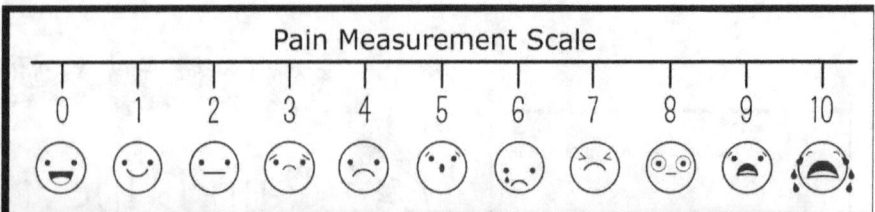

Highlight All Painful Areas

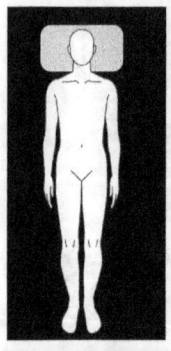 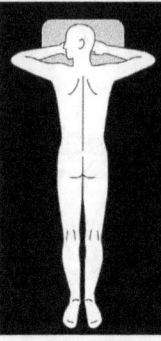 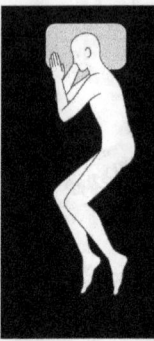 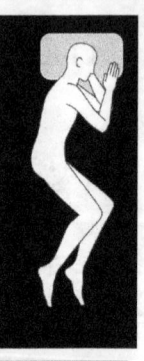

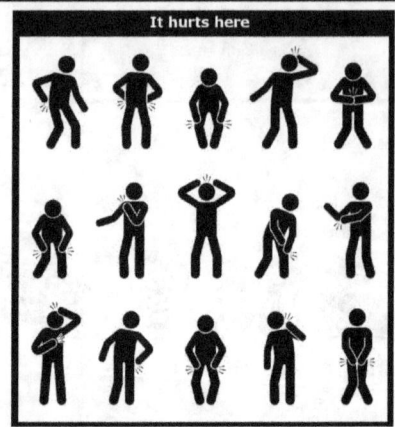

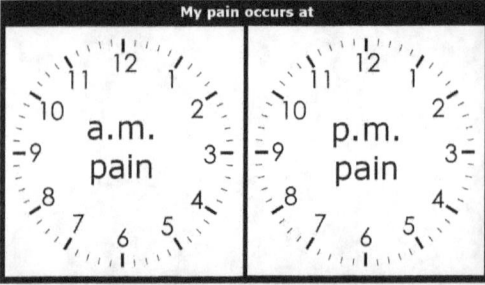

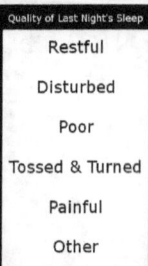

Quality of Last Night's Sleep
- Restful
- Disturbed
- Poor
- Tossed & Turned
- Painful
- Other

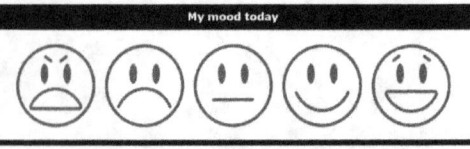

Today's Weather

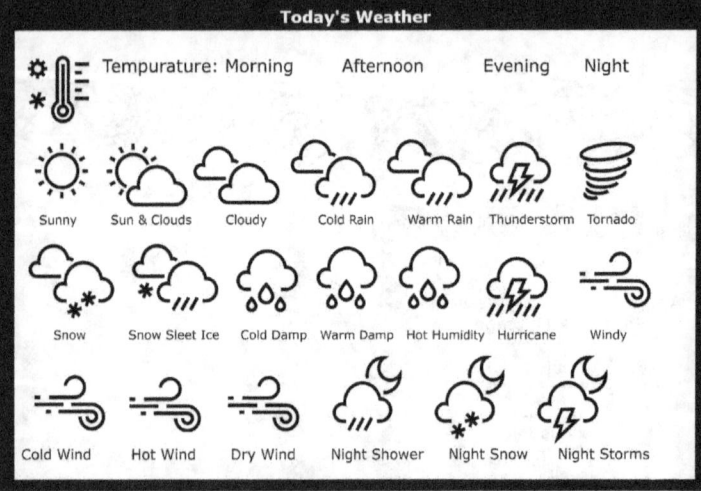

My pain is
Hot
Burning
Cold
Stabbing
Throbbing
Fixed
Moving Traveling
Constant
On & Off

Breakfast

Lunch

Dinner

Snacks

Alcohol

Food Allergy Triggers

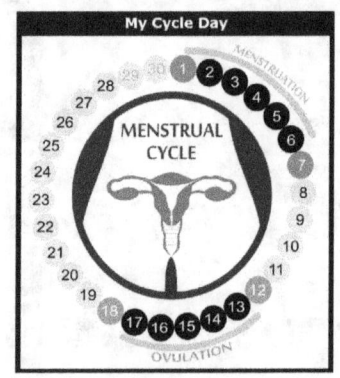

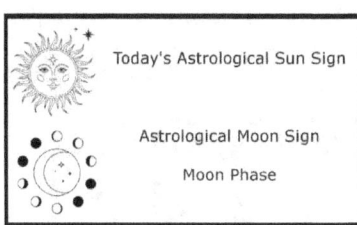

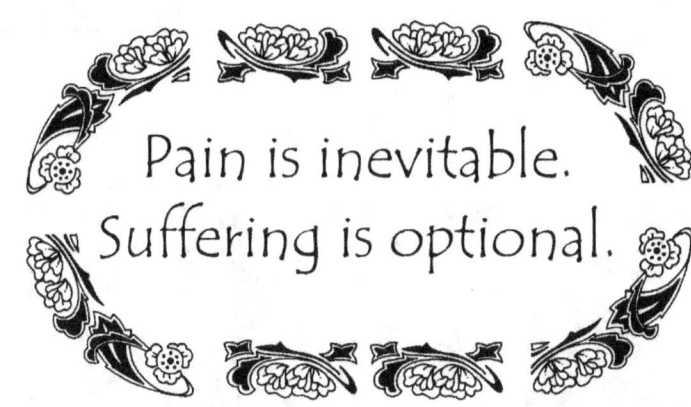

Pain is inevitable.
Suffering is optional.

Notes

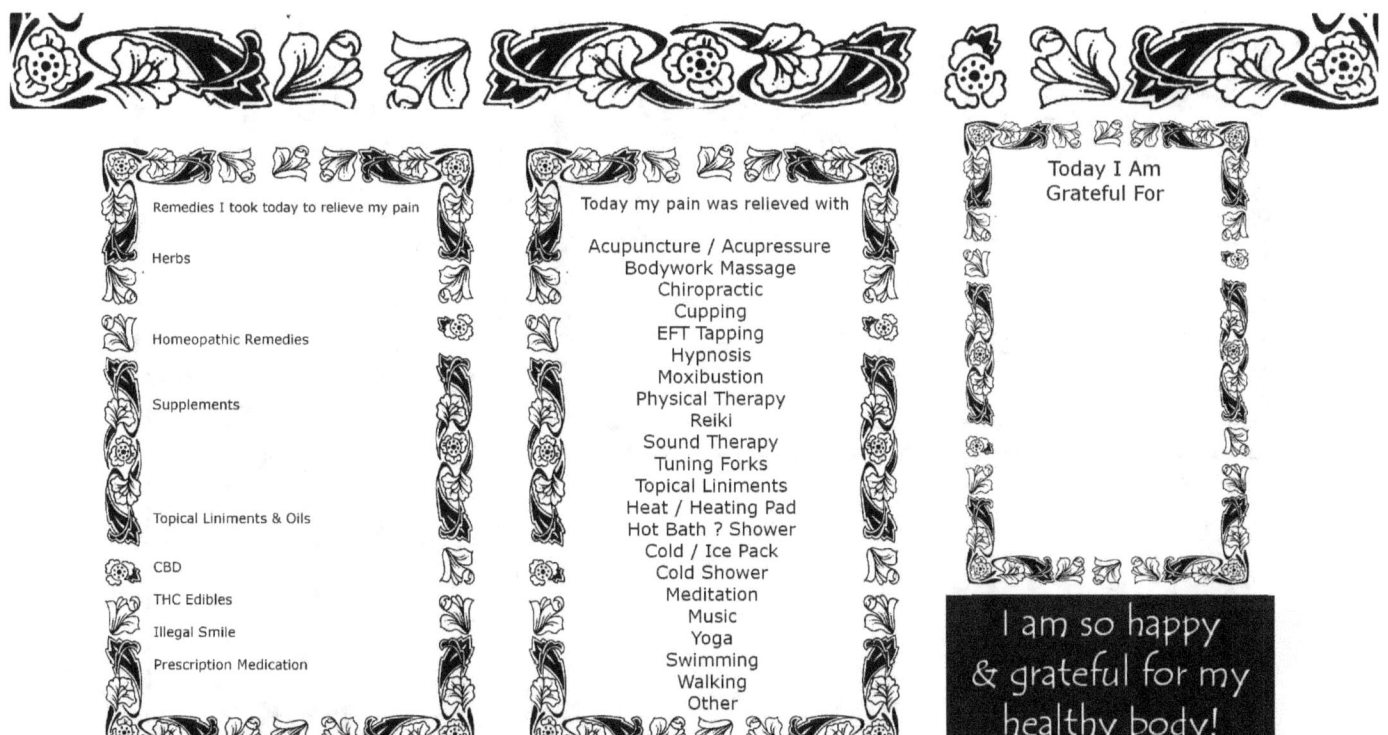

Remedies I took today to relieve my pain

- Herbs
- Homeopathic Remedies
- Supplements
- Topical Liniments & Oils
- CBD
- THC Edibles
- Illegal Smile
- Prescription Medication

Today my pain was relieved with

Acupuncture / Acupressure
Bodywork Massage
Chiropractic
Cupping
EFT Tapping
Hypnosis
Moxibustion
Physical Therapy
Reiki
Sound Therapy
Tuning Forks
Topical Liniments
Heat / Heating Pad
Hot Bath ? Shower
Cold / Ice Pack
Cold Shower
Meditation
Music
Yoga
Swimming
Walking
Other

Today I Am Grateful For

I am so happy & grateful for my healthy body!

Today's Day & Date

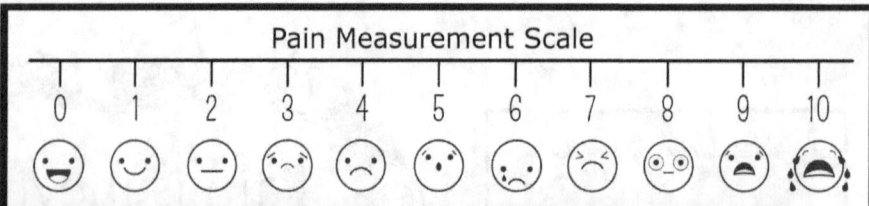

Highlight All Painful Areas

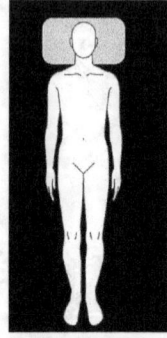 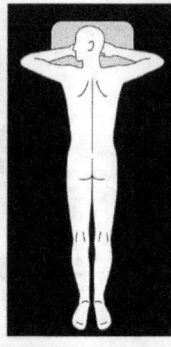 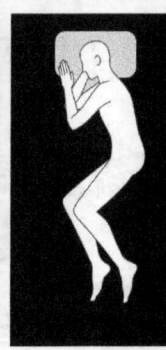 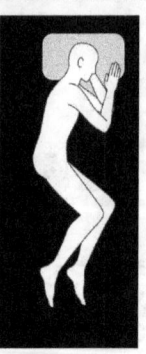

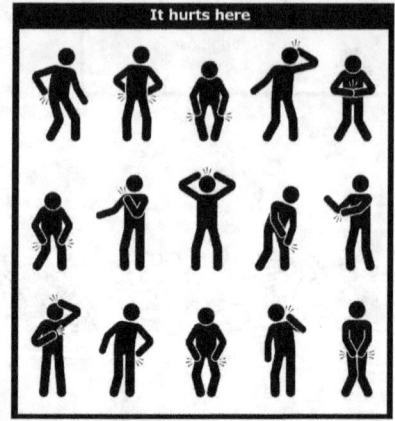
It hurts here

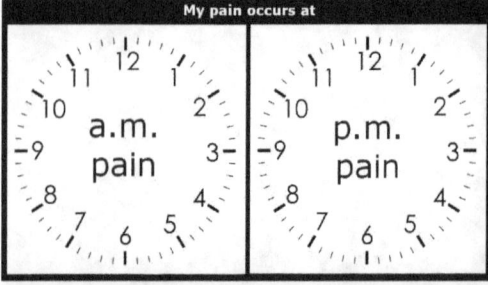
My pain occurs at — a.m. pain / p.m. pain

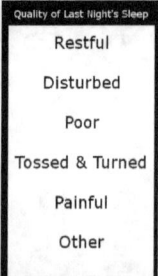

Quality of Last Night's Sleep
- Restful
- Disturbed
- Poor
- Tossed & Turned
- Painful
- Other

My mood today

My pain is
Hot
Burning
Cold
Stabbing
Throbbing
Fixed
Moving Traveling
Constant
On & Off

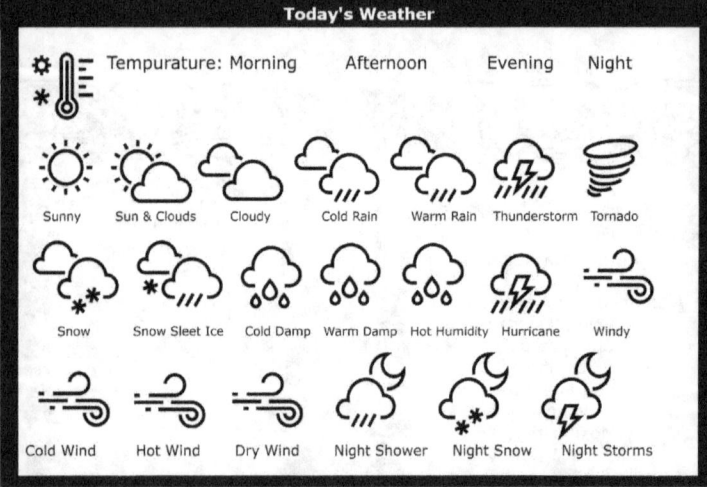
Today's Weather — Temperature: Morning, Afternoon, Evening, Night

Sunny, Sun & Clouds, Cloudy, Cold Rain, Warm Rain, Thunderstorm, Tornado
Snow, Snow Sleet Ice, Cold Damp, Warm Damp, Hot Humidity, Hurricane, Windy
Cold Wind, Hot Wind, Dry Wind, Night Shower, Night Snow, Night Storms

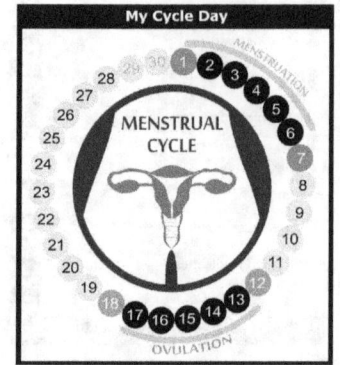
My Cycle Day

Breakfast

Lunch

Dinner

Snacks

Alcohol

Food Allergy Triggers

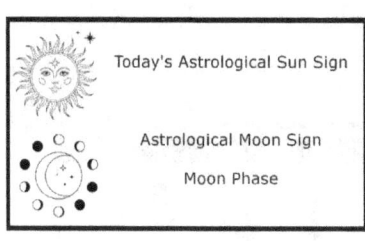

Today's Astrological Sun Sign

Astrological Moon Sign

Moon Phase

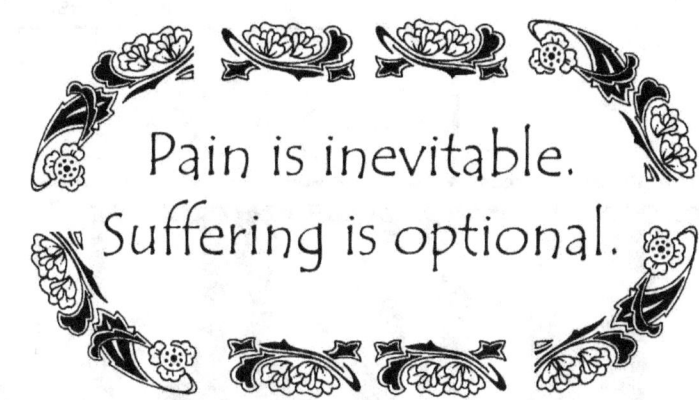

Pain is inevitable.
Suffering is optional.

Notes

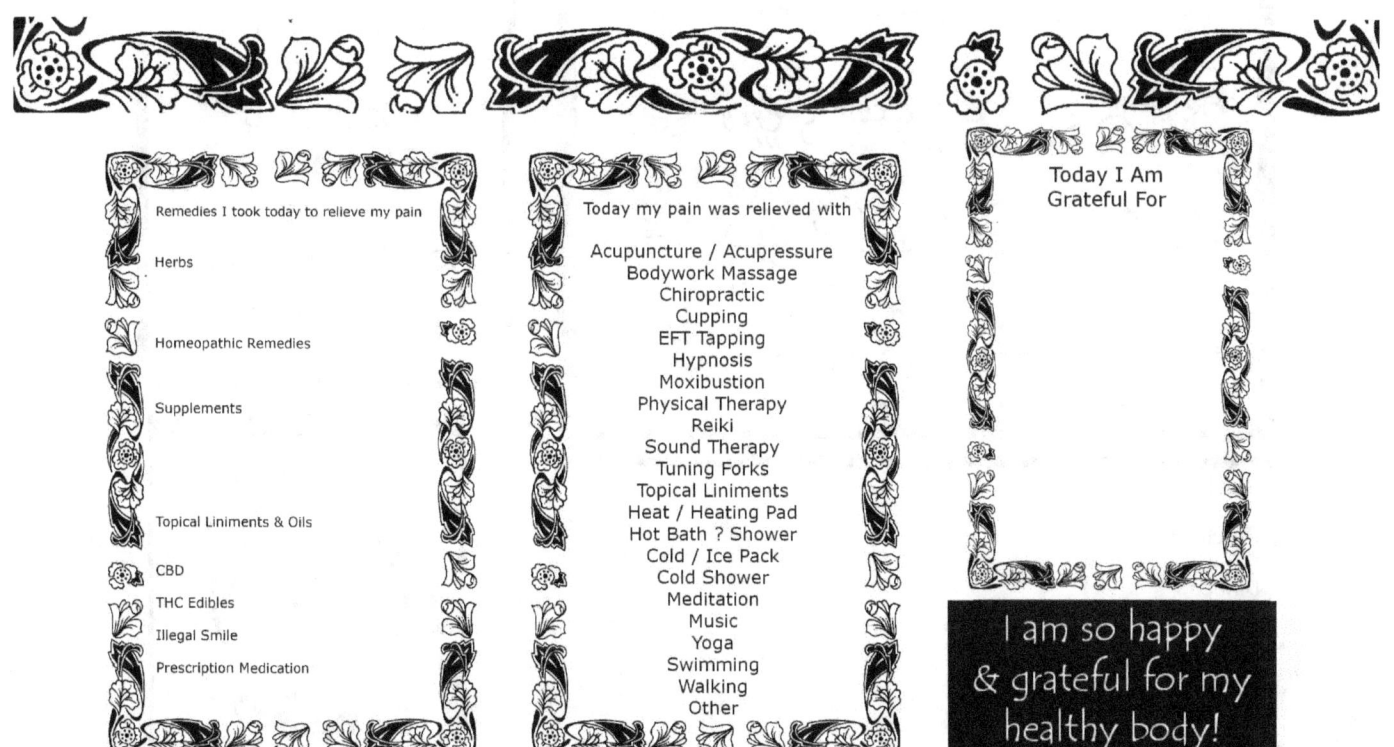

Remedies I took today to relieve my pain

Herbs

Homeopathic Remedies

Supplements

Topical Liniments & Oils

CBD
THC Edibles
Illegal Smile
Prescription Medication

Today my pain was relieved with

Acupuncture / Acupressure
Bodywork Massage
Chiropractic
Cupping
EFT Tapping
Hypnosis
Moxibustion
Physical Therapy
Reiki
Sound Therapy
Tuning Forks
Topical Liniments
Heat / Heating Pad
Hot Bath ? Shower
Cold / Ice Pack
Cold Shower
Meditation
Music
Yoga
Swimming
Walking
Other

Today I Am Grateful For

I am so happy & grateful for my healthy body!

Today's Day & Date

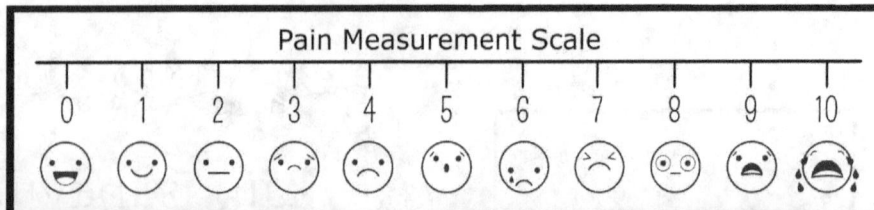

Highlight All Painful Areas

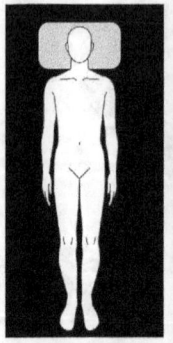 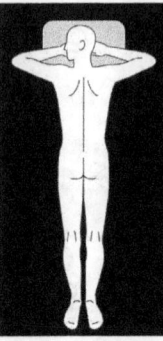 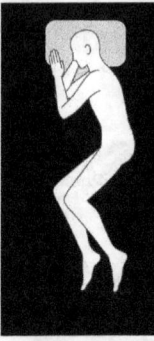 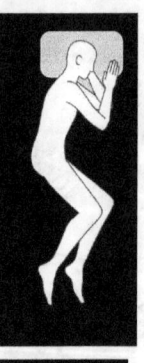

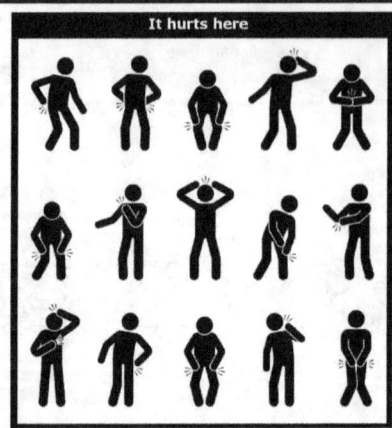
It hurts here

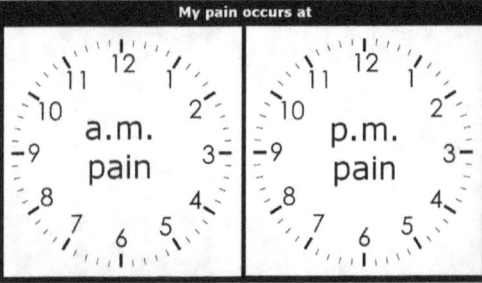
My pain occurs at — a.m. pain / p.m. pain

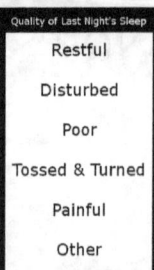

Quality of Last Night's Sleep
- Restful
- Disturbed
- Poor
- Tossed & Turned
- Painful
- Other

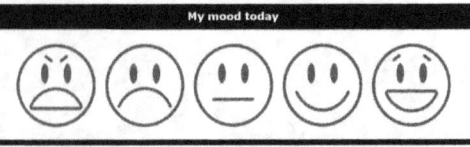
My mood today

My pain is
Hot
Burning
Cold
Stabbing
Throbbing
Fixed
Moving Traveling
Constant
On & Off

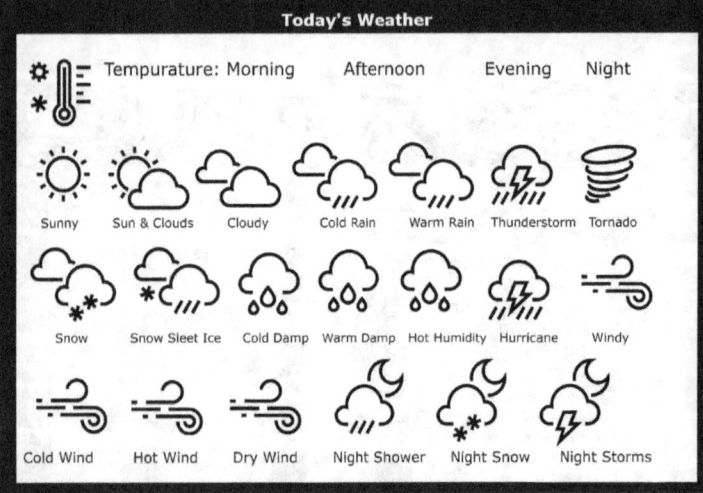
Today's Weather — Temperature: Morning, Afternoon, Evening, Night

Sunny, Sun & Clouds, Cloudy, Cold Rain, Warm Rain, Thunderstorm, Tornado, Snow, Snow Sleet Ice, Cold Damp, Warm Damp, Hot Humidity, Hurricane, Windy, Cold Wind, Hot Wind, Dry Wind, Night Shower, Night Snow, Night Storms

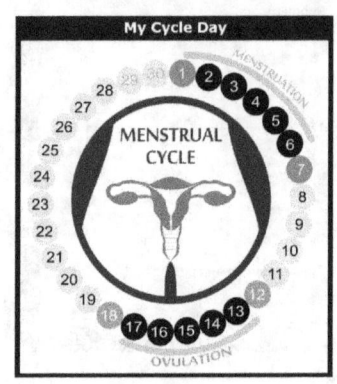
My Cycle Day

Breakfast

Lunch

Dinner

Snacks

Alcohol

Food Allergy Triggers

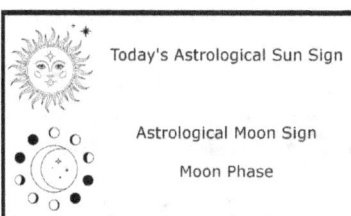

Today's Astrological Sun Sign

Astrological Moon Sign
Moon Phase

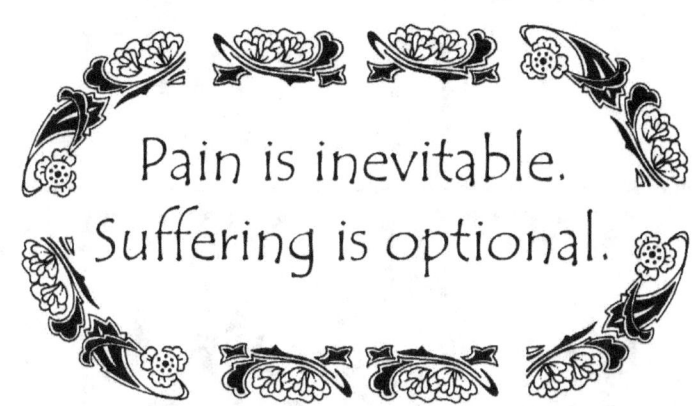

Pain is inevitable.
Suffering is optional.

Notes

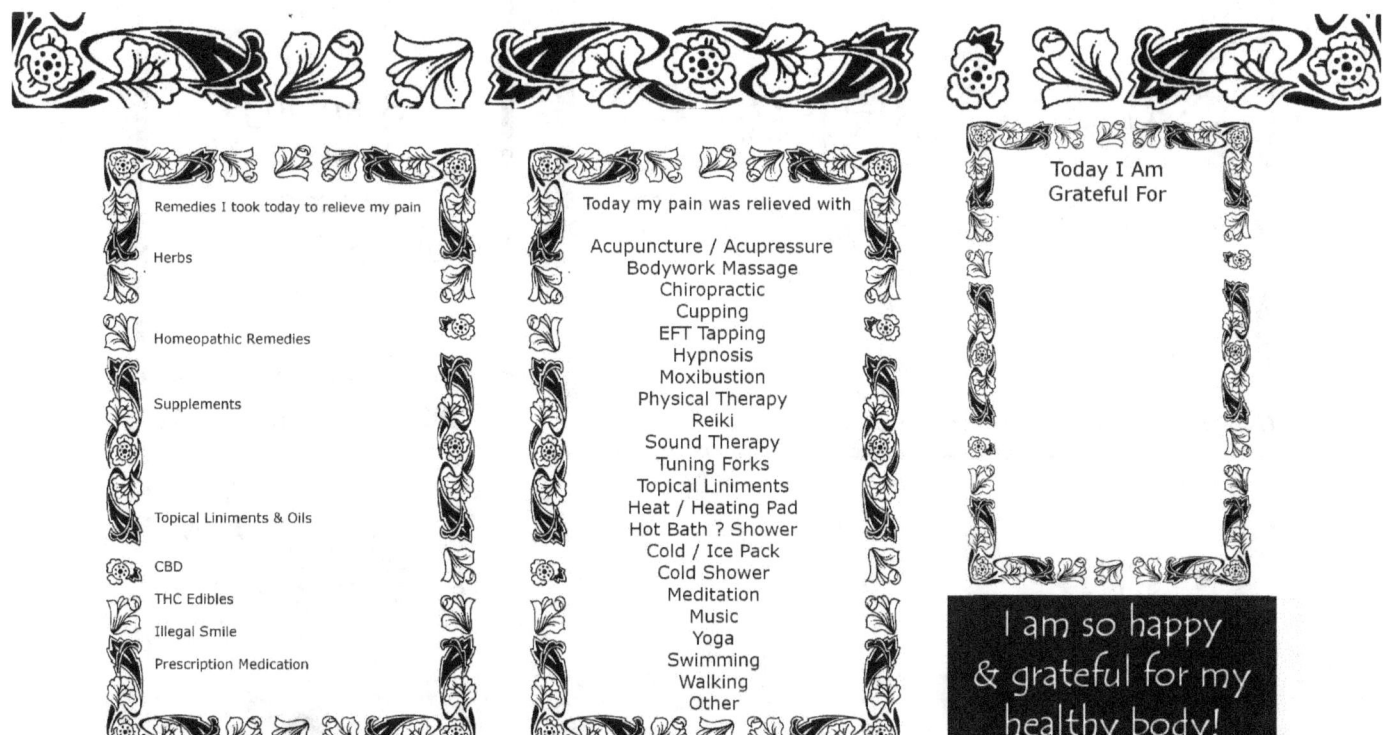

Remedies I took today to relieve my pain

Herbs

Homeopathic Remedies

Supplements

Topical Liniments & Oils

CBD
THC Edibles
Illegal Smile
Prescription Medication

Today my pain was relieved with

Acupuncture / Acupressure
Bodywork Massage
Chiropractic
Cupping
EFT Tapping
Hypnosis
Moxibustion
Physical Therapy
Reiki
Sound Therapy
Tuning Forks
Topical Liniments
Heat / Heating Pad
Hot Bath ? Shower
Cold / Ice Pack
Cold Shower
Meditation
Music
Yoga
Swimming
Walking
Other

Today I Am Grateful For

I am so happy & grateful for my healthy body!

Today's Day & Date

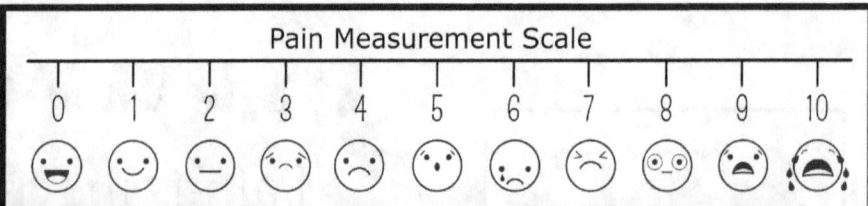

Highlight All Painful Areas

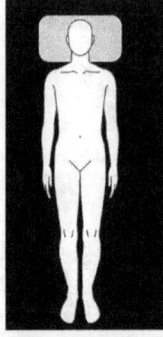 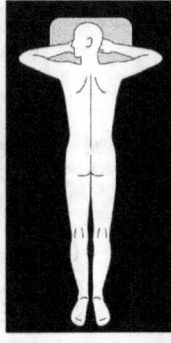 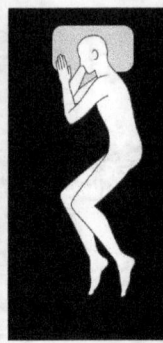 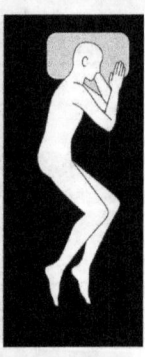

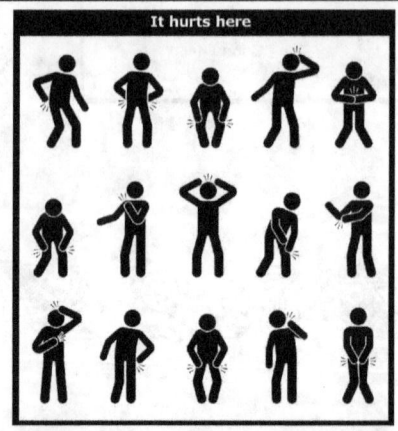
It hurts here

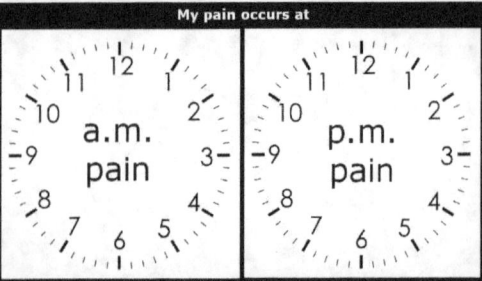
My pain occurs at — a.m. pain / p.m. pain

Quality of Last Night's Sleep
- Restful
- Disturbed
- Poor
- Tossed & Turned
- Painful
- Other

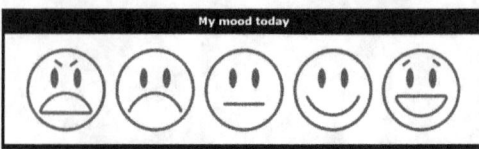
My mood today

My pain is
Hot
Burning
Cold
Stabbing
Throbbing
Fixed
Moving Traveling
Constant
On & Off

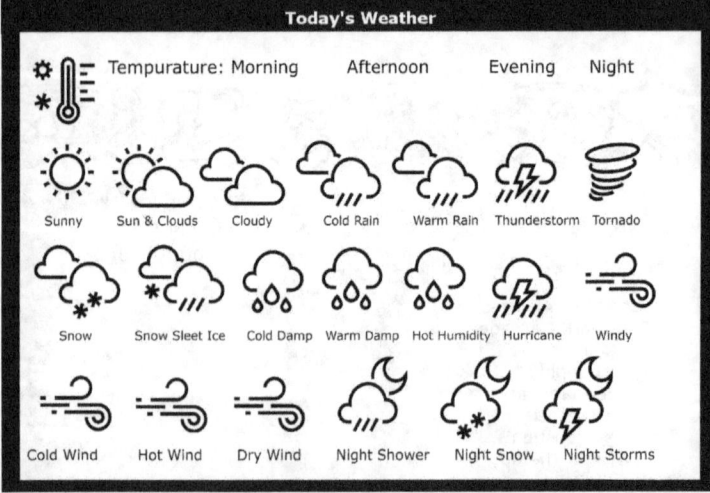
Today's Weather

Breakfast

Lunch

Dinner

Snacks

Alcohol

Food Allergy Triggers

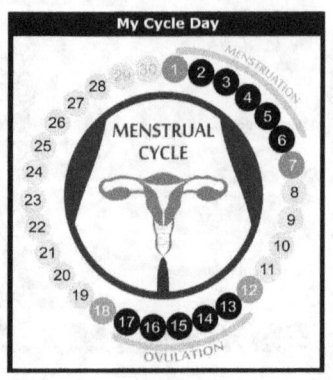
My Cycle Day

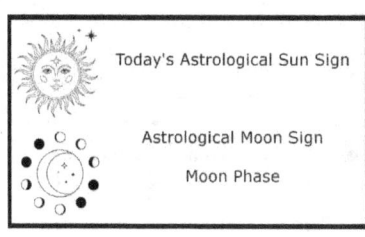

Today's Astrological Sun Sign

Astrological Moon Sign

Moon Phase

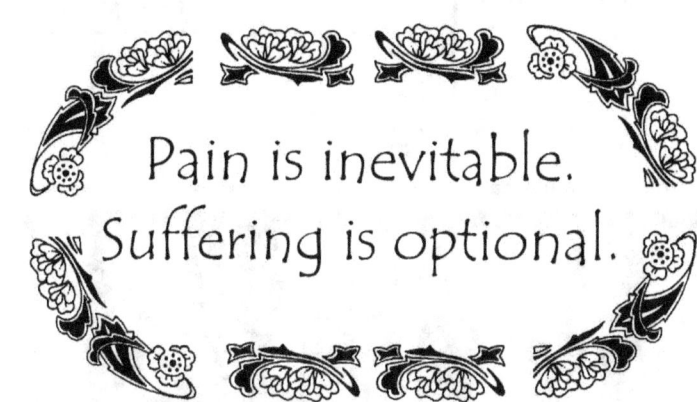

Pain is inevitable. Suffering is optional.

Notes

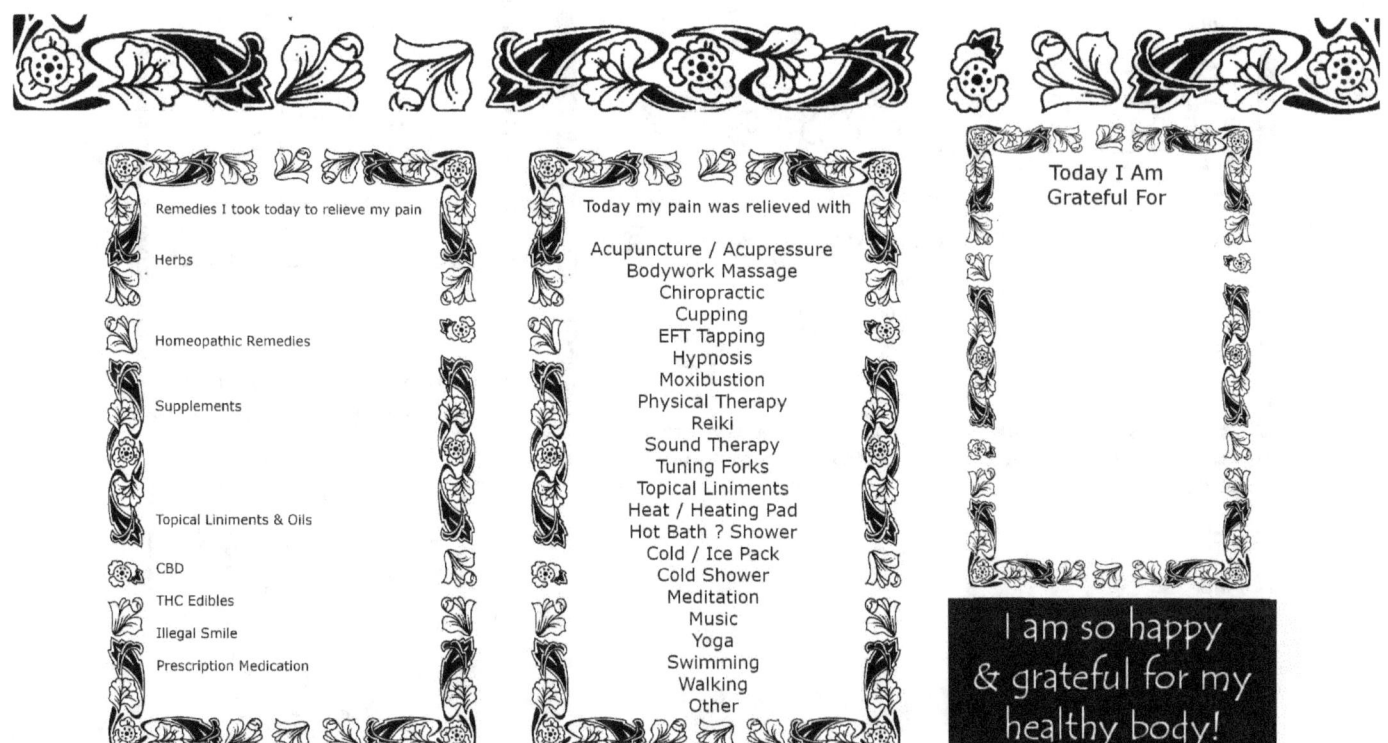

Remedies I took today to relieve my pain

Herbs

Homeopathic Remedies

Supplements

Topical Liniments & Oils

CBD

THC Edibles

Illegal Smile

Prescription Medication

Today my pain was relieved with

Acupuncture / Acupressure
Bodywork Massage
Chiropractic
Cupping
EFT Tapping
Hypnosis
Moxibustion
Physical Therapy
Reiki
Sound Therapy
Tuning Forks
Topical Liniments
Heat / Heating Pad
Hot Bath ? Shower
Cold / Ice Pack
Cold Shower
Meditation
Music
Yoga
Swimming
Walking
Other

Today I Am Grateful For

I am so happy & grateful for my healthy body!

Today's Day & Date

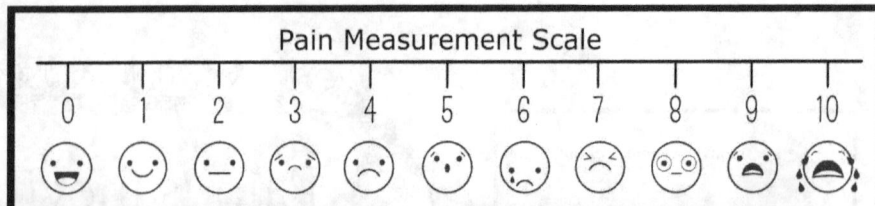

Highlight All Painful Areas

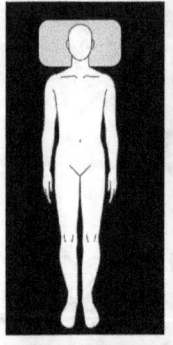
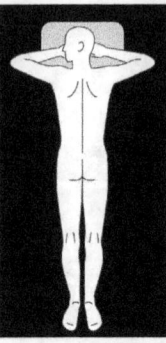
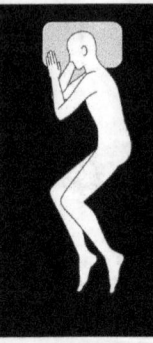
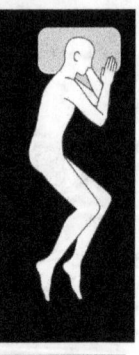

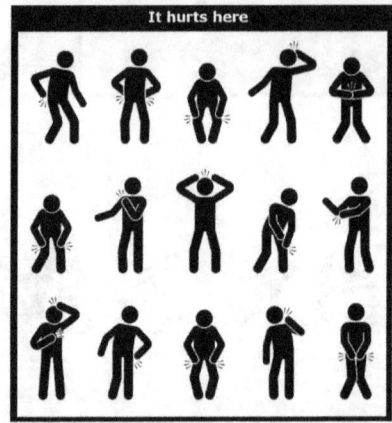
It hurts here

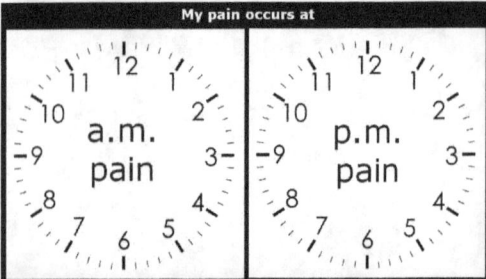
My pain occurs at — a.m. pain / p.m. pain

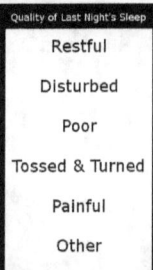

Quality of Last Night's Sleep
- Restful
- Disturbed
- Poor
- Tossed & Turned
- Painful
- Other

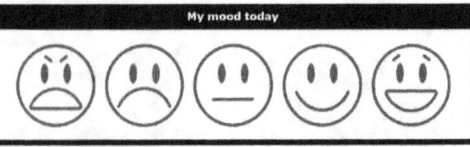
My mood today

My pain is
Hot
Burning
Cold
Stabbing
Throbbing
Fixed
Moving Traveling
Constant
On & Off

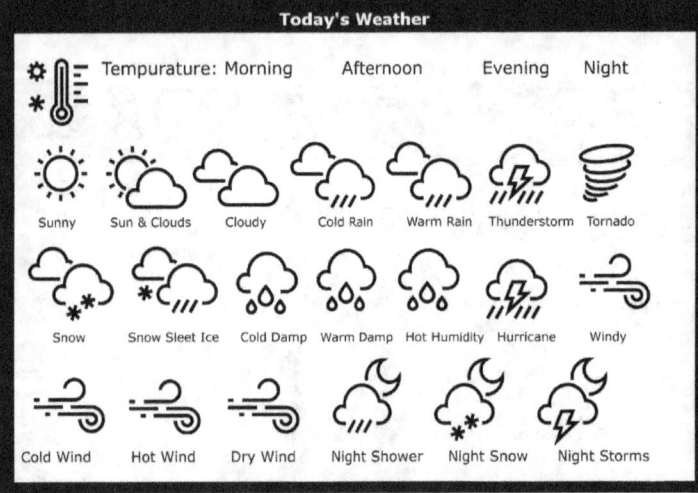
Today's Weather — Temperature: Morning, Afternoon, Evening, Night

Sunny, Sun & Clouds, Cloudy, Cold Rain, Warm Rain, Thunderstorm, Tornado
Snow, Snow Sleet Ice, Cold Damp, Warm Damp, Hot Humidity, Hurricane, Windy
Cold Wind, Hot Wind, Dry Wind, Night Shower, Night Snow, Night Storms

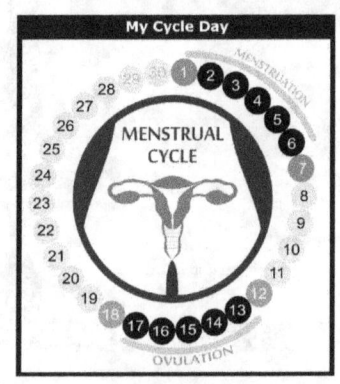
My Cycle Day

Breakfast

Lunch

Dinner

Snacks

Alcohol

Food Allergy Triggers

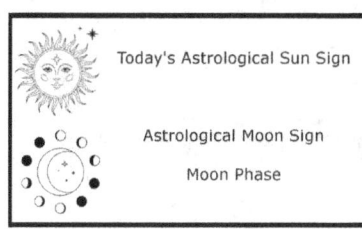

Today's Astrological Sun Sign

Astrological Moon Sign

Moon Phase

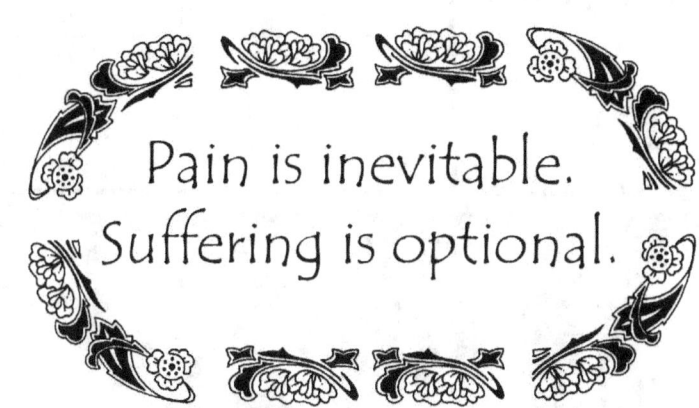

Pain is inevitable.
Suffering is optional.

Notes

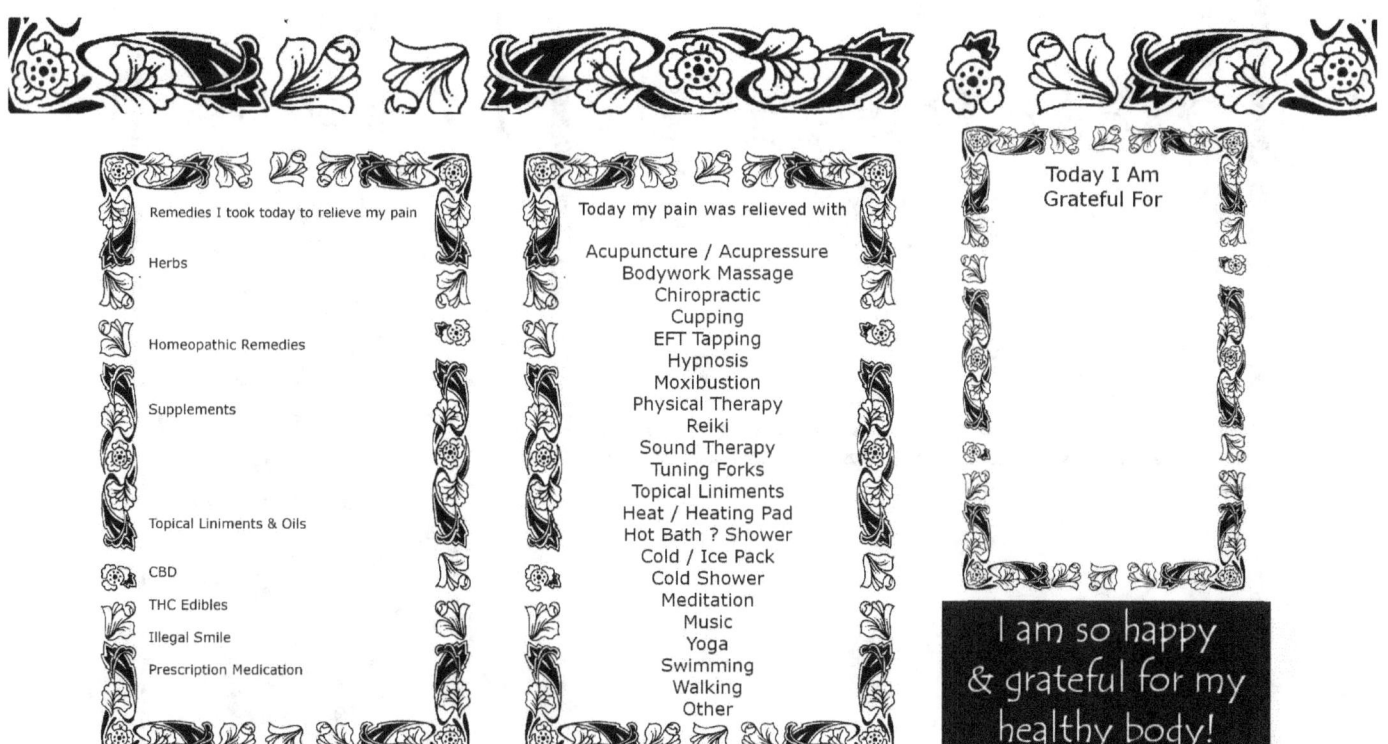

Remedies I took today to relieve my pain

Herbs

Homeopathic Remedies

Supplements

Topical Liniments & Oils

CBD

THC Edibles

Illegal Smile

Prescription Medication

Today my pain was relieved with

Acupuncture / Acupressure
Bodywork Massage
Chiropractic
Cupping
EFT Tapping
Hypnosis
Moxibustion
Physical Therapy
Reiki
Sound Therapy
Tuning Forks
Topical Liniments
Heat / Heating Pad
Hot Bath ? Shower
Cold / Ice Pack
Cold Shower
Meditation
Music
Yoga
Swimming
Walking
Other

Today I Am Grateful For

I am so happy & grateful for my healthy body!

Today's Day & Date

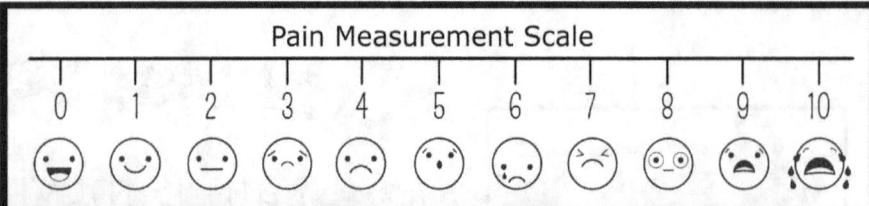

Highlight All Painful Areas

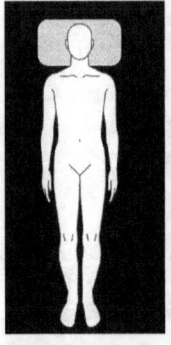 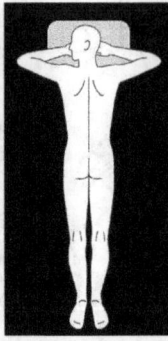 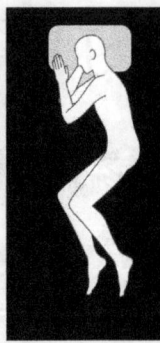 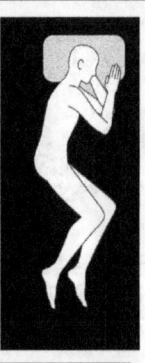

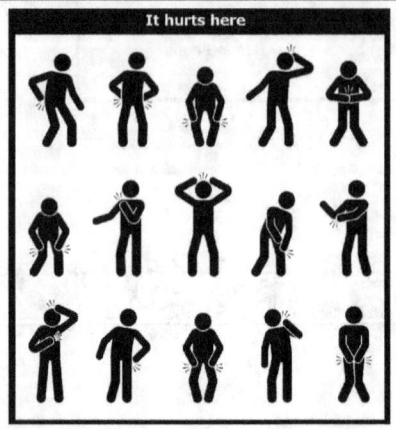
It hurts here

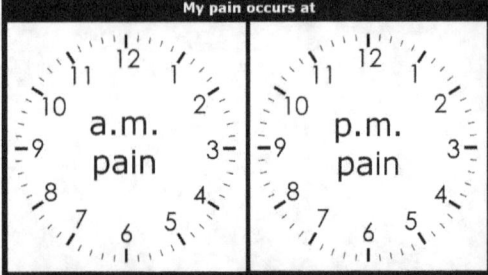
My pain occurs at — a.m. pain / p.m. pain

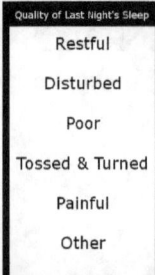

Quality of Last Night's Sleep
- Restful
- Disturbed
- Poor
- Tossed & Turned
- Painful
- Other

My mood today

My pain is
Hot
Burning
Cold
Stabbing
Throbbing
Fixed
Moving Traveling
Constant
On & Off

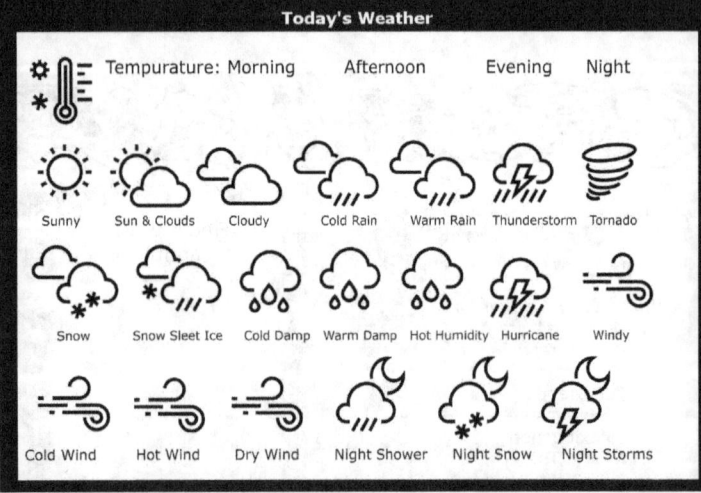
Today's Weather — Temperature: Morning, Afternoon, Evening, Night

Breakfast

Lunch

Dinner

Snacks

Alcohol

Food Allergy Triggers

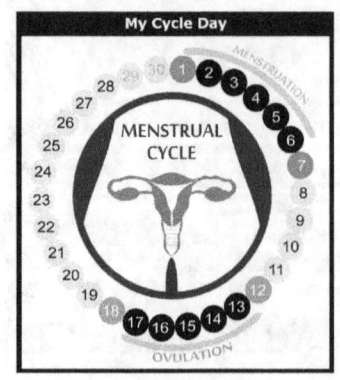
My Cycle Day

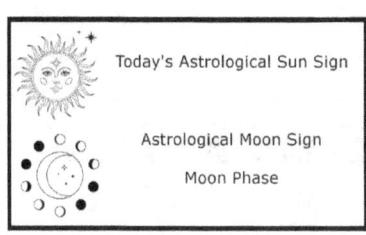

Today's Astrological Sun Sign

Astrological Moon Sign

Moon Phase

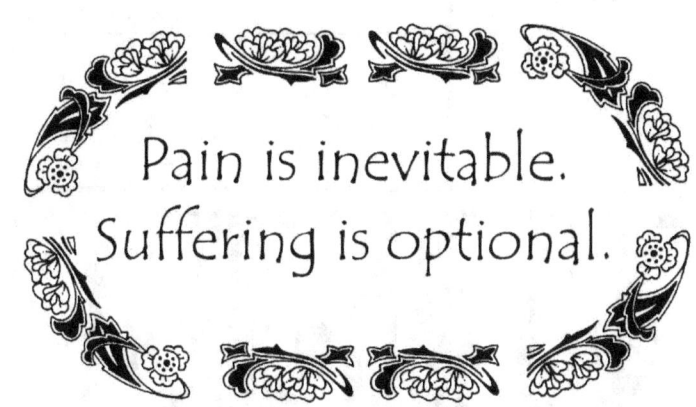

Pain is inevitable.
Suffering is optional.

Notes

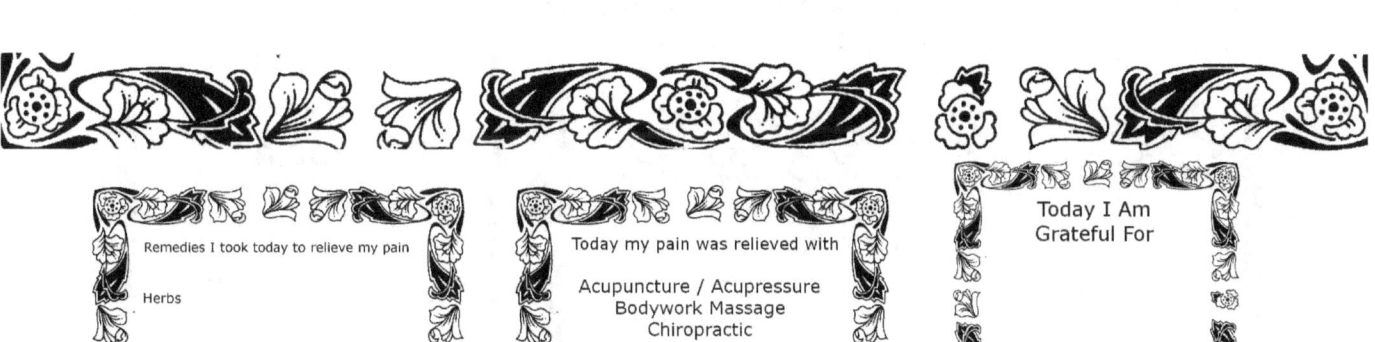

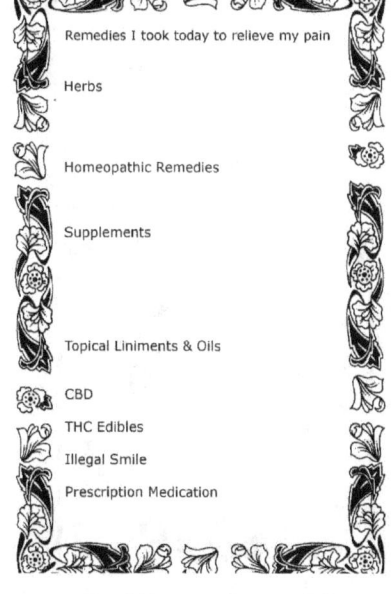

Remedies I took today to relieve my pain

Herbs

Homeopathic Remedies

Supplements

Topical Liniments & Oils

CBD

THC Edibles

Illegal Smile

Prescription Medication

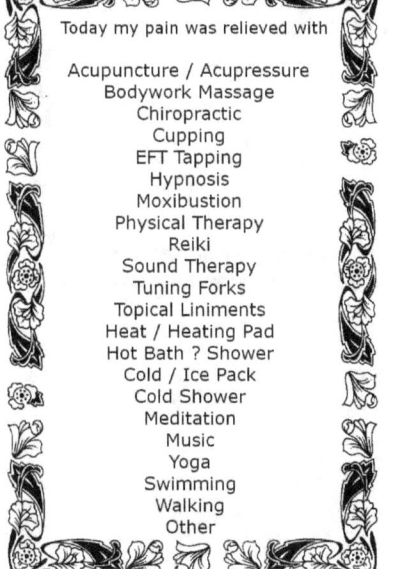

Today my pain was relieved with

Acupuncture / Acupressure
Bodywork Massage
Chiropractic
Cupping
EFT Tapping
Hypnosis
Moxibustion
Physical Therapy
Reiki
Sound Therapy
Tuning Forks
Topical Liniments
Heat / Heating Pad
Hot Bath ? Shower
Cold / Ice Pack
Cold Shower
Meditation
Music
Yoga
Swimming
Walking
Other

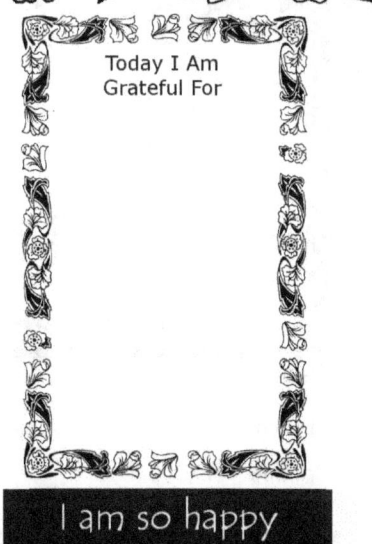

Today I Am Grateful For

I am so happy & grateful for my healthy body!

Today's Day & Date

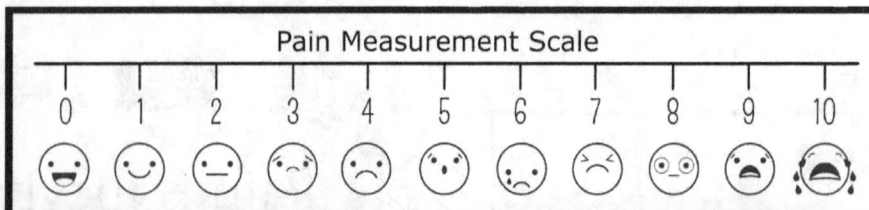

Highlight All Painful Areas

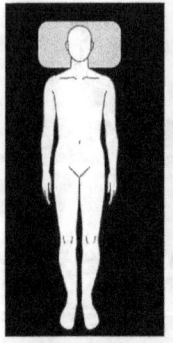 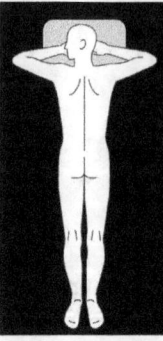 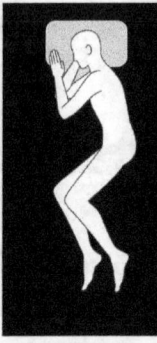 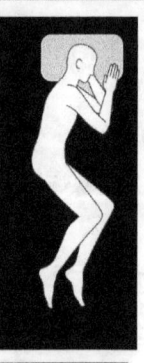

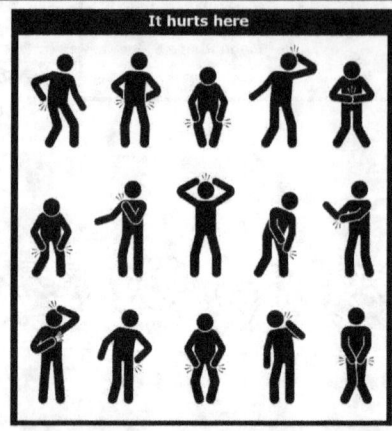

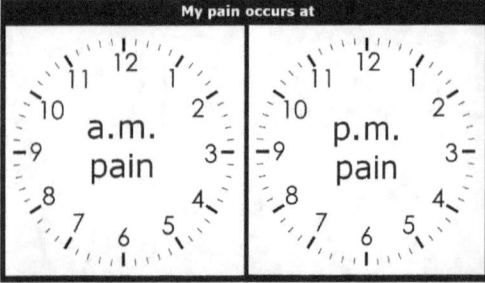

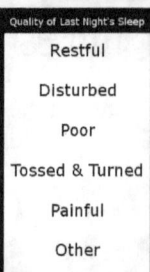

Quality of Last Night's Sleep
- Restful
- Disturbed
- Poor
- Tossed & Turned
- Painful
- Other

My pain is
Hot
Burning
Cold
Stabbing
Throbbing
Fixed
Moving Traveling
Constant
On & Off

Today's Weather

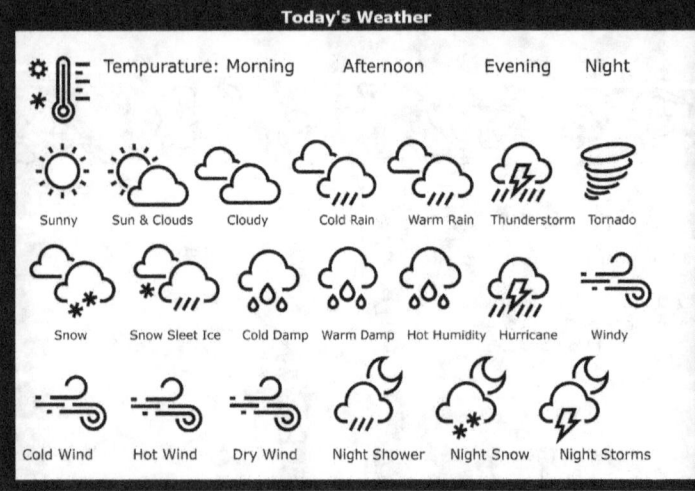

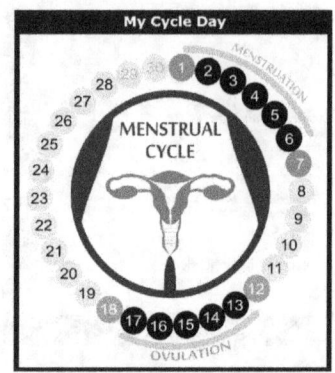

Breakfast

Lunch

Dinner

Snacks

Alcohol

Food Allergy Triggers

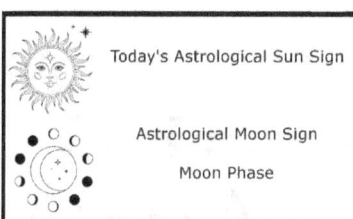

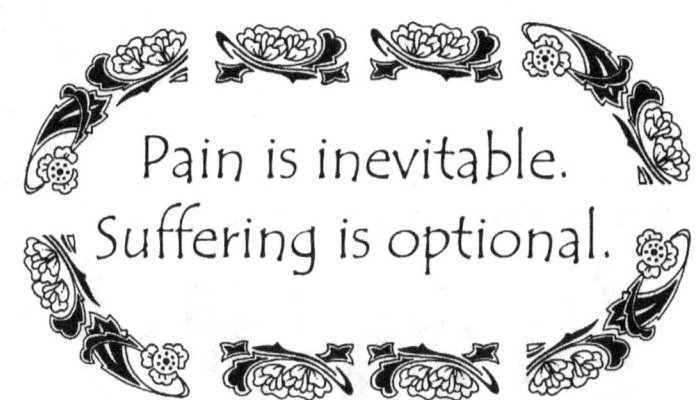

Notes

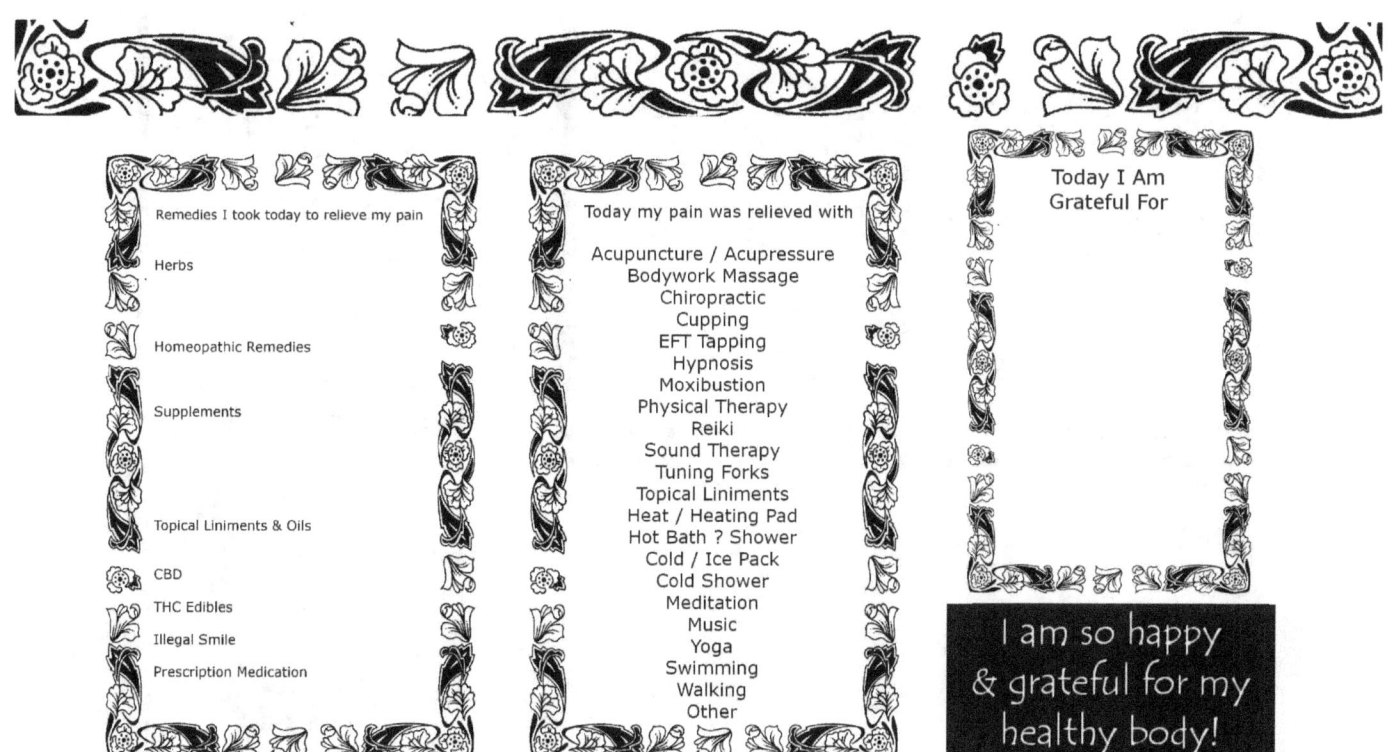

Remedies I took today to relieve my pain

Herbs

Homeopathic Remedies

Supplements

Topical Liniments & Oils

CBD

THC Edibles

Illegal Smile

Prescription Medication

Today my pain was relieved with

Acupuncture / Acupressure
Bodywork Massage
Chiropractic
Cupping
EFT Tapping
Hypnosis
Moxibustion
Physical Therapy
Reiki
Sound Therapy
Tuning Forks
Topical Liniments
Heat / Heating Pad
Hot Bath ? Shower
Cold / Ice Pack
Cold Shower
Meditation
Music
Yoga
Swimming
Walking
Other

Today I Am Grateful For

I am so happy & grateful for my healthy body!

Today's Day & Date

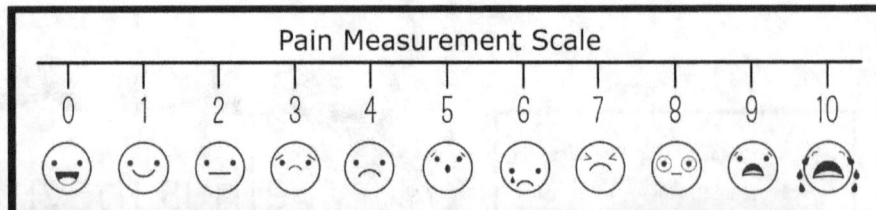

Pain Measurement Scale
0 1 2 3 4 5 6 7 8 9 10

Highlight All Painful Areas

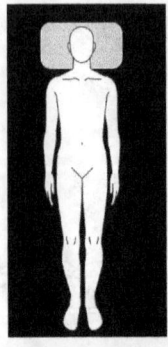 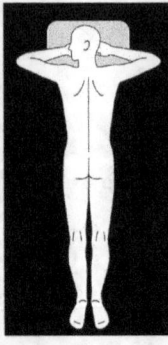 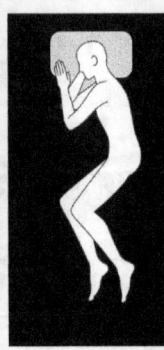 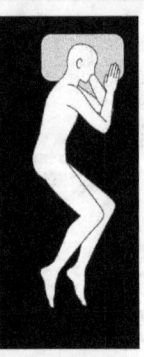

It hurts here

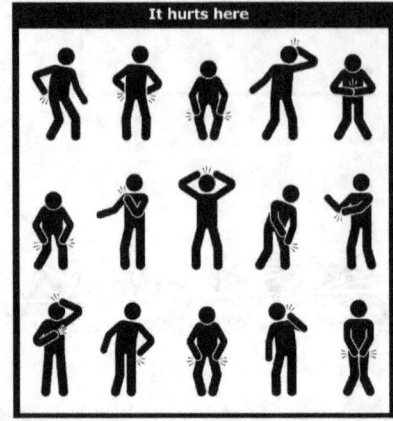

My pain occurs at

a.m. pain | p.m. pain

Quality of Last Night's Sleep

- Restful
- Disturbed
- Poor
- Tossed & Turned
- Painful
- Other

My mood today

My pain is

Hot
Burning
Cold
Stabbing
Throbbing
Fixed
Moving Traveling
Constant
On & Off

Today's Weather

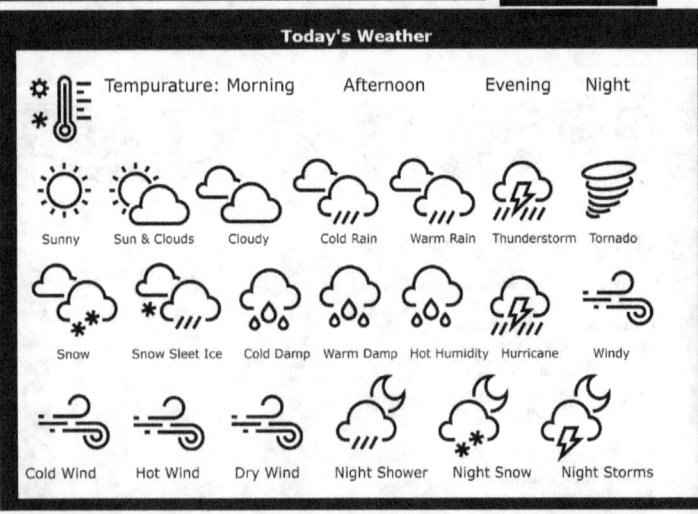

Tempurature: Morning   Afternoon   Evening   Night

Sunny · Sun & Clouds · Cloudy · Cold Rain · Warm Rain · Thunderstorm · Tornado
Snow · Snow Sleet Ice · Cold Damp · Warm Damp · Hot Humidity · Hurricane · Windy
Cold Wind · Hot Wind · Dry Wind · Night Shower · Night Snow · Night Storms

Breakfast

Lunch

Dinner

Snacks

Alcohol

Food Allergy Triggers

My Cycle Day

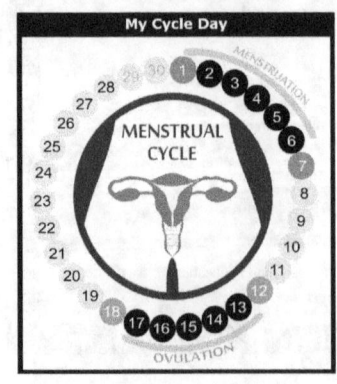

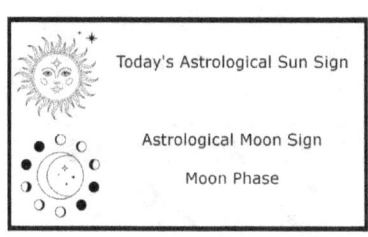

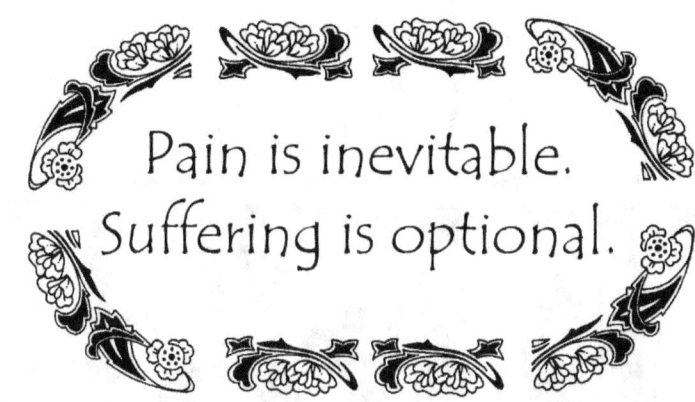

Today's Astrological Sun Sign

Astrological Moon Sign

Moon Phase

Pain is inevitable.
Suffering is optional.

Notes

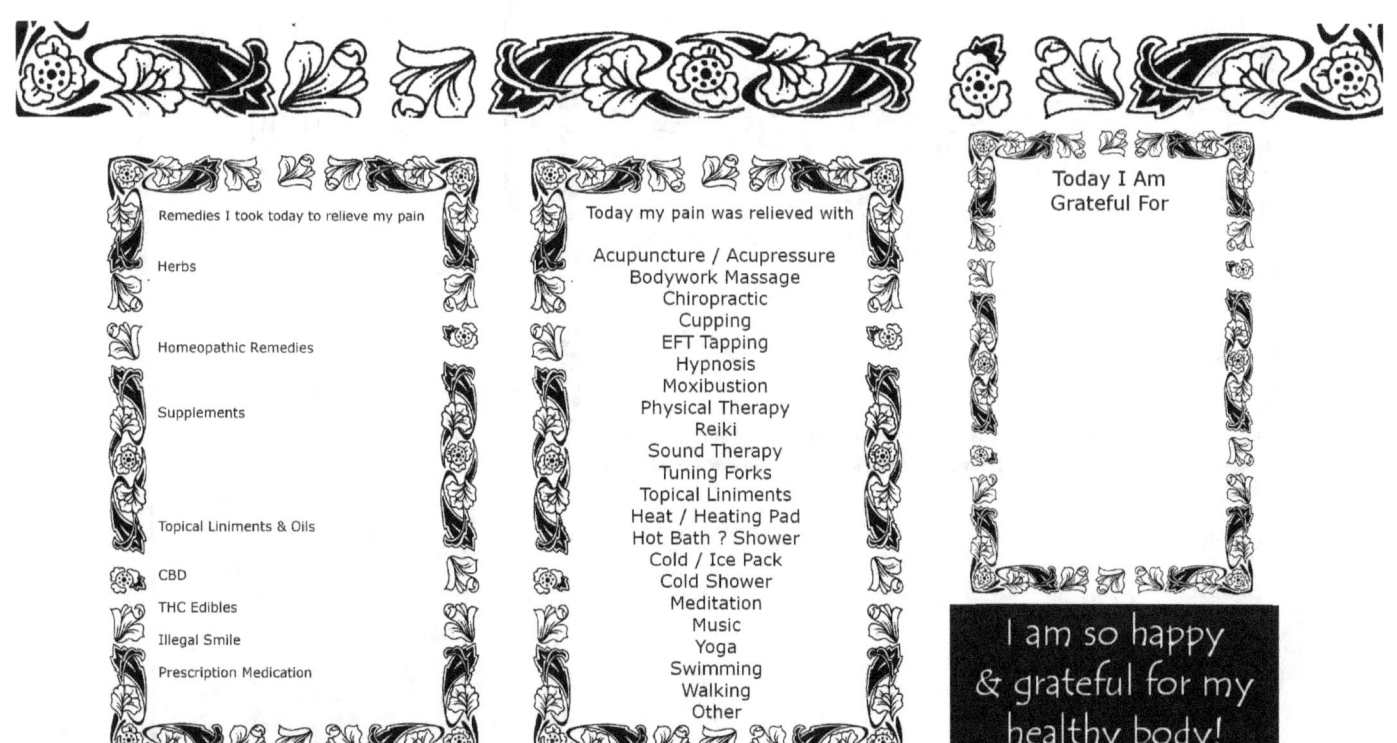

Remedies I took today to relieve my pain

Herbs

Homeopathic Remedies

Supplements

Topical Liniments & Oils

CBD

THC Edibles

Illegal Smile

Prescription Medication

Today my pain was relieved with

Acupuncture / Acupressure
Bodywork Massage
Chiropractic
Cupping
EFT Tapping
Hypnosis
Moxibustion
Physical Therapy
Reiki
Sound Therapy
Tuning Forks
Topical Liniments
Heat / Heating Pad
Hot Bath ? Shower
Cold / Ice Pack
Cold Shower
Meditation
Music
Yoga
Swimming
Walking
Other

Today I Am Grateful For

I am so happy & grateful for my healthy body!

Today's Day & Date

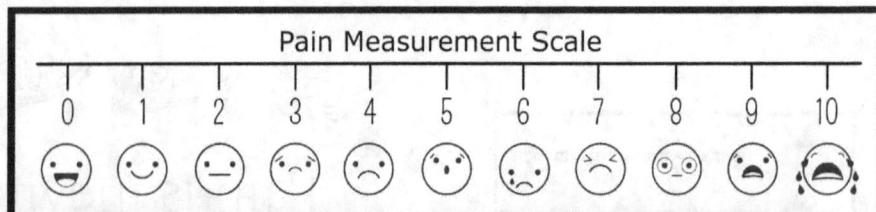

Highlight All Painful Areas

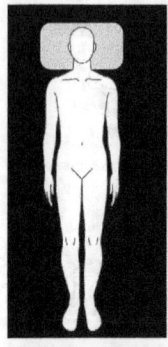 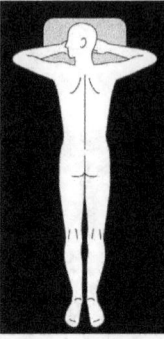 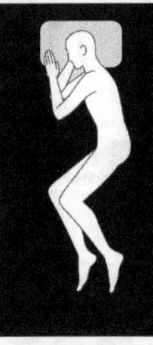 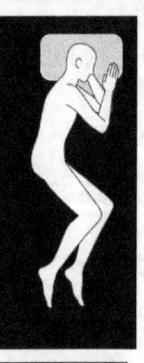

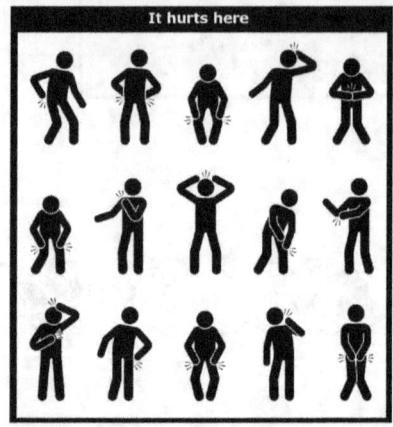

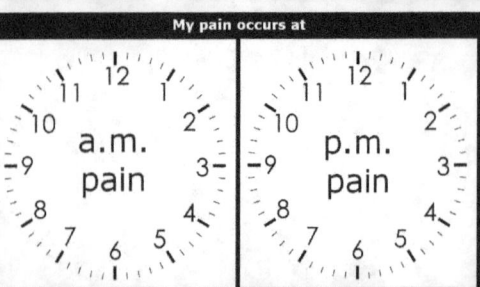

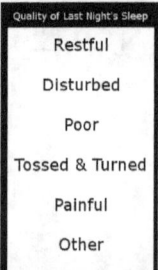

Quality of Last Night's Sleep
- Restful
- Disturbed
- Poor
- Tossed & Turned
- Painful
- Other

My pain is
Hot
Burning
Cold
Stabbing
Throbbing
Fixed
Moving Traveling
Constant
On & Off

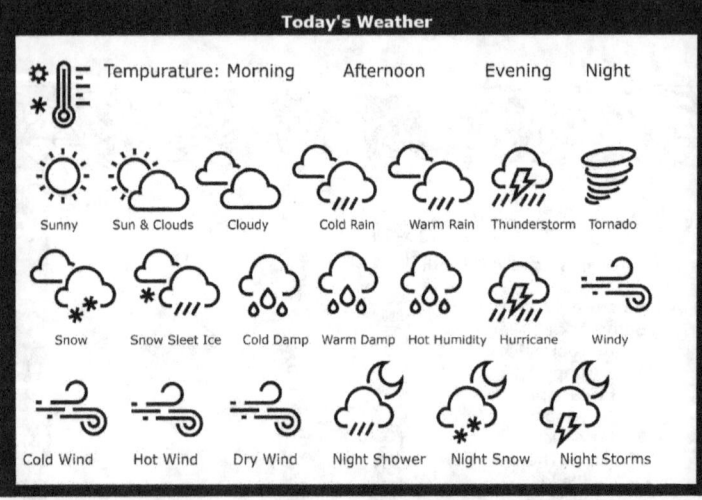

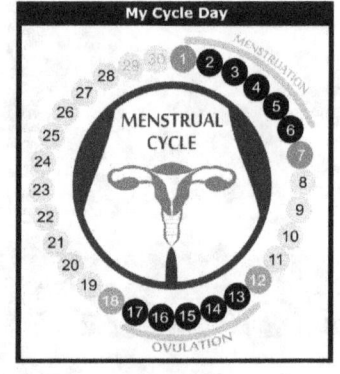

Breakfast

Lunch

Dinner

Snacks

Alcohol

Food Allergy Triggers

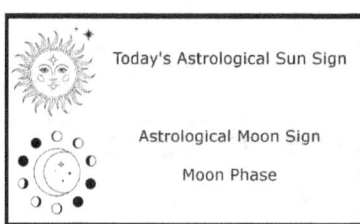

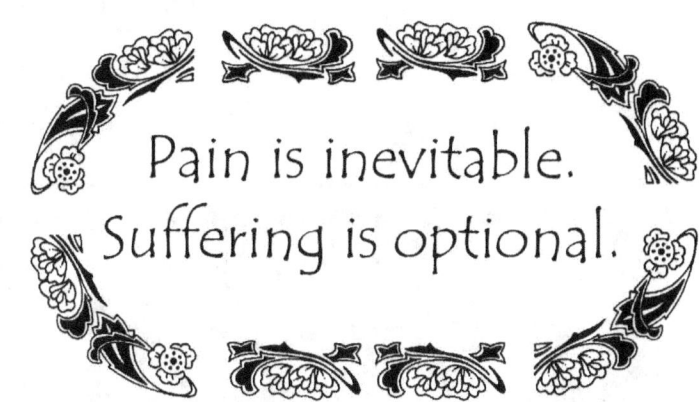

Pain is inevitable.
Suffering is optional.

Notes

Remedies I took today to relieve my pain

- Herbs
- Homeopathic Remedies
- Supplements
- Topical Liniments & Oils
- CBD
- THC Edibles
- Illegal Smile
- Prescription Medication

Today my pain was relieved with

- Acupuncture / Acupressure
- Bodywork Massage
- Chiropractic
- Cupping
- EFT Tapping
- Hypnosis
- Moxibustion
- Physical Therapy
- Reiki
- Sound Therapy
- Tuning Forks
- Topical Liniments
- Heat / Heating Pad
- Hot Bath ? Shower
- Cold / Ice Pack
- Cold Shower
- Meditation
- Music
- Yoga
- Swimming
- Walking
- Other

Today I Am Grateful For

I am so happy & grateful for my healthy body!

Today's Day & Date

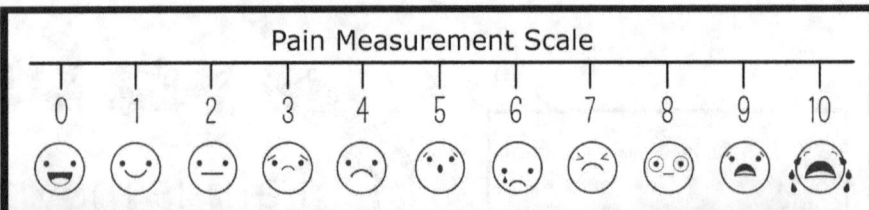

Highlight All Painful Areas

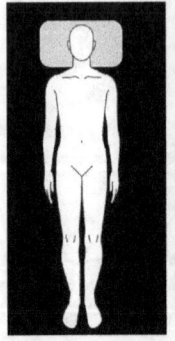 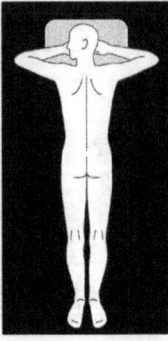 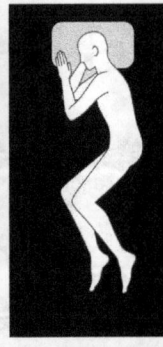 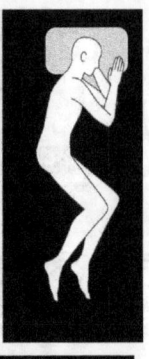

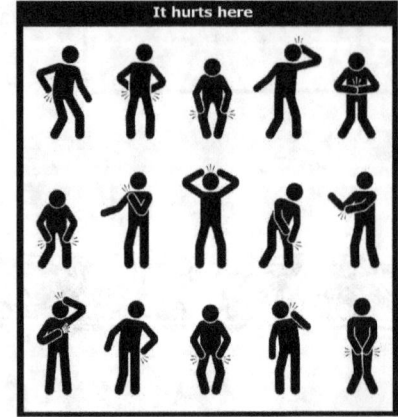
It hurts here

My pain occurs at

a.m. pain | p.m. pain

Quality of Last Night's Sleep
- Restful
- Disturbed
- Poor
- Tossed & Turned
- Painful
- Other

My mood today

My pain is

Hot
Burning
Cold
Stabbing
Throbbing
Fixed
Moving Traveling
Constant
On & Off

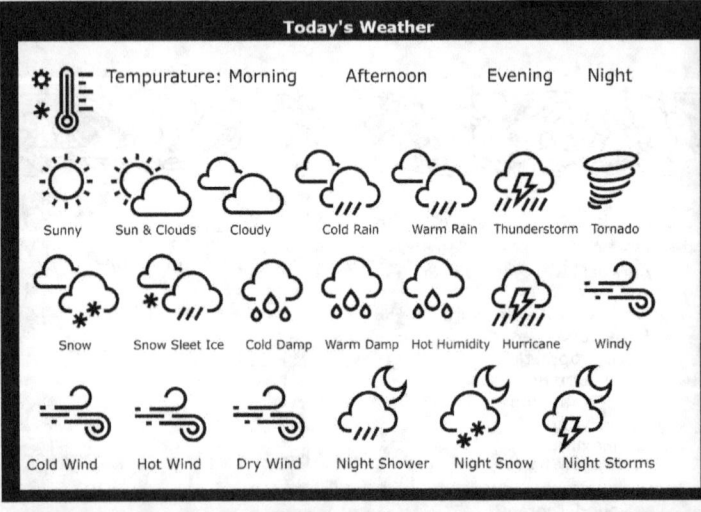
Today's Weather

Tempurature: Morning   Afternoon   Evening   Night

Sunny | Sun & Clouds | Cloudy | Cold Rain | Warm Rain | Thunderstorm | Tornado
Snow | Snow Sleet Ice | Cold Damp | Warm Damp | Hot Humidity | Hurricane | Windy
Cold Wind | Hot Wind | Dry Wind | Night Shower | Night Snow | Night Storms

Breakfast

Lunch

Dinner

Snacks

Alcohol

Food Allergy Triggers

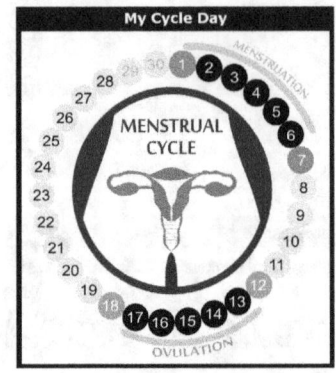
My Cycle Day

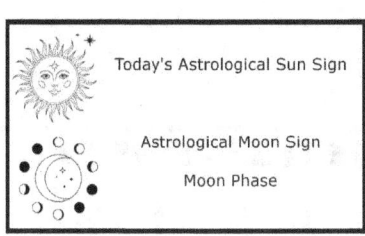

Today's Astrological Sun Sign

Astrological Moon Sign

Moon Phase

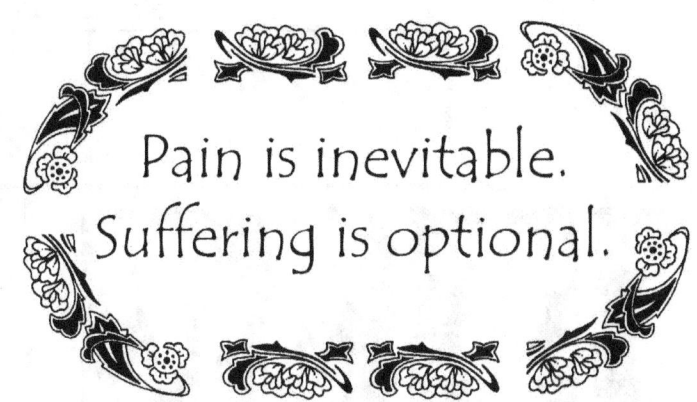

Pain is inevitable.
Suffering is optional.

Notes

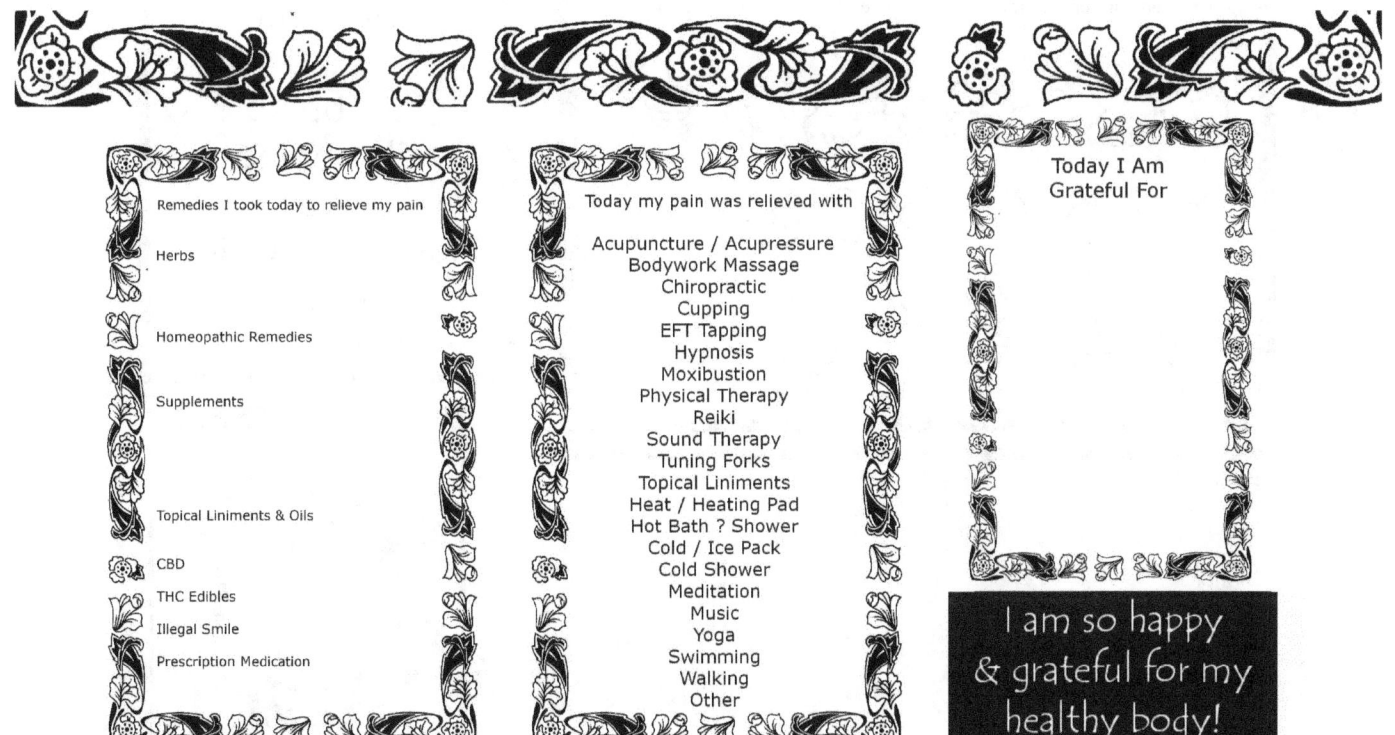

Remedies I took today to relieve my pain

Herbs

Homeopathic Remedies

Supplements

Topical Liniments & Oils

CBD
THC Edibles
Illegal Smile
Prescription Medication

Today my pain was relieved with

Acupuncture / Acupressure
Bodywork Massage
Chiropractic
Cupping
EFT Tapping
Hypnosis
Moxibustion
Physical Therapy
Reiki
Sound Therapy
Tuning Forks
Topical Liniments
Heat / Heating Pad
Hot Bath ? Shower
Cold / Ice Pack
Cold Shower
Meditation
Music
Yoga
Swimming
Walking
Other

Today I Am Grateful For

I am so happy & grateful for my healthy body!

Today's Day & Date

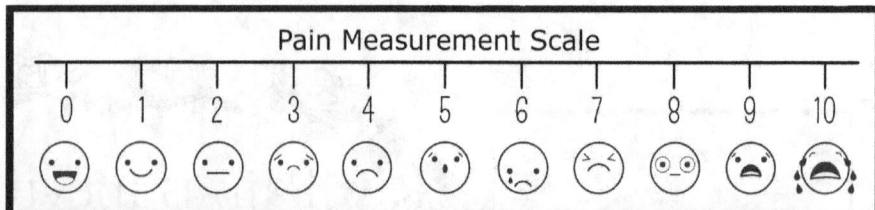

Highlight All Painful Areas

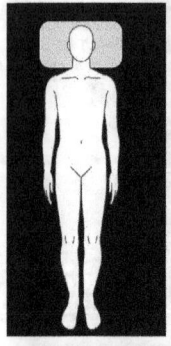 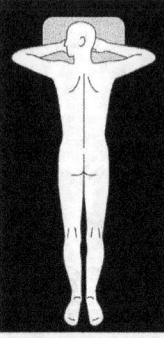 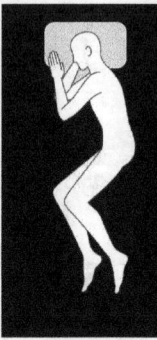 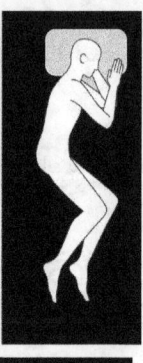

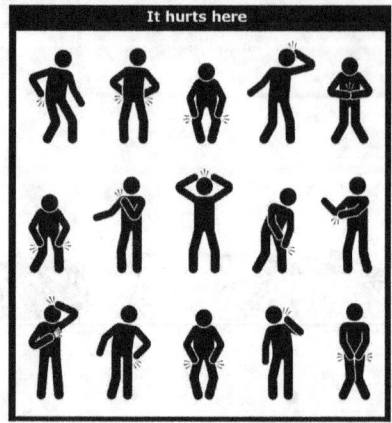
It hurts here

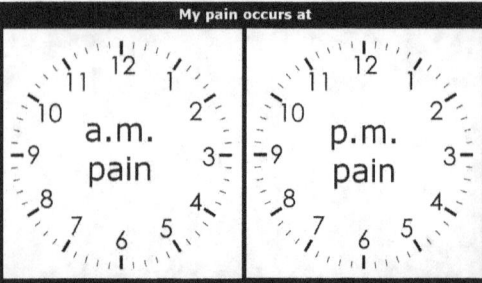
My pain occurs at — a.m. pain / p.m. pain

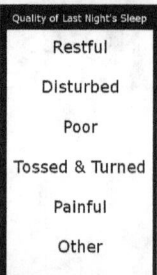
Quality of Last Night's Sleep
- Restful
- Disturbed
- Poor
- Tossed & Turned
- Painful
- Other

My mood today

My pain is

Hot
Burning
Cold
Stabbing
Throbbing
Fixed
Moving Traveling
Constant
On & Off

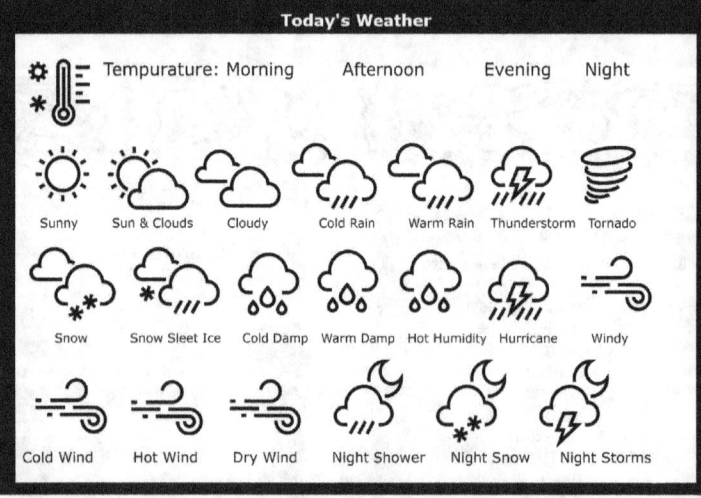
Today's Weather

Tempurature: Morning Afternoon Evening Night

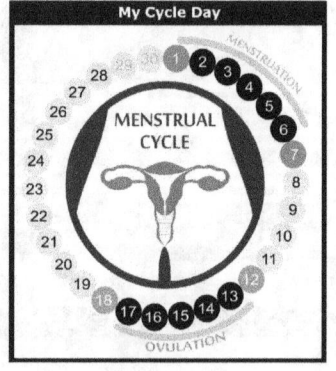
My Cycle Day

Breakfast

Lunch

Dinner

Snacks

Alcohol

Food Allergy Triggers

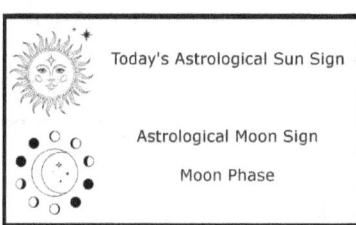

Today's Astrological Sun Sign

Astrological Moon Sign

Moon Phase

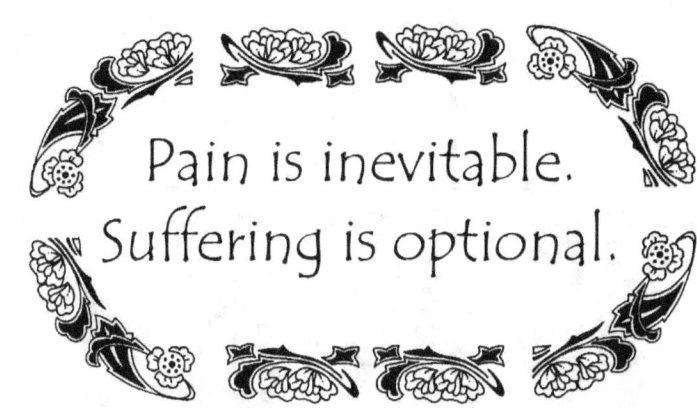

Pain is inevitable.
Suffering is optional.

Notes

Remedies I took today to relieve my pain

Herbs

Homeopathic Remedies

Supplements

Topical Liniments & Oils

CBD

THC Edibles

Illegal Smile

Prescription Medication

Today my pain was relieved with

Acupuncture / Acupressure
Bodywork Massage
Chiropractic
Cupping
EFT Tapping
Hypnosis
Moxibustion
Physical Therapy
Reiki
Sound Therapy
Tuning Forks
Topical Liniments
Heat / Heating Pad
Hot Bath ? Shower
Cold / Ice Pack
Cold Shower
Meditation
Music
Yoga
Swimming
Walking
Other

Today I Am Grateful For

I am so happy & grateful for my healthy body!

Today's Day & Date

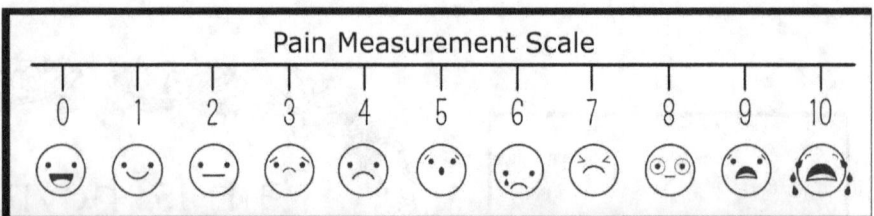

Highlight All Painful Areas

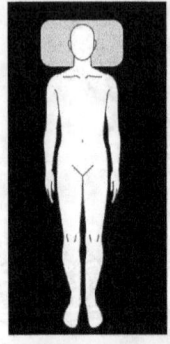 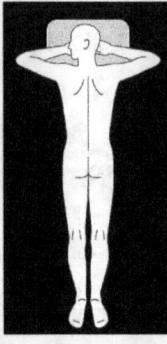 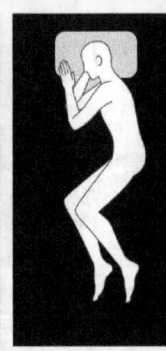 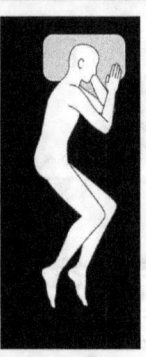

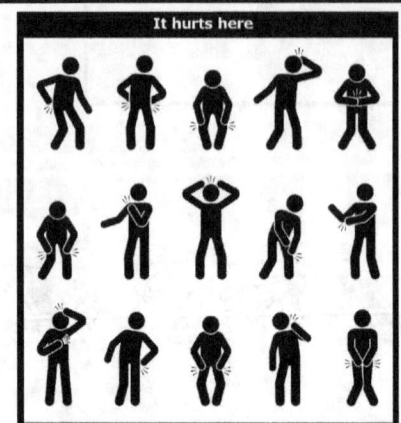
It hurts here

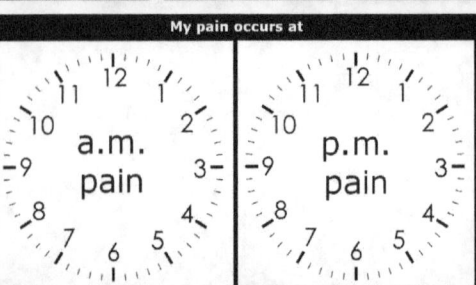
My pain occurs at — a.m. pain / p.m. pain

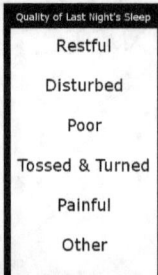

Quality of Last Night's Sleep
- Restful
- Disturbed
- Poor
- Tossed & Turned
- Painful
- Other

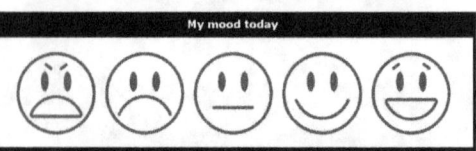
My mood today

My pain is
Hot
Burning
Cold
Stabbing
Throbbing
Fixed
Moving Traveling
Constant
On & Off

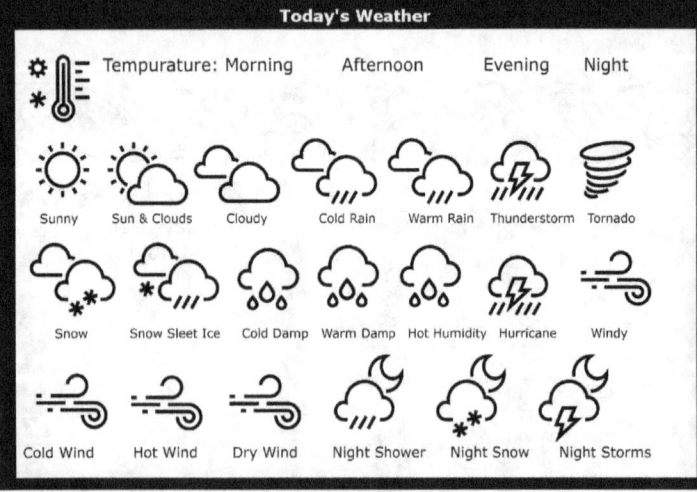
Today's Weather — Tempurature: Morning, Afternoon, Evening, Night

Breakfast

Lunch

Dinner

Snacks

Alcohol

Food Allergy Triggers

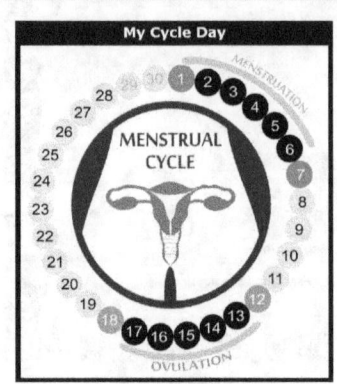
My Cycle Day

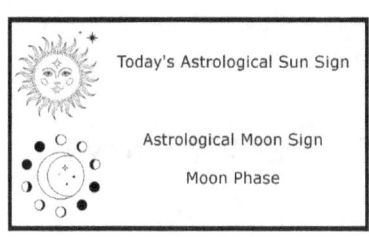

Today's Astrological Sun Sign

Astrological Moon Sign

Moon Phase

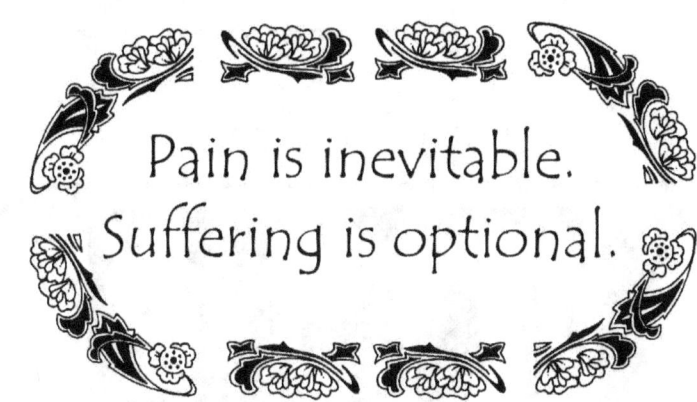

Pain is inevitable.
Suffering is optional.

Notes

Remedies I took today to relieve my pain

Herbs

Homeopathic Remedies

Supplements

Topical Liniments & Oils

CBD
THC Edibles
Illegal Smile
Prescription Medication

Today my pain was relieved with

Acupuncture / Acupressure
Bodywork Massage
Chiropractic
Cupping
EFT Tapping
Hypnosis
Moxibustion
Physical Therapy
Reiki
Sound Therapy
Tuning Forks
Topical Liniments
Heat / Heating Pad
Hot Bath ? Shower
Cold / Ice Pack
Cold Shower
Meditation
Music
Yoga
Swimming
Walking
Other

Today I Am Grateful For

I am so happy & grateful for my healthy body!

Today's Day & Date

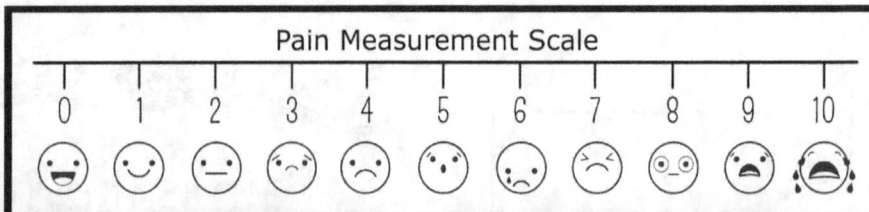

Highlight All Painful Areas

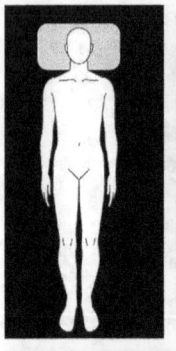 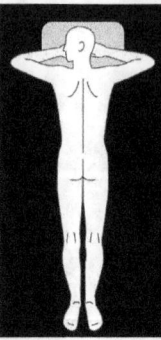 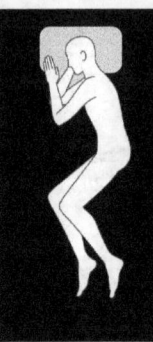 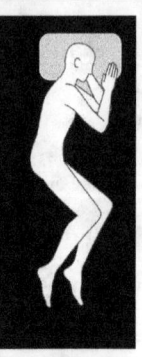

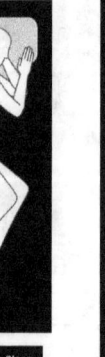

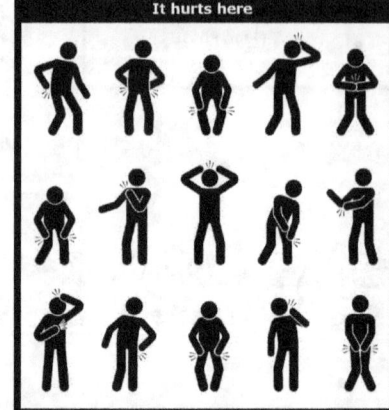

It hurts here

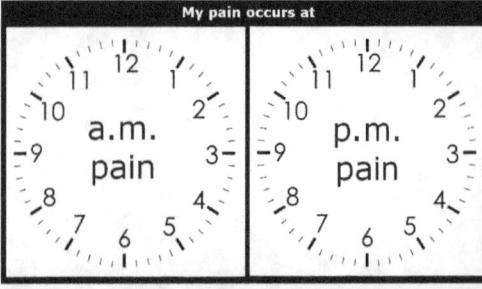

My pain occurs at — a.m. pain / p.m. pain

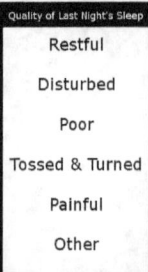

Quality of Last Night's Sleep
- Restful
- Disturbed
- Poor
- Tossed & Turned
- Painful
- Other

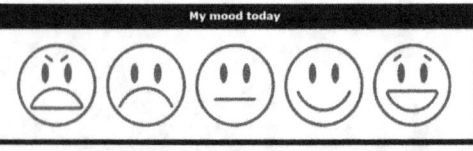

My mood today

My pain is
Hot
Burning
Cold
Stabbing
Throbbing
Fixed
Moving Traveling
Constant
On & Off

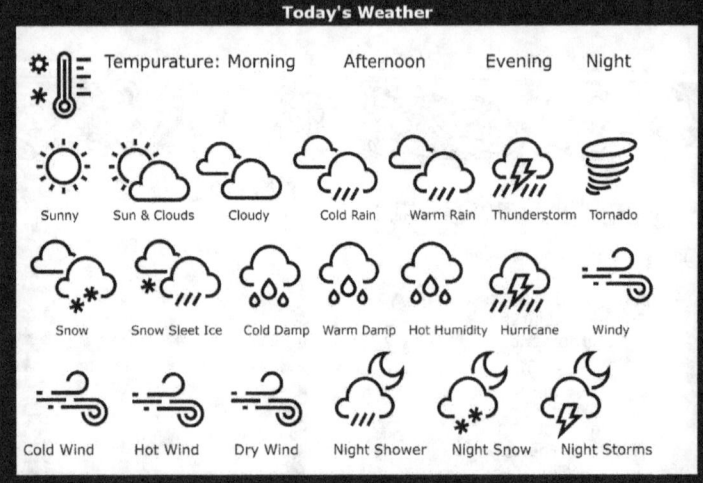

Today's Weather — Temperature: Morning, Afternoon, Evening, Night

Sunny, Sun & Clouds, Cloudy, Cold Rain, Warm Rain, Thunderstorm, Tornado, Snow, Snow Sleet Ice, Cold Damp, Warm Damp, Hot Humidity, Hurricane, Windy, Cold Wind, Hot Wind, Dry Wind, Night Shower, Night Snow, Night Storms

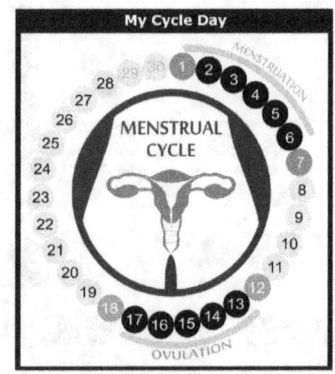

My Cycle Day

Breakfast

Lunch

Dinner

Snacks

Alcohol

Food Allergy Triggers

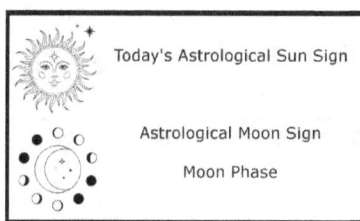

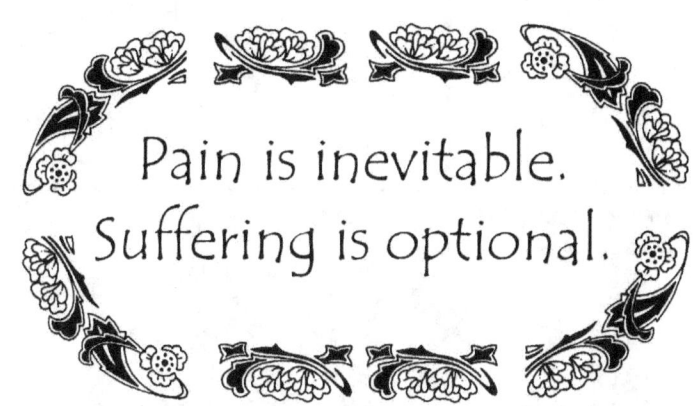

Pain is inevitable. Suffering is optional.

Notes

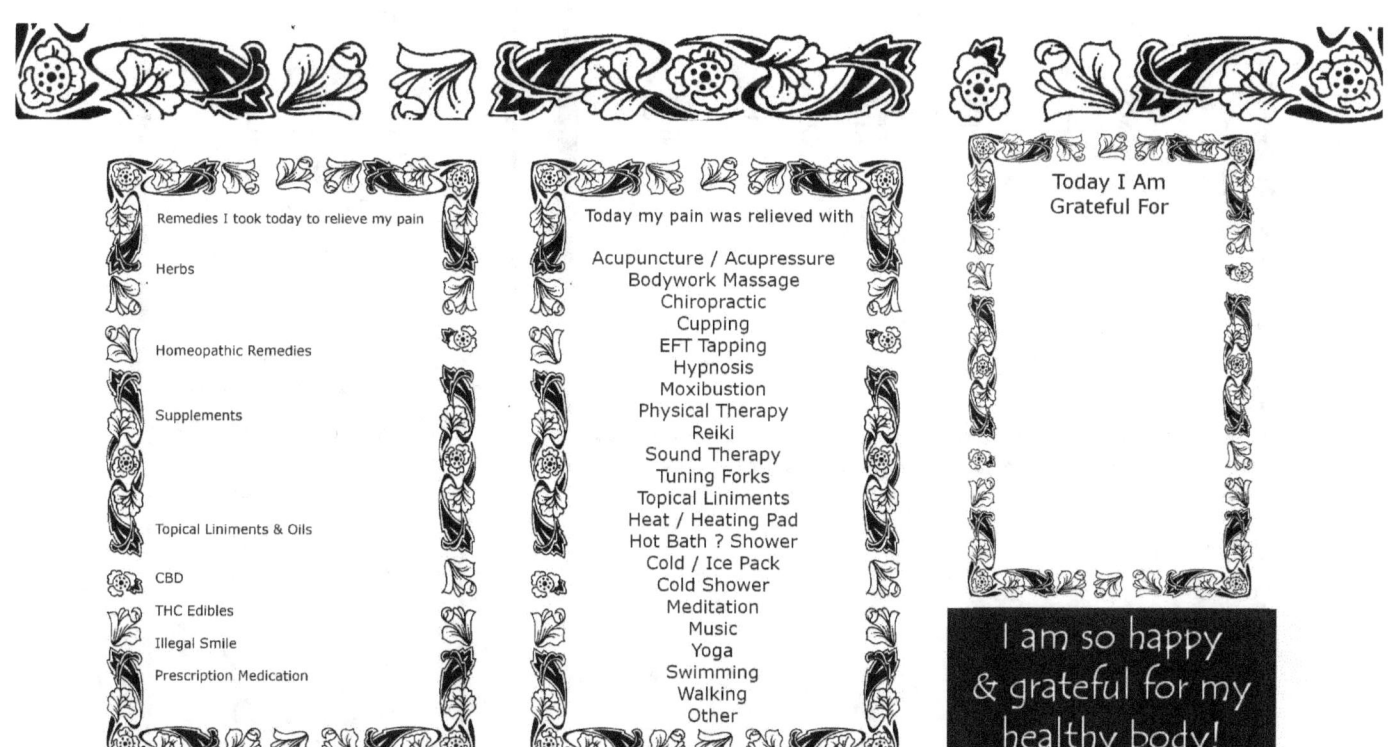

Remedies I took today to relieve my pain

Herbs

Homeopathic Remedies

Supplements

Topical Liniments & Oils

CBD

THC Edibles

Illegal Smile

Prescription Medication

Today my pain was relieved with

Acupuncture / Acupressure
Bodywork Massage
Chiropractic
Cupping
EFT Tapping
Hypnosis
Moxibustion
Physical Therapy
Reiki
Sound Therapy
Tuning Forks
Topical Liniments
Heat / Heating Pad
Hot Bath ? Shower
Cold / Ice Pack
Cold Shower
Meditation
Music
Yoga
Swimming
Walking
Other

Today I Am Grateful For

I am so happy & grateful for my healthy body!

Today's Day & Date

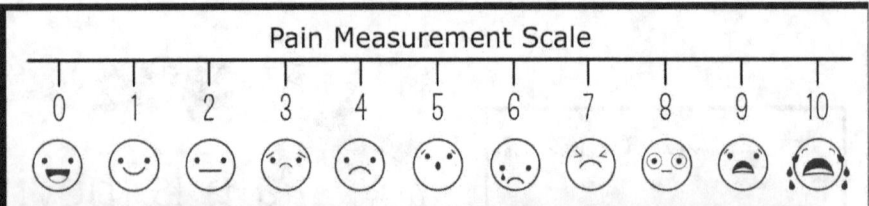

Highlight All Painful Areas

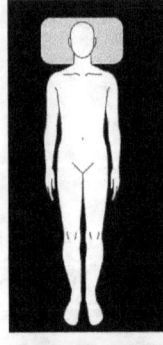 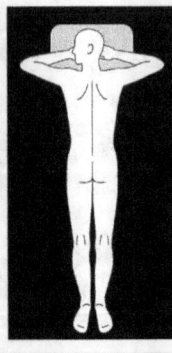 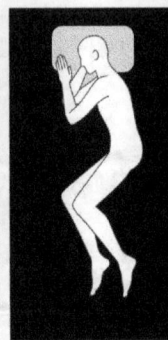 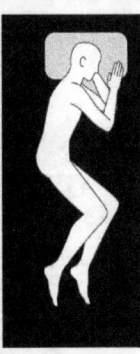

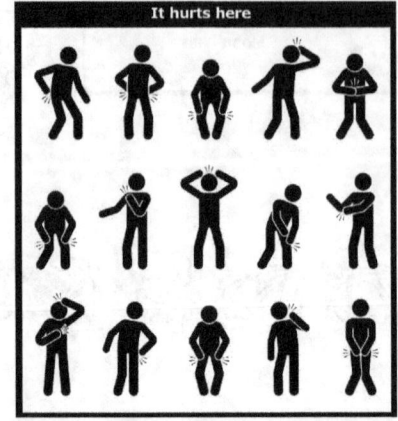
It hurts here

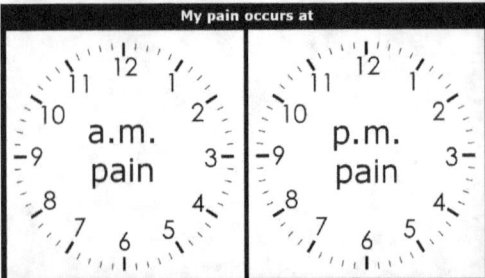
My pain occurs at

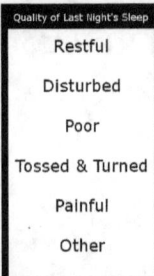
Quality of Last Night's Sleep
- Restful
- Disturbed
- Poor
- Tossed & Turned
- Painful
- Other

My mood today

My pain is
Hot
Burning
Cold
Stabbing
Throbbing
Fixed
Moving Traveling
Constant
On & Off

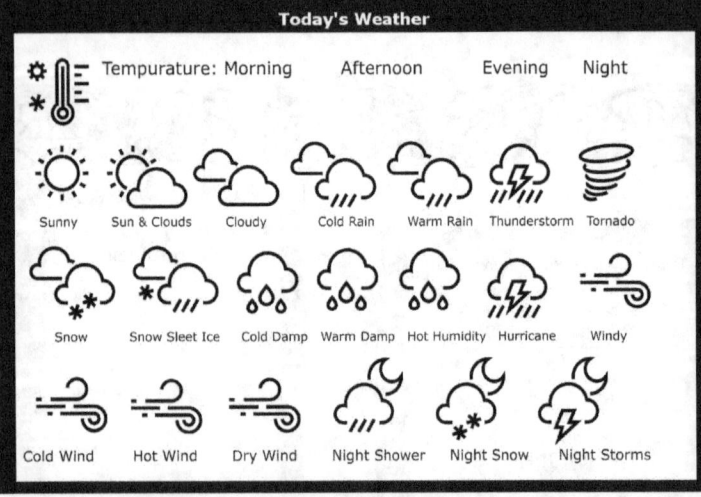
Today's Weather

Breakfast

Lunch

Dinner

Snacks

Alcohol

Food Allergy Triggers

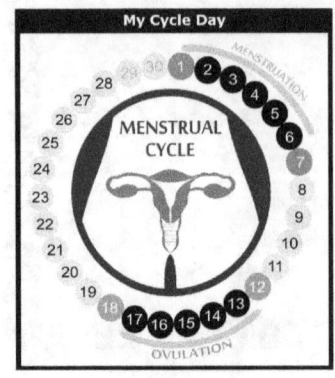
My Cycle Day

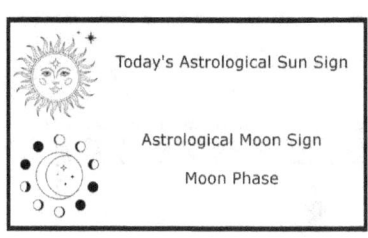

Today's Astrological Sun Sign

Astrological Moon Sign

Moon Phase

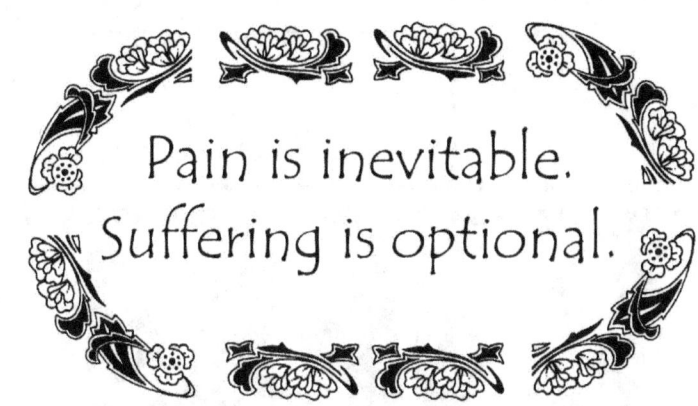

Pain is inevitable.
Suffering is optional.

Notes

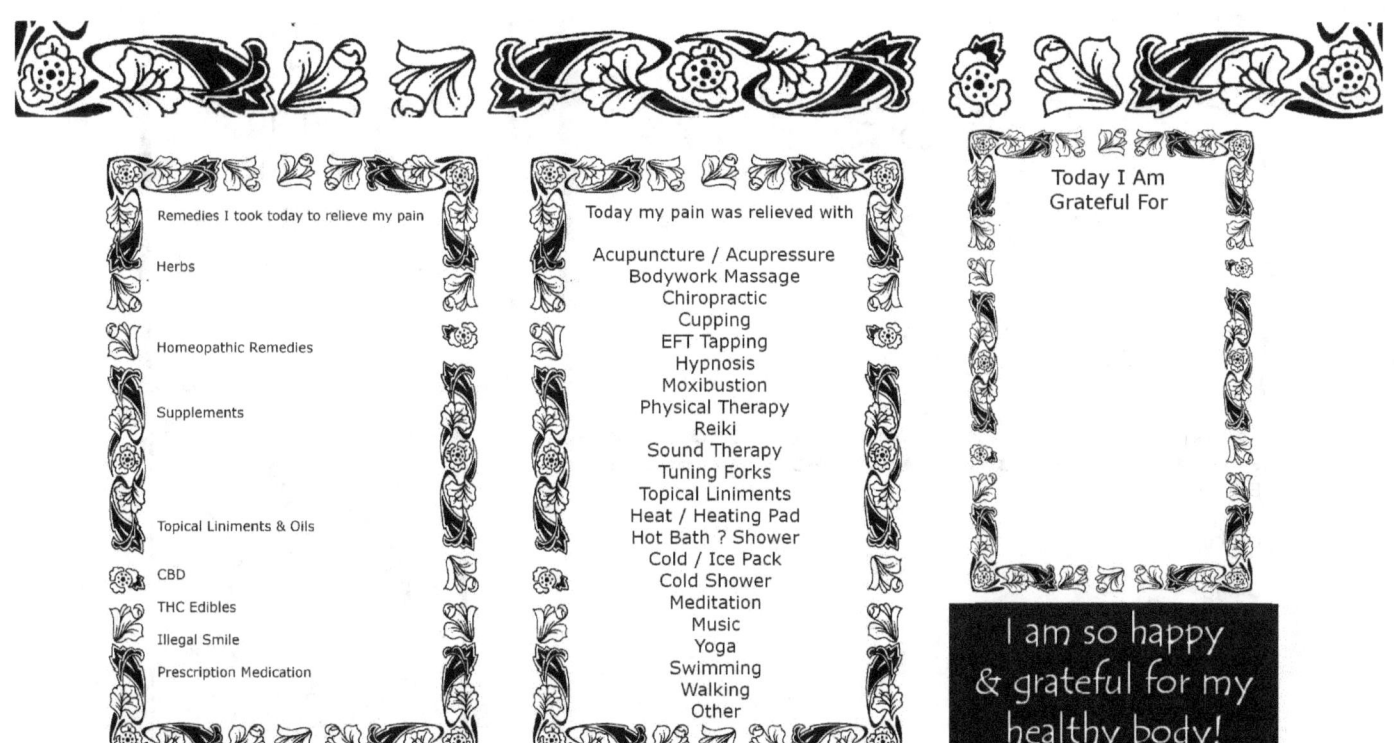

Remedies I took today to relieve my pain

Herbs

Homeopathic Remedies

Supplements

Topical Liniments & Oils

CBD

THC Edibles

Illegal Smile

Prescription Medication

Today my pain was relieved with

Acupuncture / Acupressure
Bodywork Massage
Chiropractic
Cupping
EFT Tapping
Hypnosis
Moxibustion
Physical Therapy
Reiki
Sound Therapy
Tuning Forks
Topical Liniments
Heat / Heating Pad
Hot Bath ? Shower
Cold / Ice Pack
Cold Shower
Meditation
Music
Yoga
Swimming
Walking
Other

Today I Am Grateful For

I am so happy & grateful for my healthy body!

Today's Day & Date

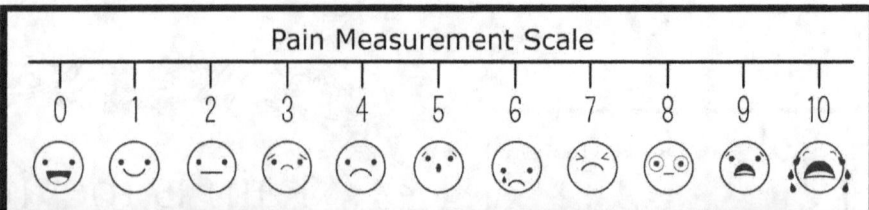

Highlight All Painful Areas

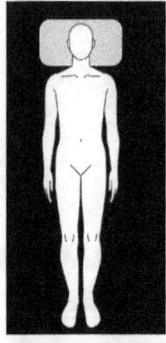 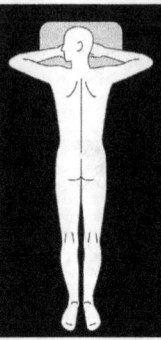 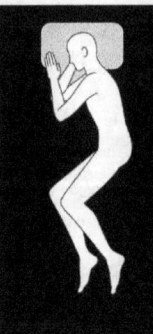 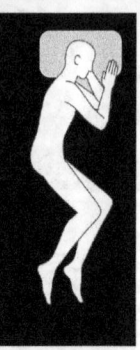

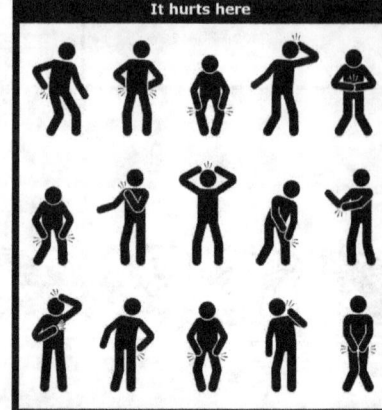

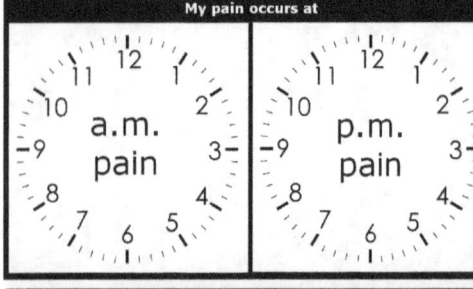

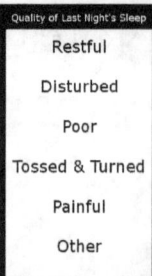

Quality of Last Night's Sleep
- Restful
- Disturbed
- Poor
- Tossed & Turned
- Painful
- Other

My mood today

My pain is
Hot
Burning
Cold
Stabbing
Throbbing
Fixed
Moving Traveling
Constant
On & Off

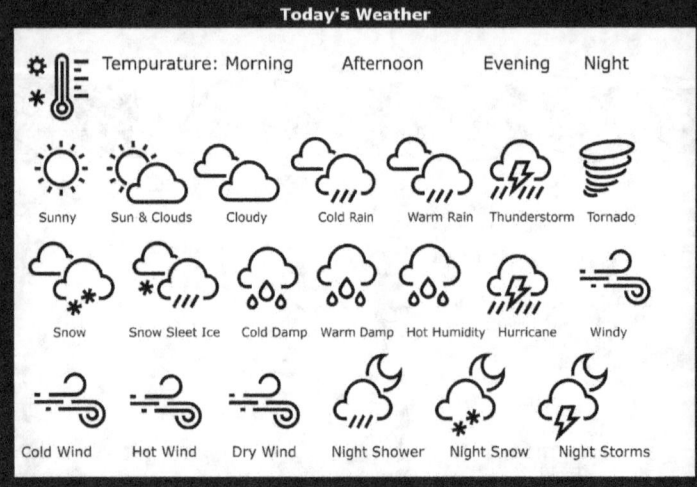

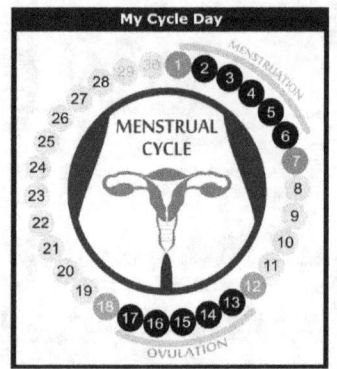

Breakfast

Lunch

Dinner

Snacks

Alcohol

Food Allergy Triggers

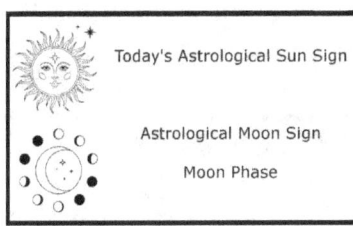

Today's Astrological Sun Sign

Astrological Moon Sign

Moon Phase

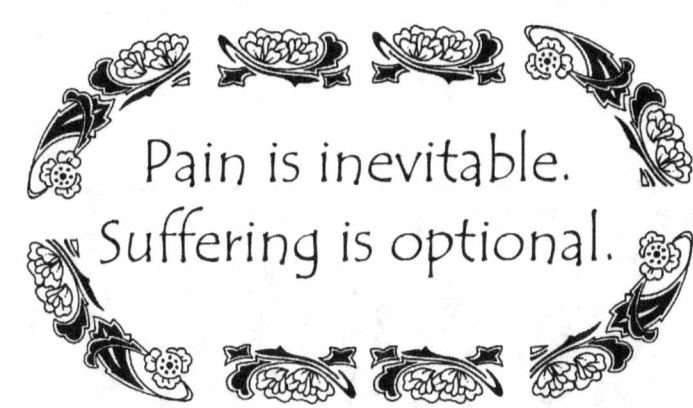

Pain is inevitable. Suffering is optional.

Notes

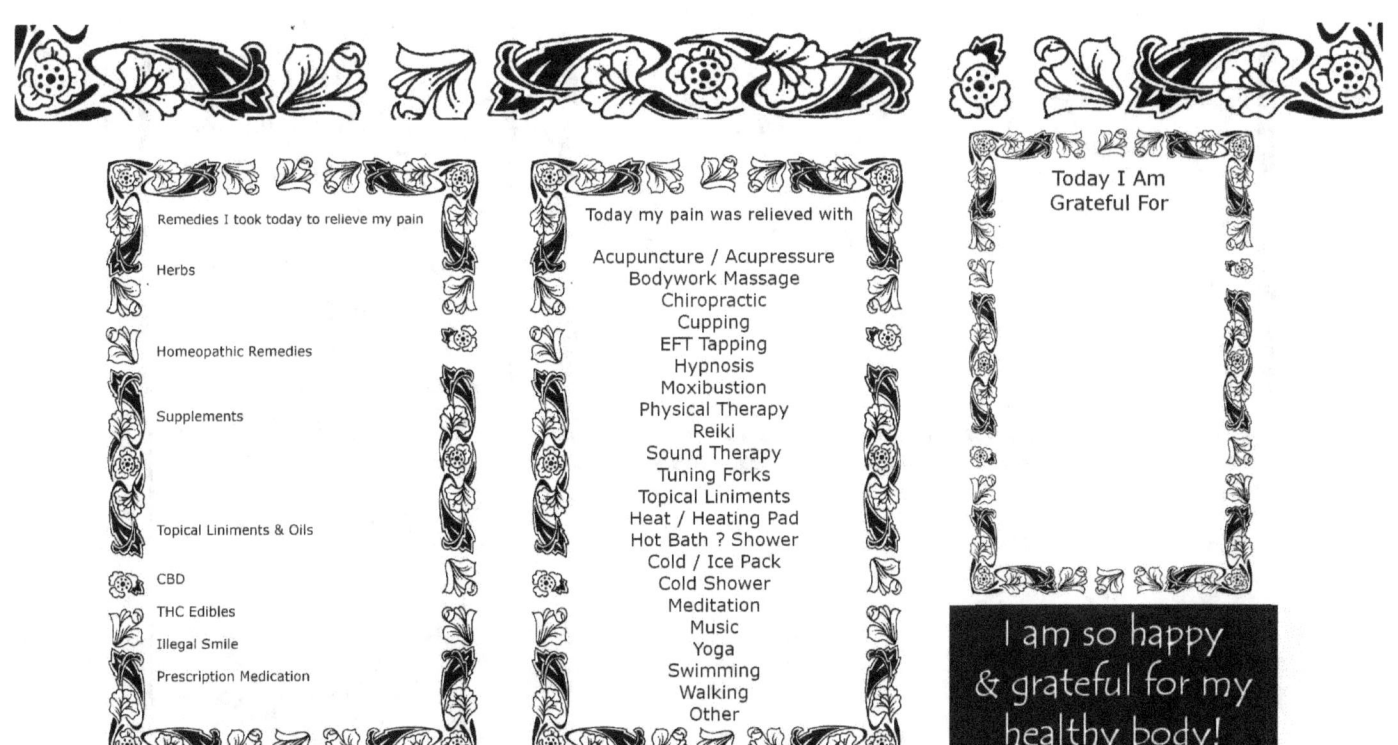

Remedies I took today to relieve my pain

Herbs

Homeopathic Remedies

Supplements

Topical Liniments & Oils

CBD
THC Edibles
Illegal Smile
Prescription Medication

Today my pain was relieved with

Acupuncture / Acupressure
Bodywork Massage
Chiropractic
Cupping
EFT Tapping
Hypnosis
Moxibustion
Physical Therapy
Reiki
Sound Therapy
Tuning Forks
Topical Liniments
Heat / Heating Pad
Hot Bath ? Shower
Cold / Ice Pack
Cold Shower
Meditation
Music
Yoga
Swimming
Walking
Other

Today I Am Grateful For

I am so happy & grateful for my healthy body!

Today's Day & Date

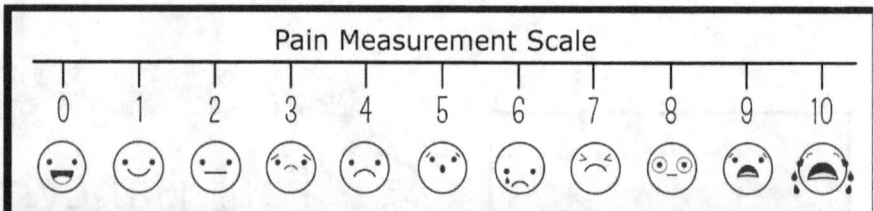

Highlight All Painful Areas

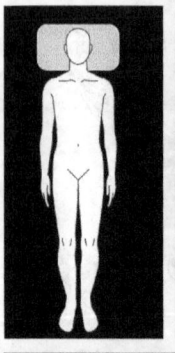 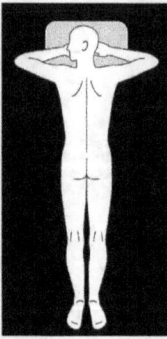 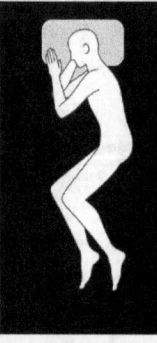 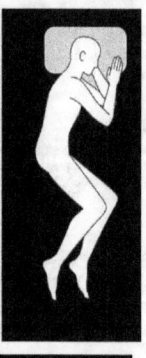 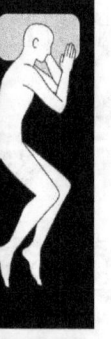

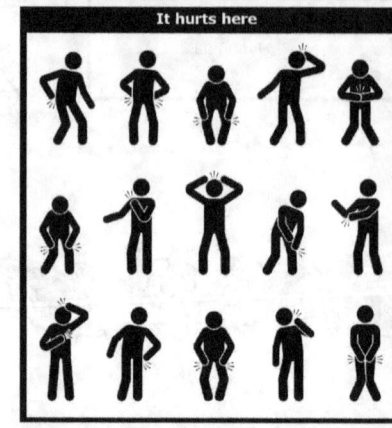
It hurts here

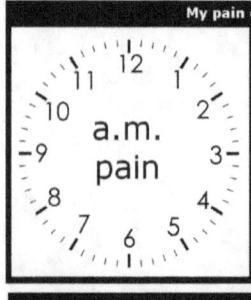
My pain occurs at — a.m. pain / p.m. pain

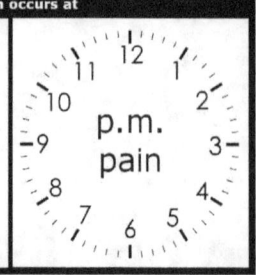

Quality of Last Night's Sleep
- Restful
- Disturbed
- Poor
- Tossed & Turned
- Painful
- Other

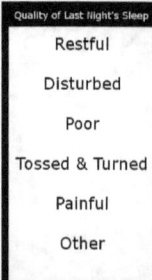

My mood today

My pain is
Hot
Burning
Cold
Stabbing
Throbbing
Fixed
Moving Traveling
Constant
On & Off

Today's Weather

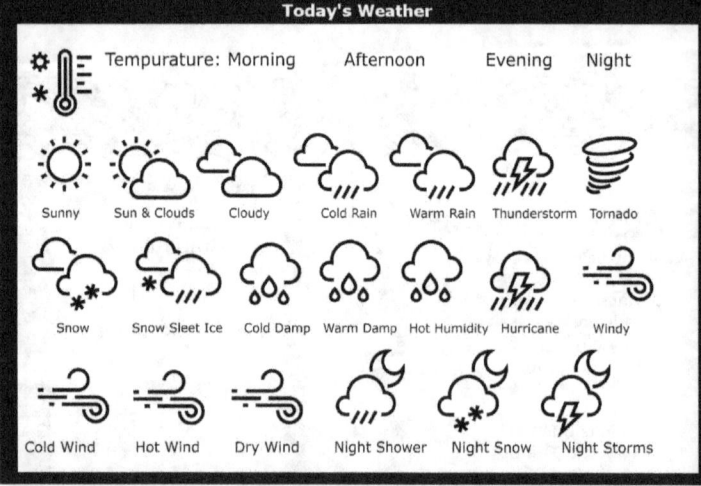

Tempurature: Morning Afternoon Evening Night

Sunny / Sun & Clouds / Cloudy / Cold Rain / Warm Rain / Thunderstorm / Tornado
Snow / Snow Sleet Ice / Cold Damp / Warm Damp / Hot Humidity / Hurricane / Windy
Cold Wind / Hot Wind / Dry Wind / Night Shower / Night Snow / Night Storms

Breakfast

Lunch

Dinner

Snacks

Alcohol

Food Allergy Triggers

My Cycle Day — MENSTRUAL CYCLE

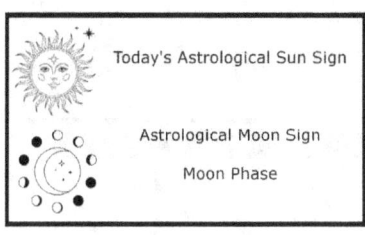

Today's Astrological Sun Sign

Astrological Moon Sign

Moon Phase

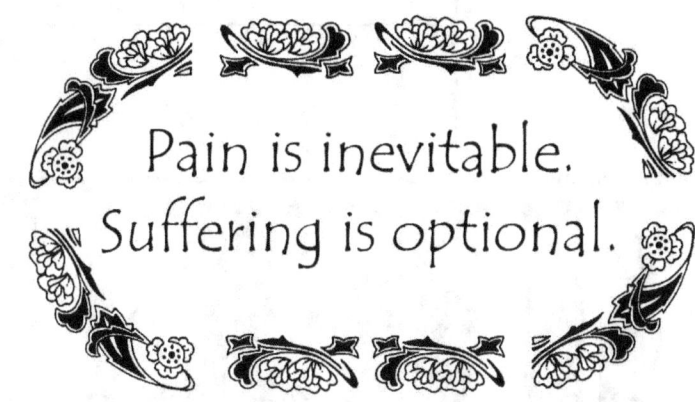

Pain is inevitable.
Suffering is optional.

Notes

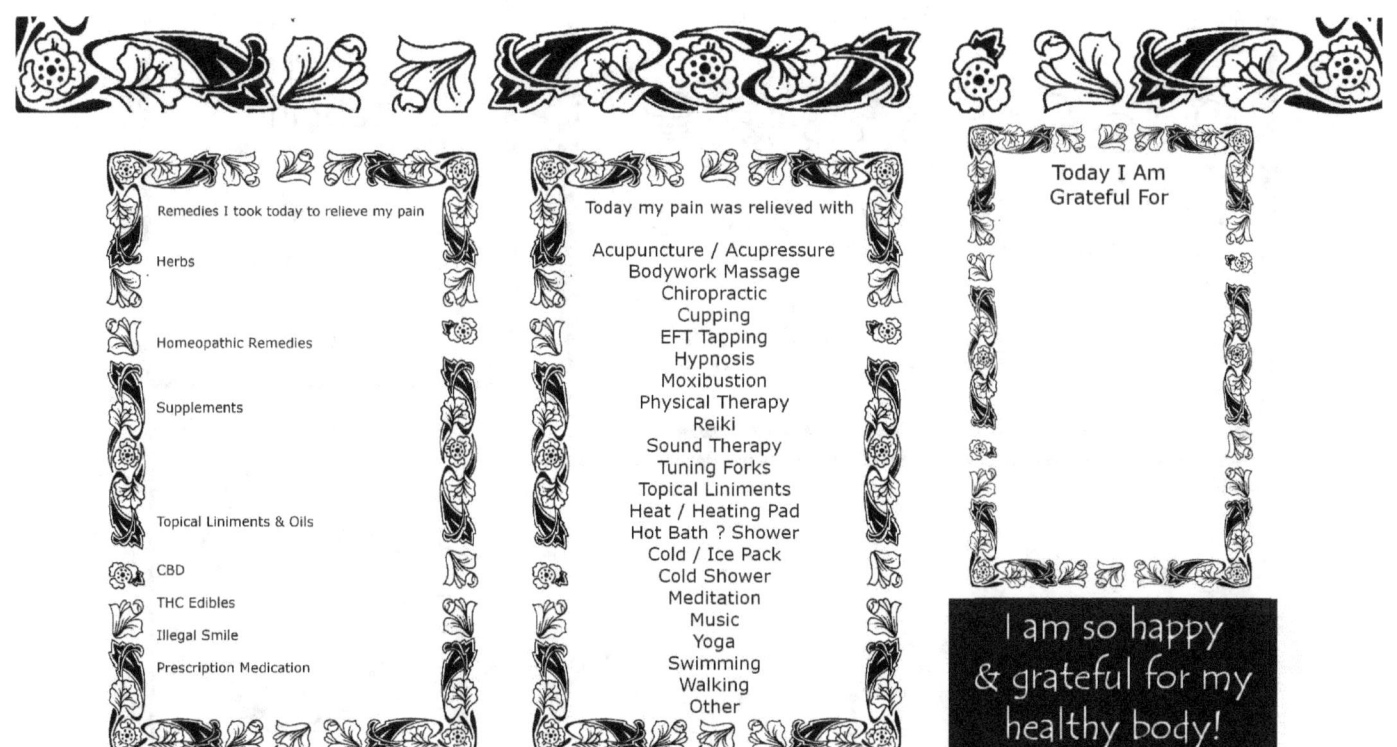

Remedies I took today to relieve my pain

Herbs

Homeopathic Remedies

Supplements

Topical Liniments & Oils

CBD
THC Edibles
Illegal Smile
Prescription Medication

Today my pain was relieved with

Acupuncture / Acupressure
Bodywork Massage
Chiropractic
Cupping
EFT Tapping
Hypnosis
Moxibustion
Physical Therapy
Reiki
Sound Therapy
Tuning Forks
Topical Liniments
Heat / Heating Pad
Hot Bath ? Shower
Cold / Ice Pack
Cold Shower
Meditation
Music
Yoga
Swimming
Walking
Other

Today I Am
Grateful For

I am so happy
& grateful for my
healthy body!

Today's Day & Date

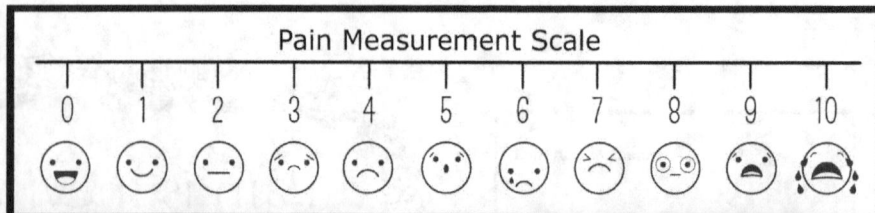

Highlight All Painful Areas

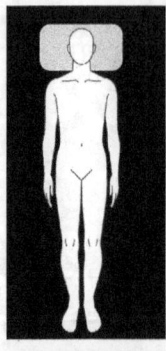 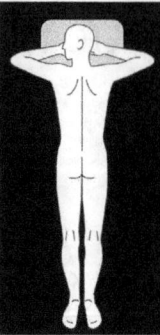 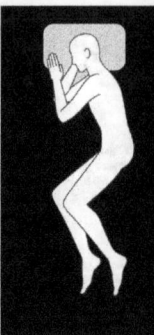 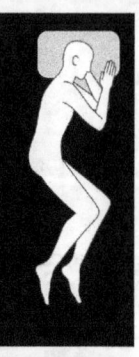

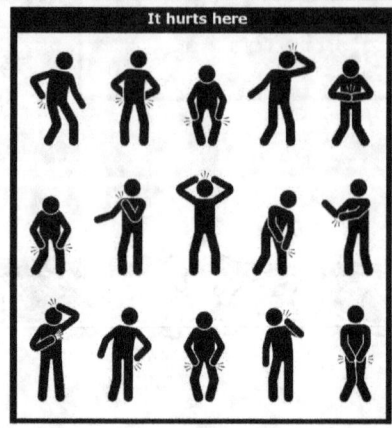
It hurts here

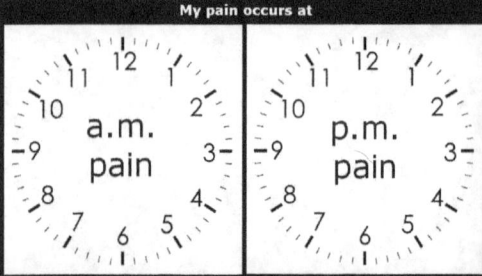

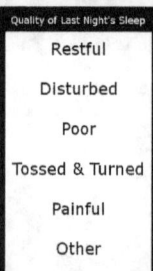

Quality of Last Night's Sleep
- Restful
- Disturbed
- Poor
- Tossed & Turned
- Painful
- Other

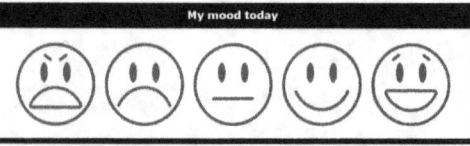
My mood today

My pain is
Hot
Burning
Cold
Stabbing
Throbbing
Fixed
Moving Traveling
Constant
On & Off

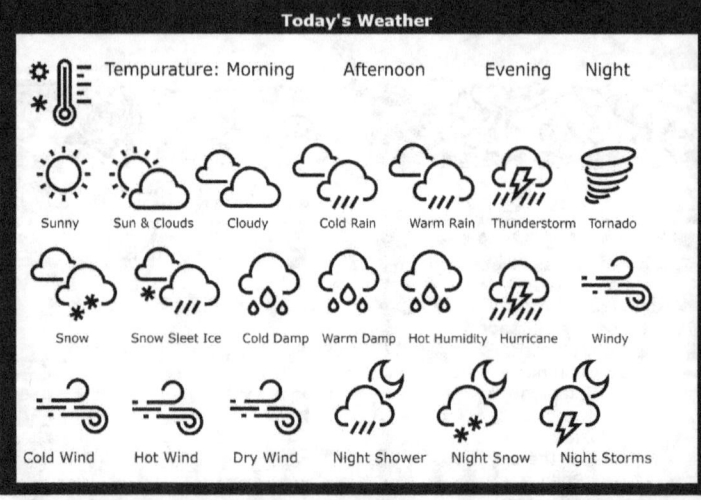

Breakfast

Lunch

Dinner

Snacks

Alcohol

Food Allergy Triggers

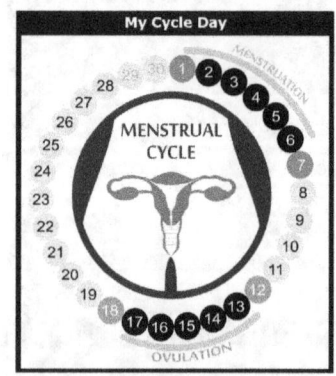
My Cycle Day

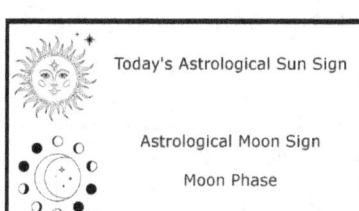

Today's Astrological Sun Sign

Astrological Moon Sign

Moon Phase

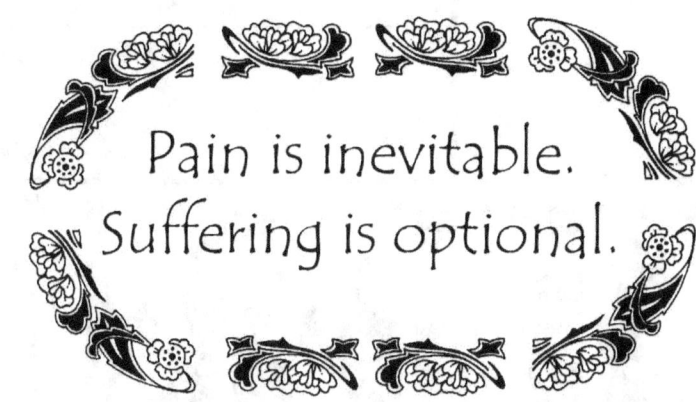

Pain is inevitable.
Suffering is optional.

Notes

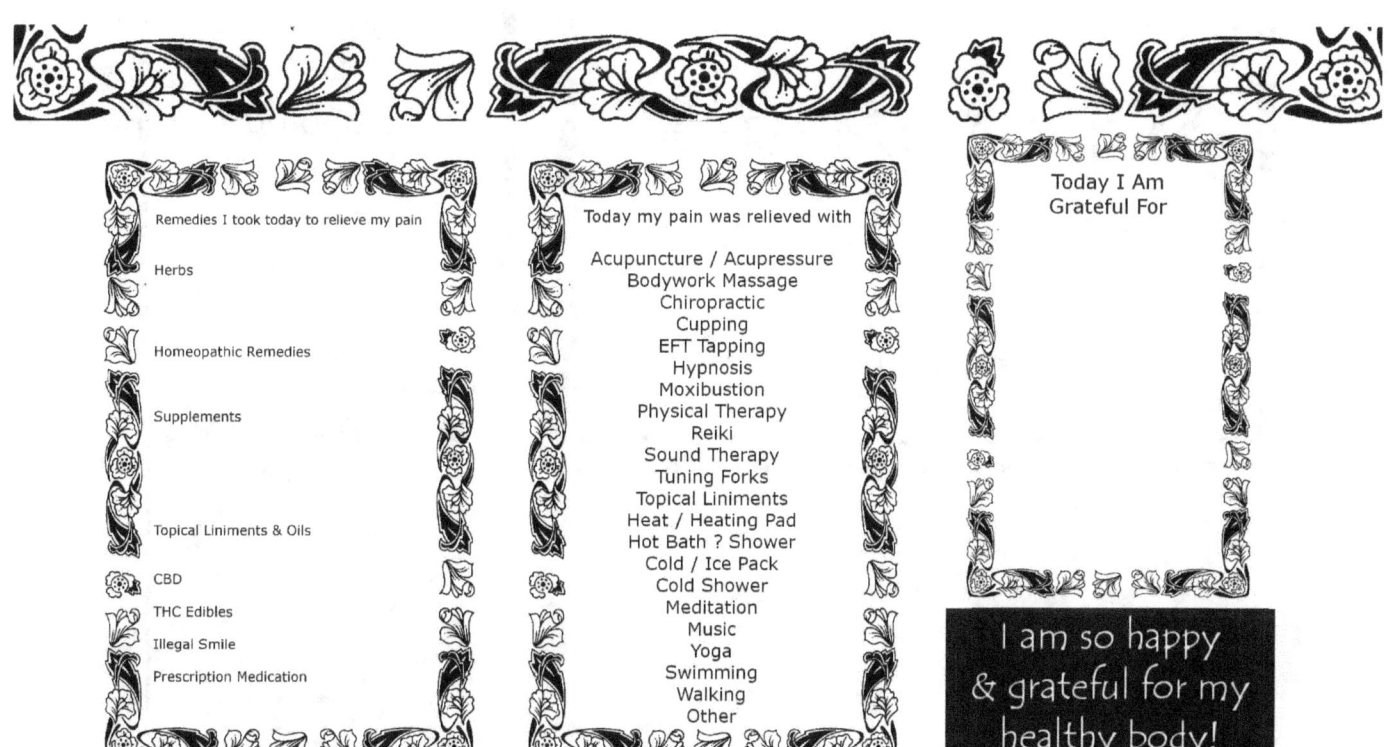

Remedies I took today to relieve my pain

Herbs

Homeopathic Remedies

Supplements

Topical Liniments & Oils

CBD

THC Edibles

Illegal Smile

Prescription Medication

Today my pain was relieved with

Acupuncture / Acupressure
Bodywork Massage
Chiropractic
Cupping
EFT Tapping
Hypnosis
Moxibustion
Physical Therapy
Reiki
Sound Therapy
Tuning Forks
Topical Liniments
Heat / Heating Pad
Hot Bath ? Shower
Cold / Ice Pack
Cold Shower
Meditation
Music
Yoga
Swimming
Walking
Other

Today I Am Grateful For

I am so happy & grateful for my healthy body!

Today's Day & Date

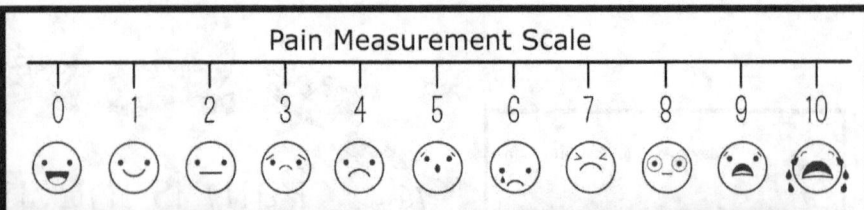
Pain Measurement Scale
0 1 2 3 4 5 6 7 8 9 10

Highlight All Painful Areas

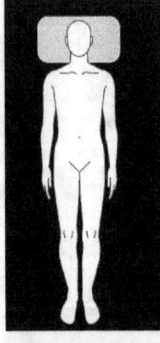 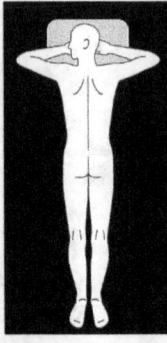 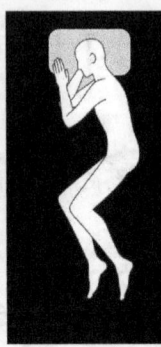 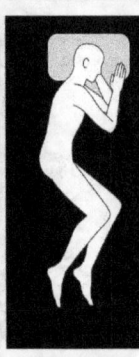

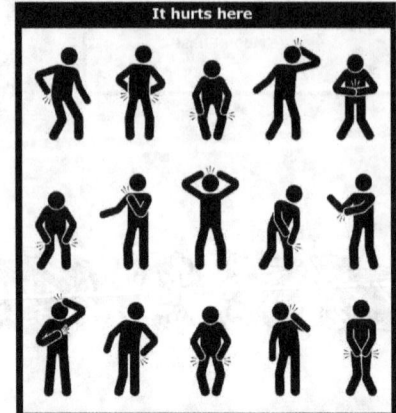
It hurts here

My pain occurs at

a.m. pain | p.m. pain

Quality of Last Night's Sleep
- Restful
- Disturbed
- Poor
- Tossed & Turned
- Painful
- Other

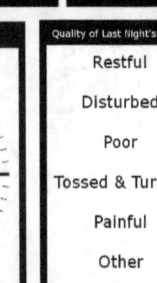

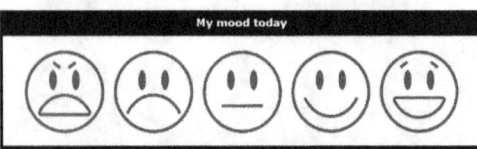
My mood today

My pain is
Hot
Burning
Cold
Stabbing
Throbbing
Fixed
Moving Traveling
Constant
On & Off

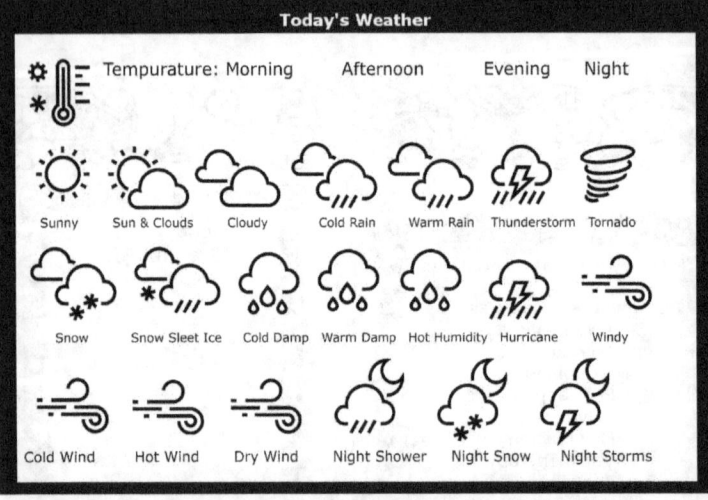
Today's Weather — Temperature: Morning, Afternoon, Evening, Night
Sunny, Sun & Clouds, Cloudy, Cold Rain, Warm Rain, Thunderstorm, Tornado
Snow, Snow Sleet Ice, Cold Damp, Warm Damp, Hot Humidity, Hurricane, Windy
Cold Wind, Hot Wind, Dry Wind, Night Shower, Night Snow, Night Storms

Breakfast

Lunch

Dinner

Snacks

Alcohol

Food Allergy Triggers

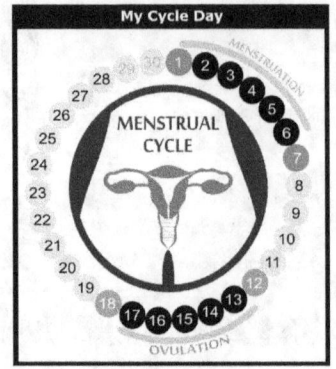
My Cycle Day

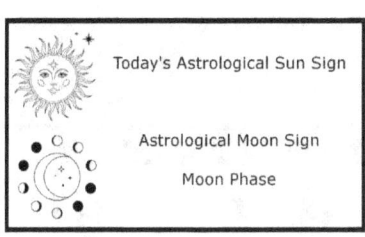

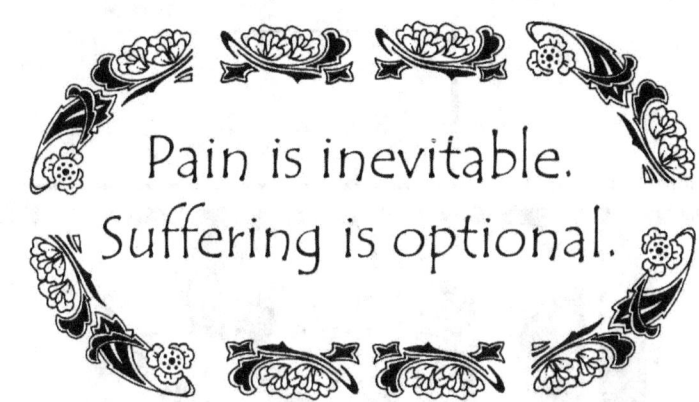

Notes

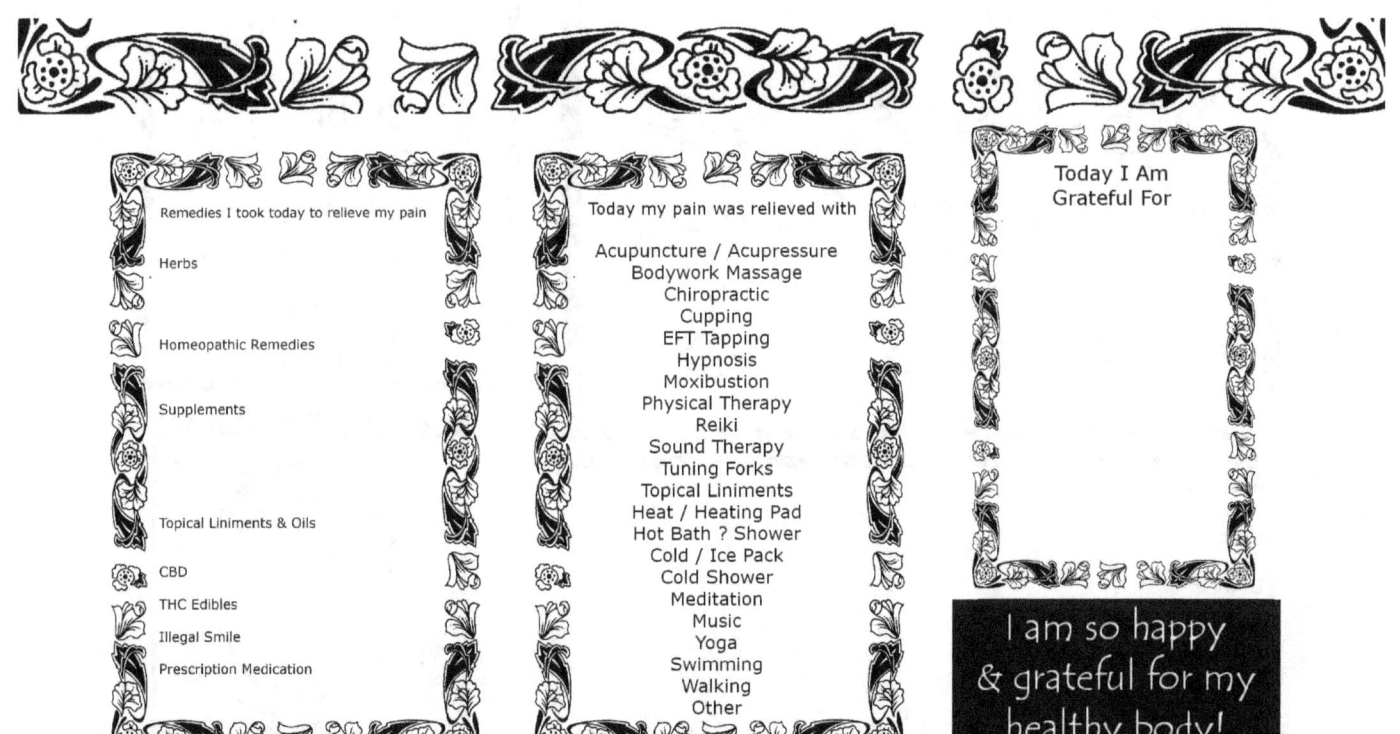

I am so happy & grateful for my healthy body!

Today's Day & Date

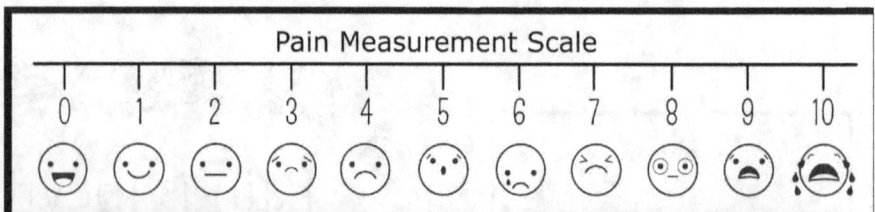

Highlight All Painful Areas

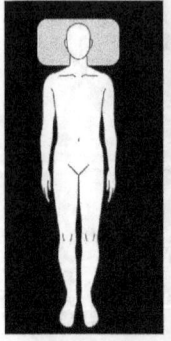 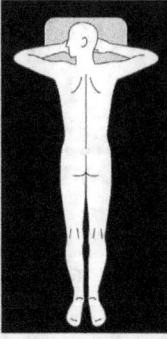 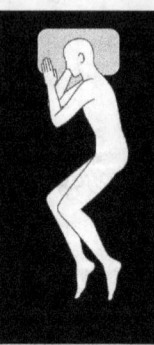 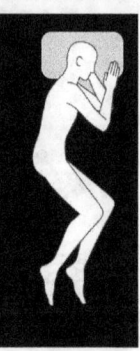

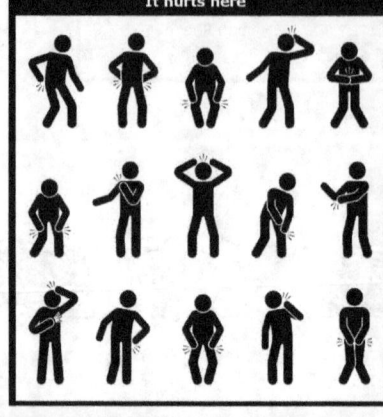

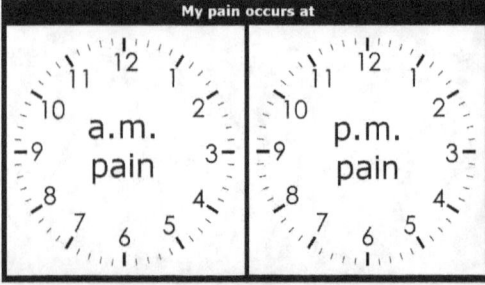

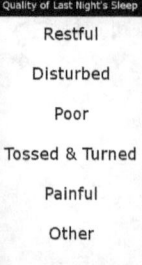

Quality of Last Night's Sleep
- Restful
- Disturbed
- Poor
- Tossed & Turned
- Painful
- Other

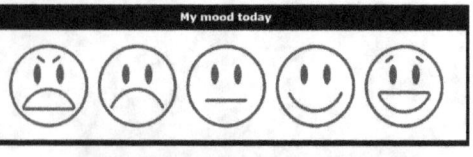

My pain is
Hot
Burning
Cold
Stabbing
Throbbing
Fixed
Moving Traveling
Constant
On & Off

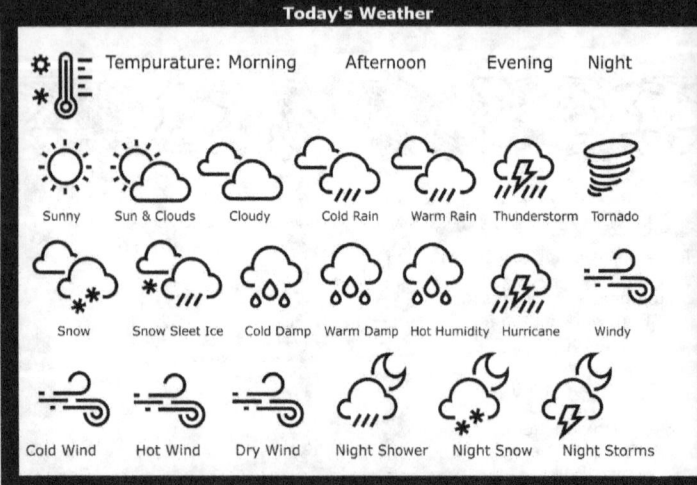

Breakfast

Lunch

Dinner

Snacks

Alcohol

Food Allergy Triggers

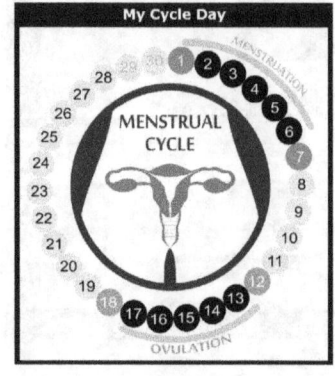

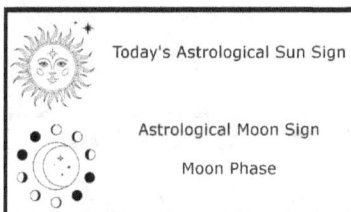

Today's Astrological Sun Sign

Astrological Moon Sign

Moon Phase

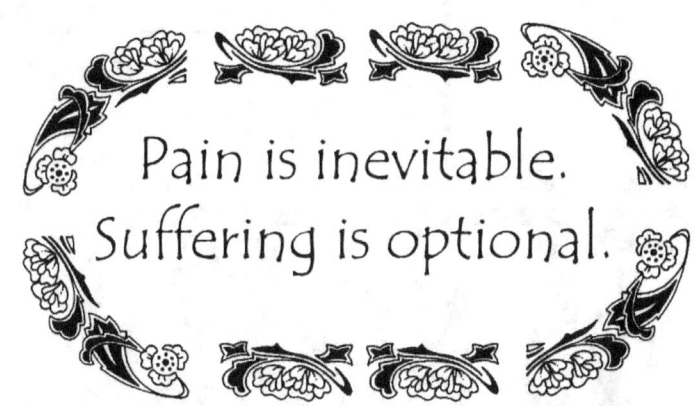

Pain is inevitable.
Suffering is optional.

Notes

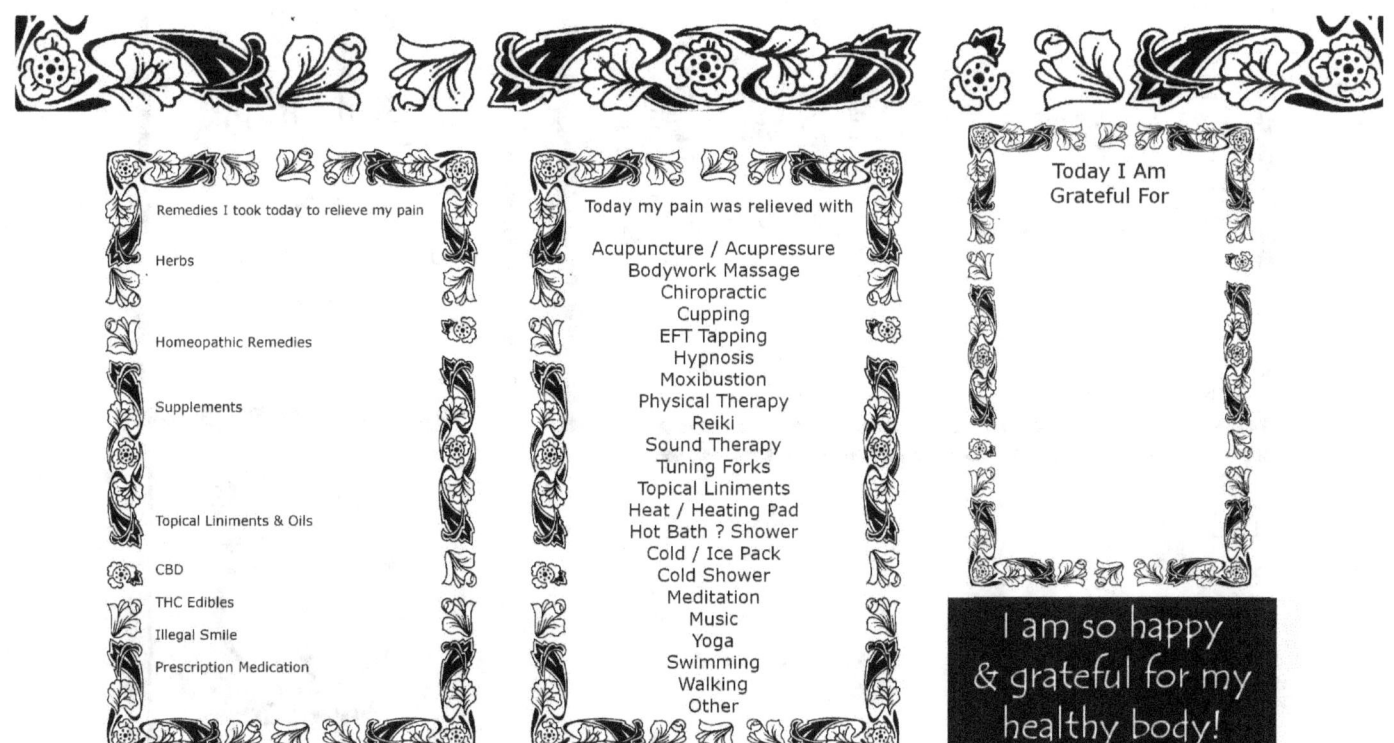

Remedies I took today to relieve my pain

Herbs

Homeopathic Remedies

Supplements

Topical Liniments & Oils

CBD

THC Edibles

Illegal Smile

Prescription Medication

Today my pain was relieved with

Acupuncture / Acupressure
Bodywork Massage
Chiropractic
Cupping
EFT Tapping
Hypnosis
Moxibustion
Physical Therapy
Reiki
Sound Therapy
Tuning Forks
Topical Liniments
Heat / Heating Pad
Hot Bath ? Shower
Cold / Ice Pack
Cold Shower
Meditation
Music
Yoga
Swimming
Walking
Other

Today I Am Grateful For

I am so happy & grateful for my healthy body!

Today's Day & Date

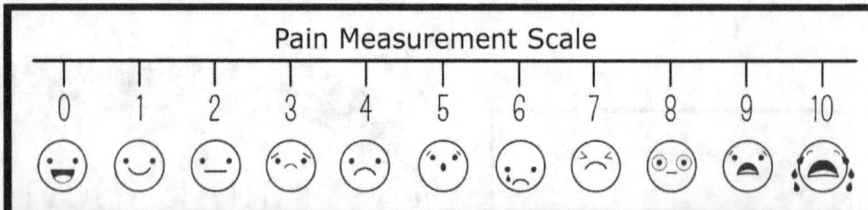

Highlight All Painful Areas

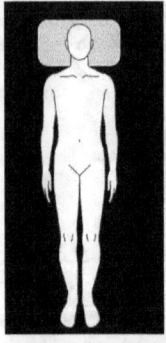
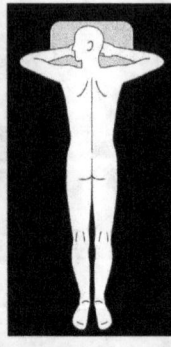
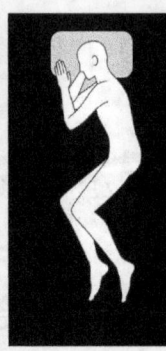
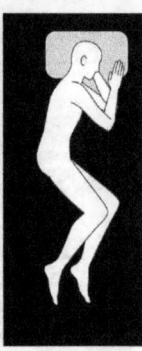

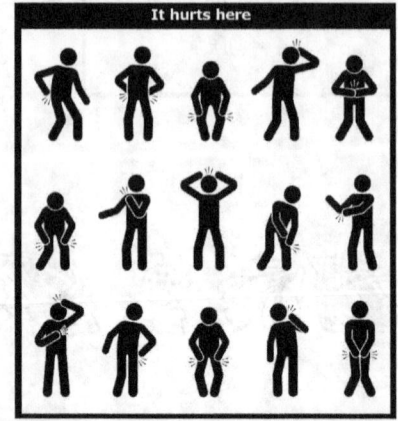

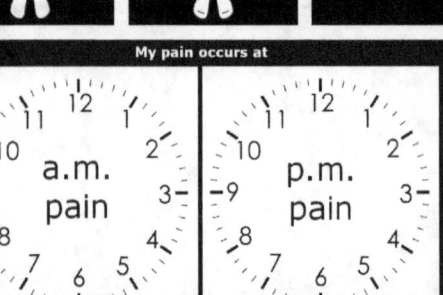

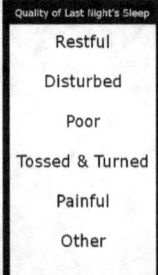

Quality of Last Night's Sleep
- Restful
- Disturbed
- Poor
- Tossed & Turned
- Painful
- Other

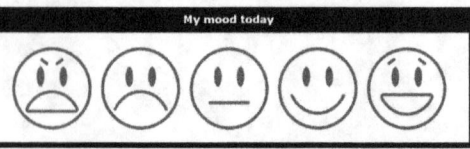

My pain is
Hot
Burning
Cold
Stabbing
Throbbing
Fixed
Moving Traveling
Constant
On & Off

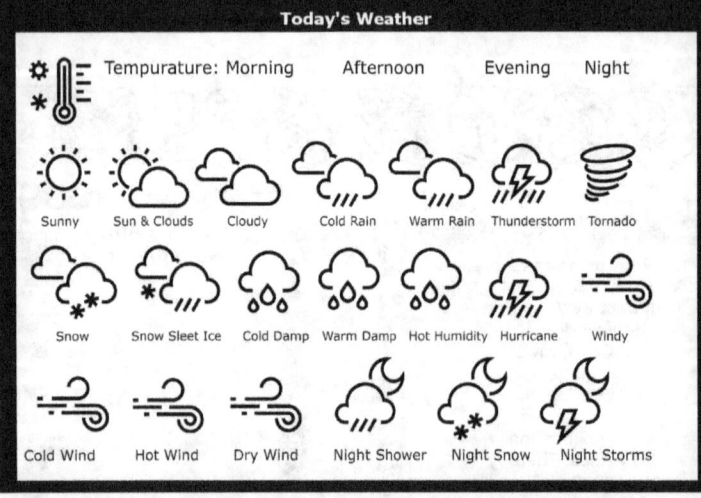

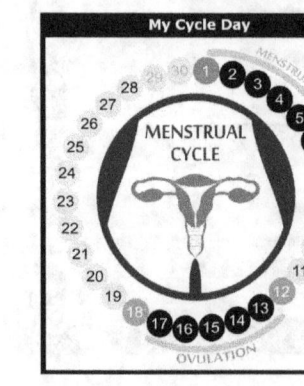

Breakfast

Lunch

Dinner

Snacks

Alcohol

Food Allergy Triggers

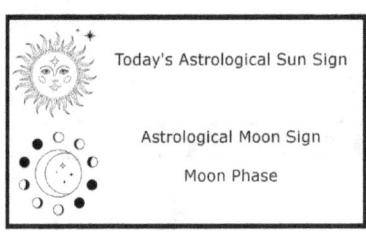

Today's Astrological Sun Sign

Astrological Moon Sign

Moon Phase

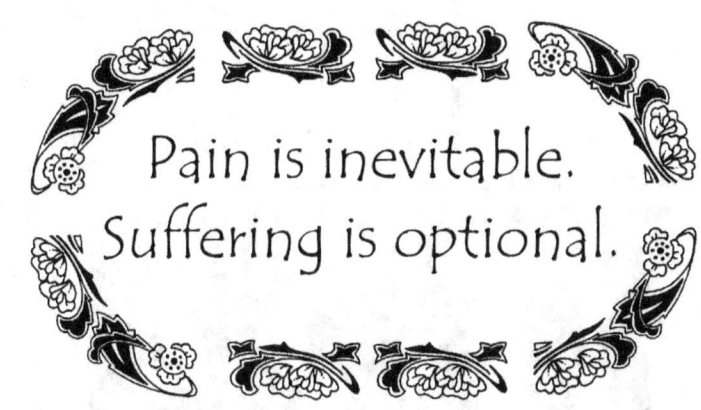

Pain is inevitable.
Suffering is optional.

Notes

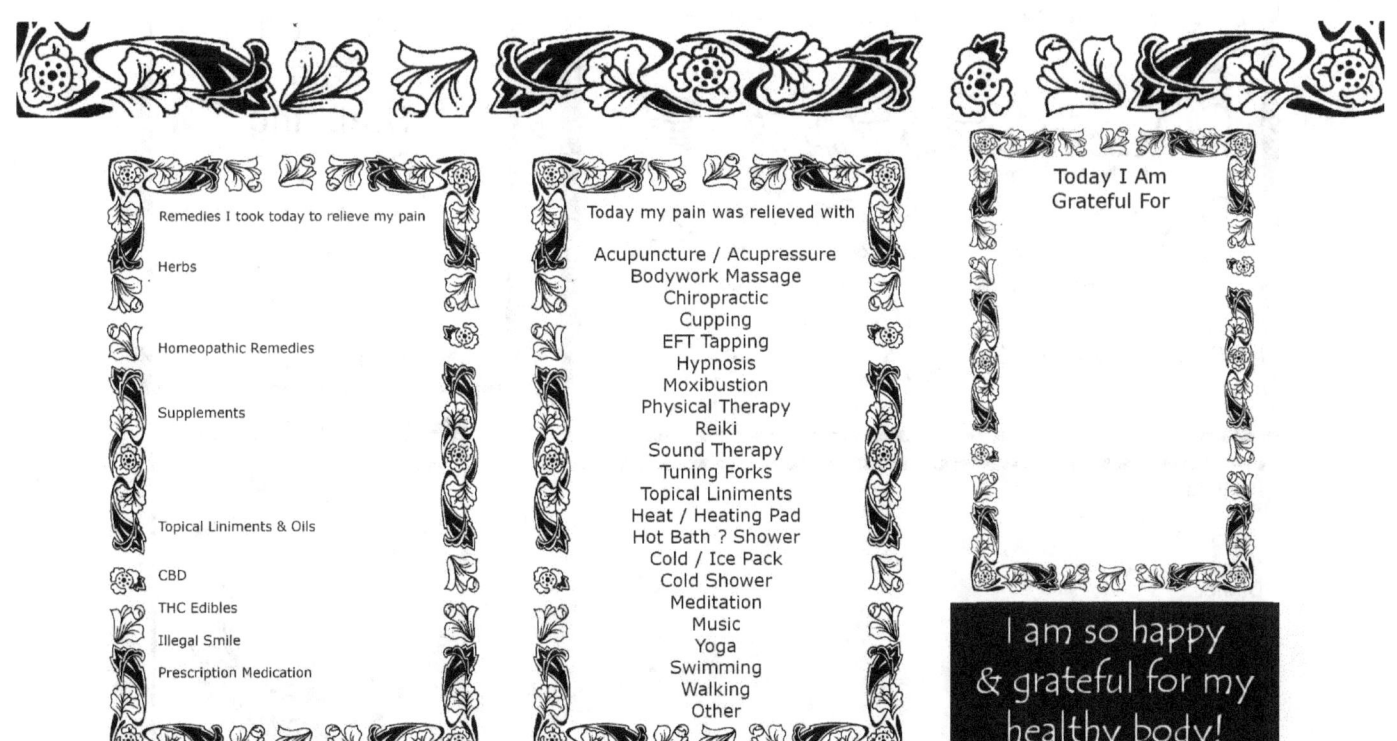

Remedies I took today to relieve my pain

Herbs

Homeopathic Remedies

Supplements

Topical Liniments & Oils

CBD

THC Edibles

Illegal Smile

Prescription Medication

Today my pain was relieved with

Acupuncture / Acupressure
Bodywork Massage
Chiropractic
Cupping
EFT Tapping
Hypnosis
Moxibustion
Physical Therapy
Reiki
Sound Therapy
Tuning Forks
Topical Liniments
Heat / Heating Pad
Hot Bath ? Shower
Cold / Ice Pack
Cold Shower
Meditation
Music
Yoga
Swimming
Walking
Other

Today I Am Grateful For

I am so happy & grateful for my healthy body!

Today's Day & Date

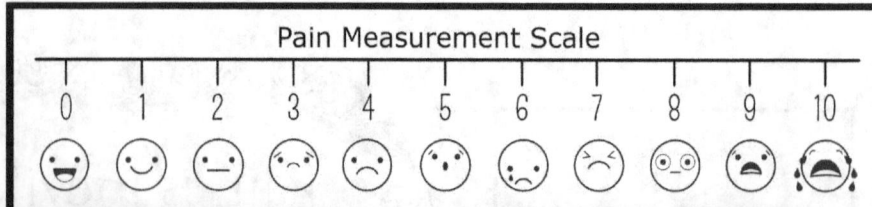

Highlight All Painful Areas

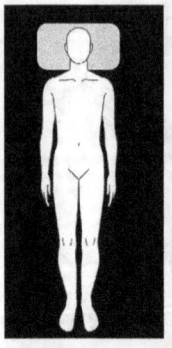 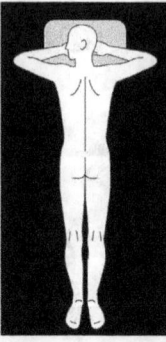 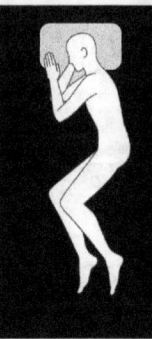 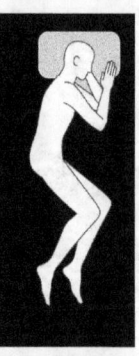

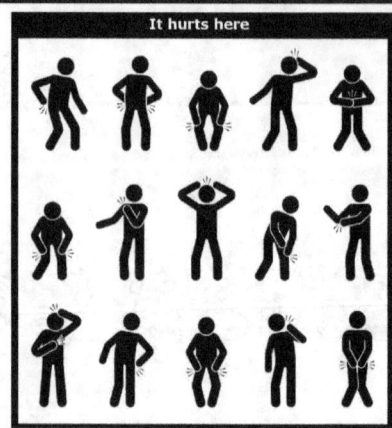
It hurts here

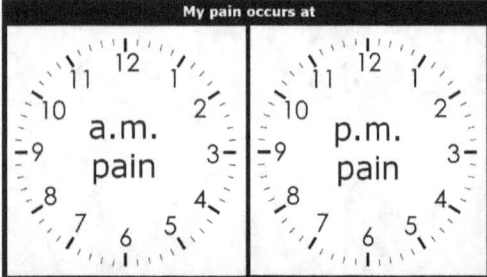
My pain occurs at — a.m. pain / p.m. pain

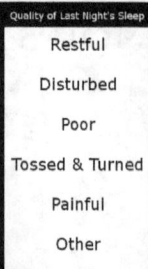
Quality of Last Night's Sleep
- Restful
- Disturbed
- Poor
- Tossed & Turned
- Painful
- Other

My mood today

My pain is

Hot
Burning
Cold
Stabbing
Throbbing
Fixed
Moving Traveling
Constant
On & Off

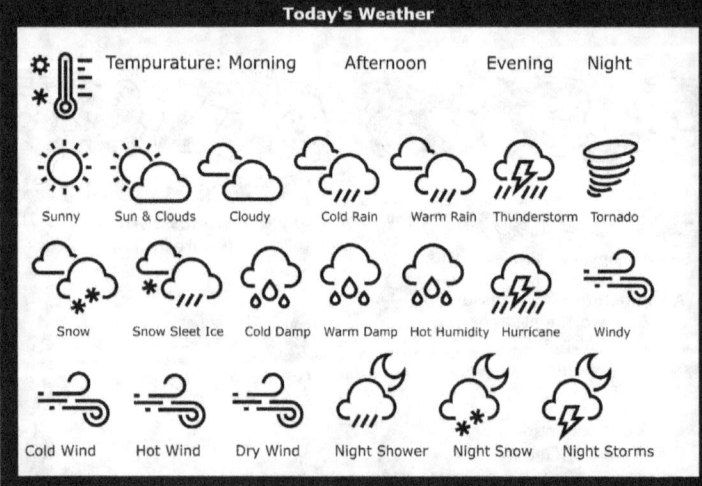
Today's Weather — Temperature: Morning, Afternoon, Evening, Night

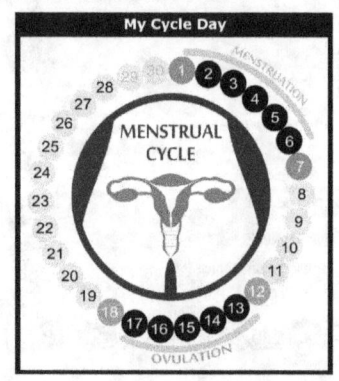
My Cycle Day

Breakfast

Lunch

Dinner

Snacks

Alcohol

Food Allergy Triggers

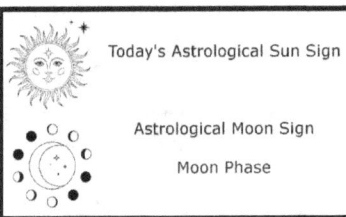

Today's Astrological Sun Sign

Astrological Moon Sign
Moon Phase

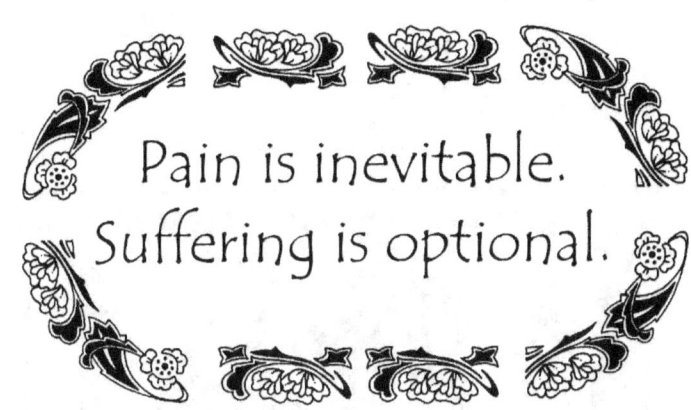

Pain is inevitable.
Suffering is optional.

Notes

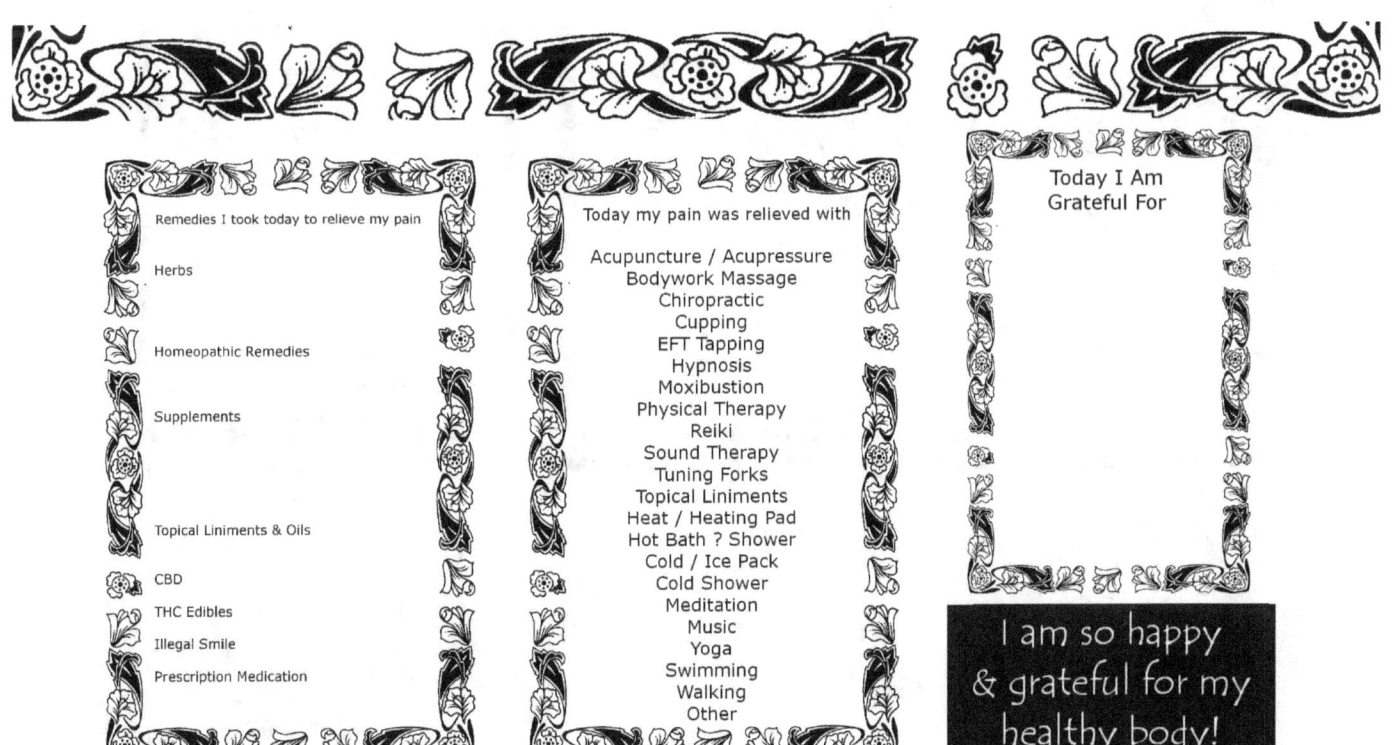

Remedies I took today to relieve my pain

Herbs

Homeopathic Remedies

Supplements

Topical Liniments & Oils

CBD
THC Edibles
Illegal Smile
Prescription Medication

Today my pain was relieved with

Acupuncture / Acupressure
Bodywork Massage
Chiropractic
Cupping
EFT Tapping
Hypnosis
Moxibustion
Physical Therapy
Reiki
Sound Therapy
Tuning Forks
Topical Liniments
Heat / Heating Pad
Hot Bath ? Shower
Cold / Ice Pack
Cold Shower
Meditation
Music
Yoga
Swimming
Walking
Other

Today I Am Grateful For

I am so happy & grateful for my healthy body!

Today's Day & Date

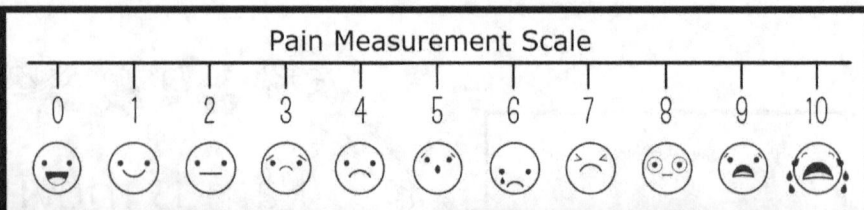
Pain Measurement Scale
0 1 2 3 4 5 6 7 8 9 10

Highlight All Painful Areas

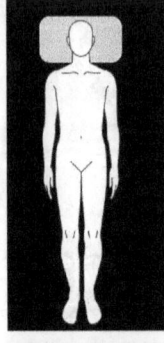 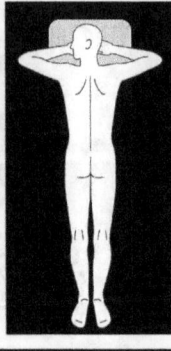 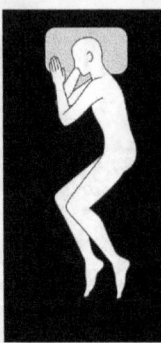 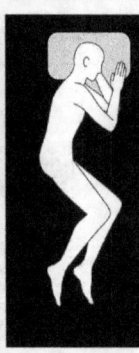

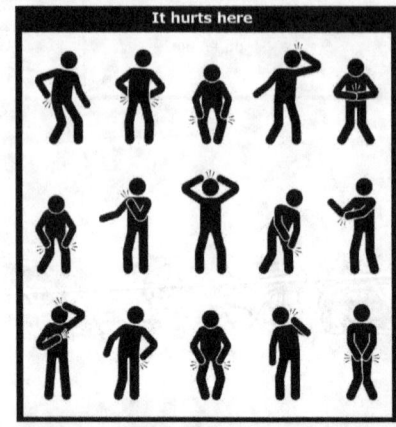
It hurts here

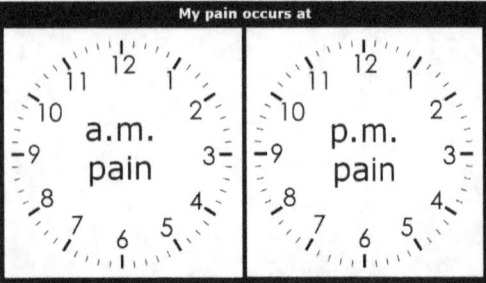
My pain occurs at — a.m. pain / p.m. pain

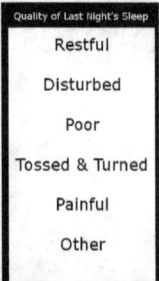

Quality of Last Night's Sleep
- Restful
- Disturbed
- Poor
- Tossed & Turned
- Painful
- Other

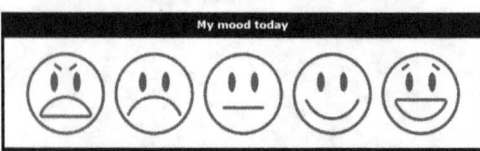
My mood today

My pain is
Hot
Burning
Cold
Stabbing
Throbbing
Fixed
Moving Traveling
Constant
On & Off

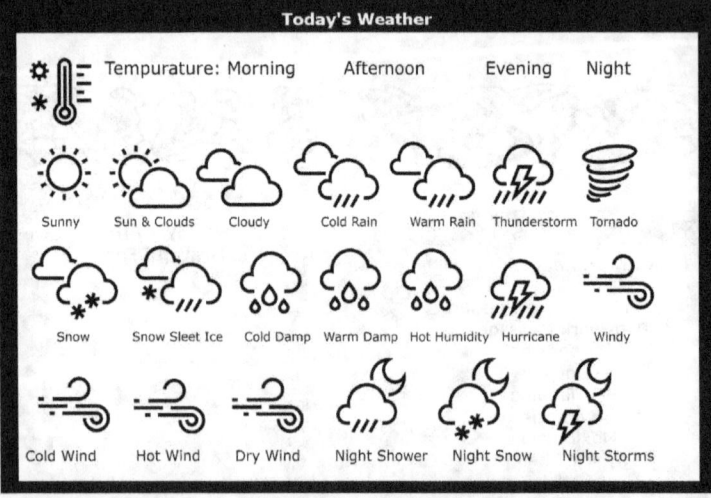
Today's Weather — Temperature: Morning, Afternoon, Evening, Night
Sunny, Sun & Clouds, Cloudy, Cold Rain, Warm Rain, Thunderstorm, Tornado
Snow, Snow Sleet Ice, Cold Damp, Warm Damp, Hot Humidity, Hurricane, Windy
Cold Wind, Hot Wind, Dry Wind, Night Shower, Night Snow, Night Storms

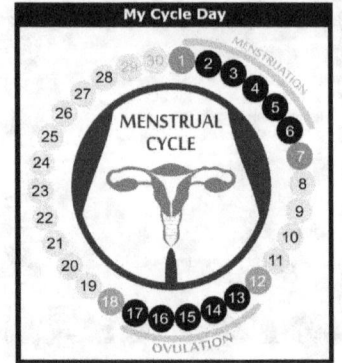
My Cycle Day

Breakfast

Lunch

Dinner

Snacks

Alcohol

Food Allergy Triggers

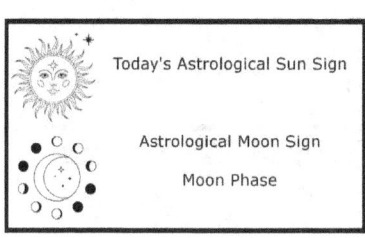

Today's Astrological Sun Sign

Astrological Moon Sign

Moon Phase

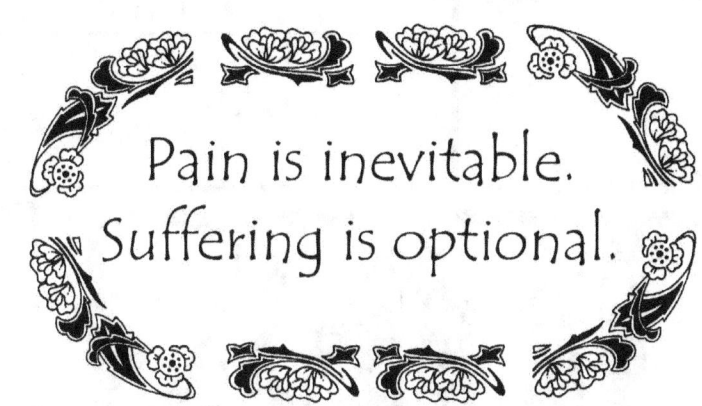

Pain is inevitable.
Suffering is optional.

Notes

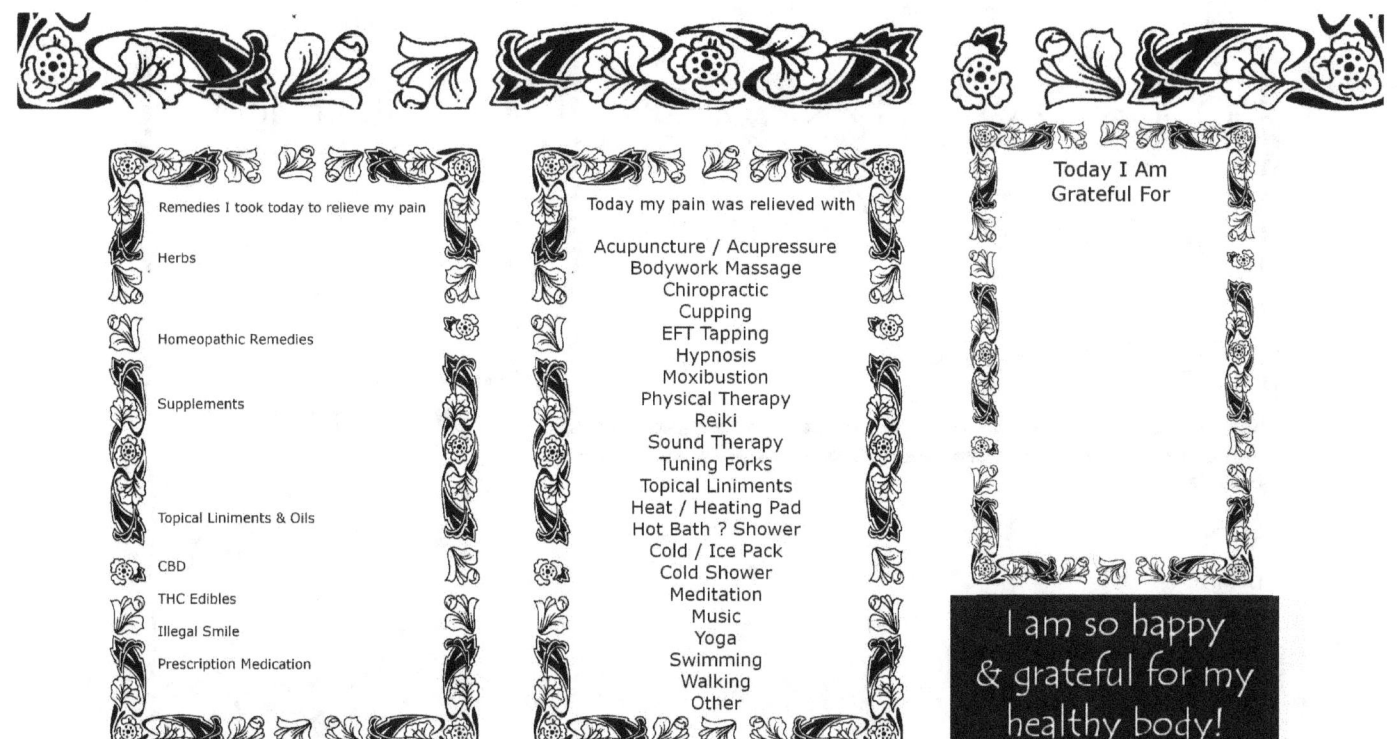

Remedies I took today to relieve my pain

Herbs

Homeopathic Remedies

Supplements

Topical Liniments & Oils

CBD

THC Edibles

Illegal Smile

Prescription Medication

Today my pain was relieved with

Acupuncture / Acupressure
Bodywork Massage
Chiropractic
Cupping
EFT Tapping
Hypnosis
Moxibustion
Physical Therapy
Reiki
Sound Therapy
Tuning Forks
Topical Liniments
Heat / Heating Pad
Hot Bath ? Shower
Cold / Ice Pack
Cold Shower
Meditation
Music
Yoga
Swimming
Walking
Other

Today I Am Grateful For

I am so happy & grateful for my healthy body!

Today's Day & Date

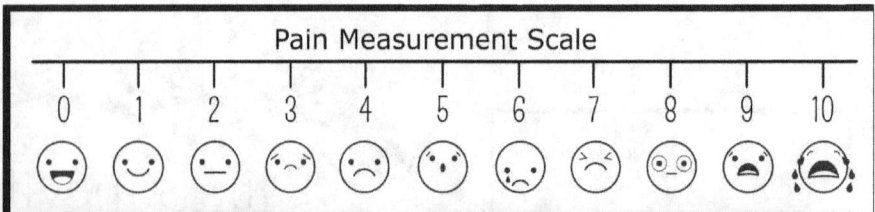

Highlight All Painful Areas

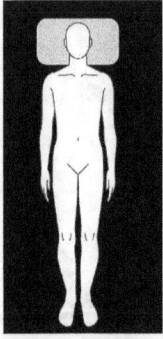
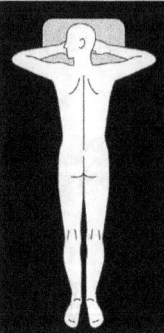
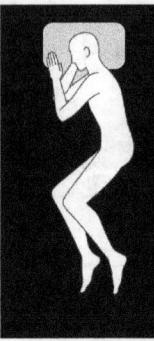
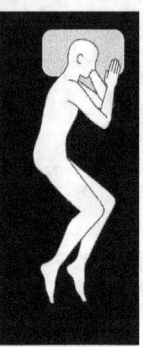

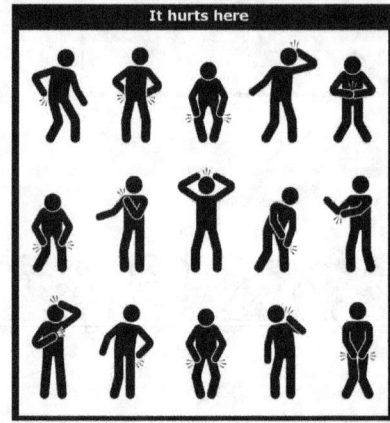
It hurts here

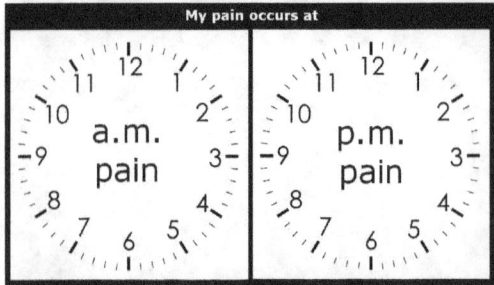
My pain occurs at — a.m. pain / p.m. pain

Quality of Last Night's Sleep
- Restful
- Disturbed
- Poor
- Tossed & Turned
- Painful
- Other

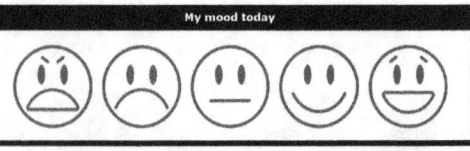
My mood today

My pain is
Hot
Burning
Cold
Stabbing
Throbbing
Fixed
Moving Traveling
Constant
On & Off

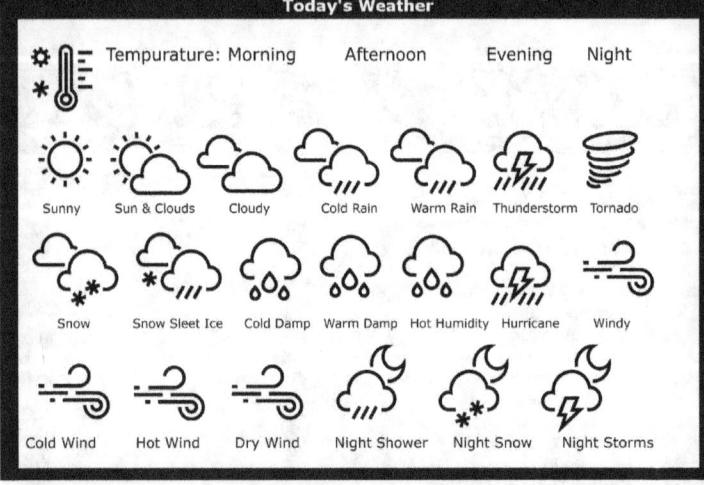
Today's Weather — Temperature: Morning, Afternoon, Evening, Night

Breakfast

Lunch

Dinner

Snacks

Alcohol

Food Allergy Triggers

My Cycle Day

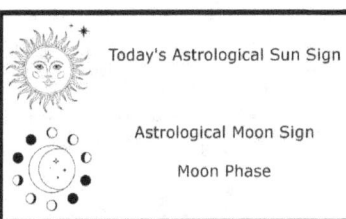

Today's Astrological Sun Sign

Astrological Moon Sign

Moon Phase

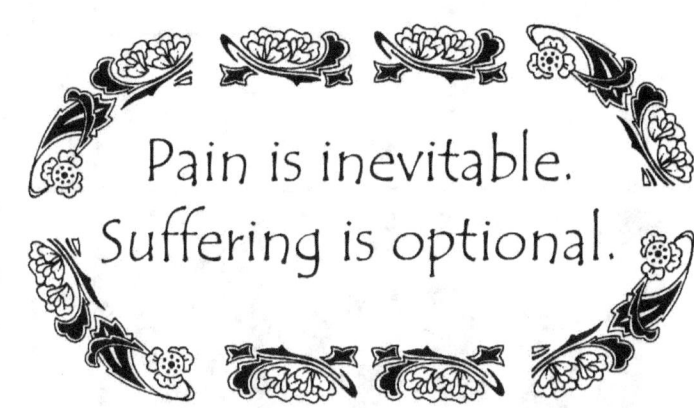

Pain is inevitable. Suffering is optional.

Notes

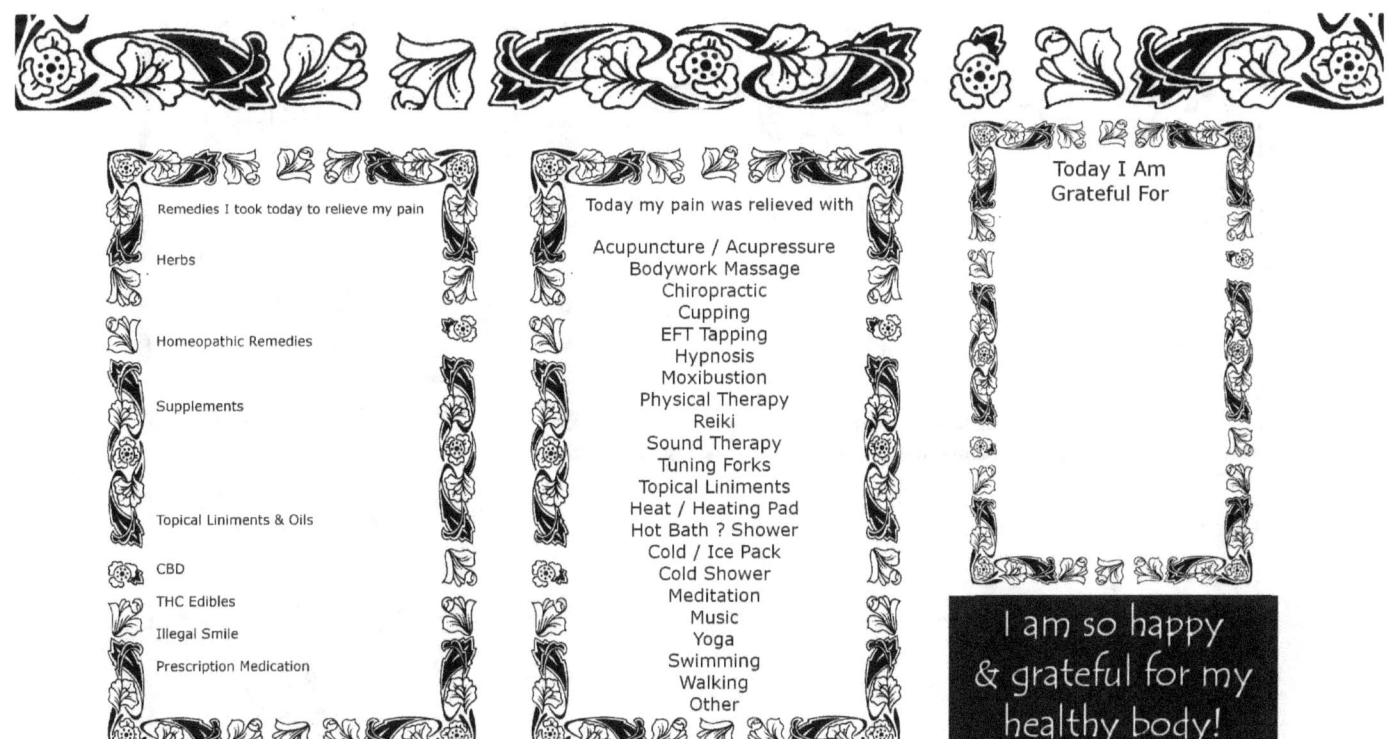

Remedies I took today to relieve my pain

Herbs

Homeopathic Remedies

Supplements

Topical Liniments & Oils

CBD

THC Edibles

Illegal Smile

Prescription Medication

Today my pain was relieved with

Acupuncture / Acupressure
Bodywork Massage
Chiropractic
Cupping
EFT Tapping
Hypnosis
Moxibustion
Physical Therapy
Reiki
Sound Therapy
Tuning Forks
Topical Liniments
Heat / Heating Pad
Hot Bath ? Shower
Cold / Ice Pack
Cold Shower
Meditation
Music
Yoga
Swimming
Walking
Other

Today I Am Grateful For

I am so happy & grateful for my healthy body!

Today's Day & Date

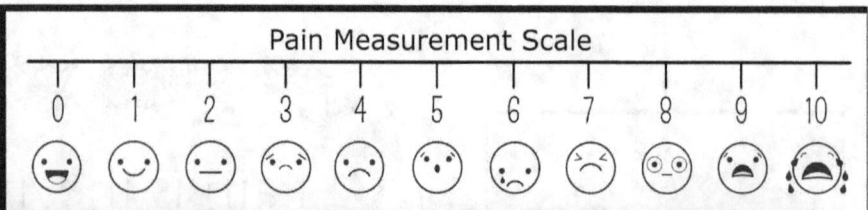

Highlight All Painful Areas

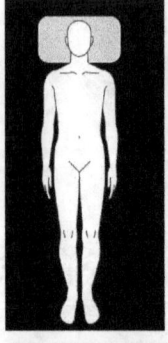 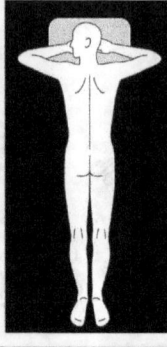 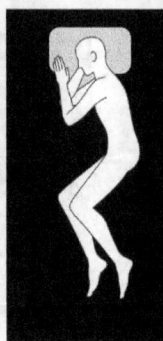 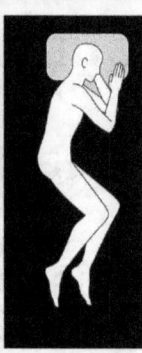

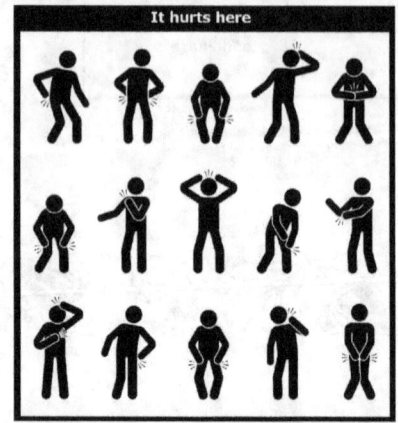

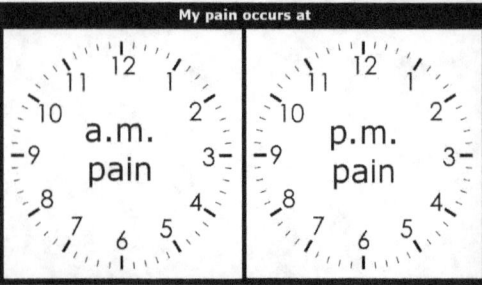

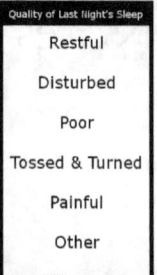

Quality of Last Night's Sleep
- Restful
- Disturbed
- Poor
- Tossed & Turned
- Painful
- Other

My pain is

Hot
Burning
Cold
Stabbing
Throbbing
Fixed
Moving Traveling
Constant
On & Off

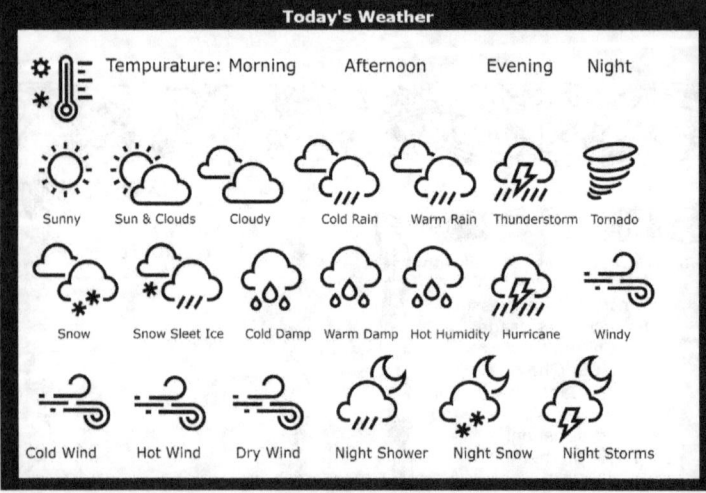

Breakfast

Lunch

Dinner

Snacks

Alcohol

Food Allergy Triggers

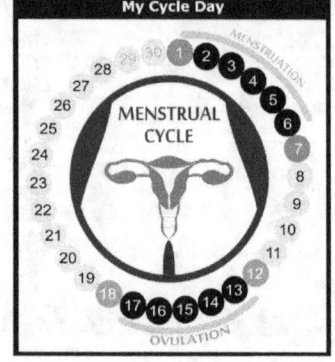

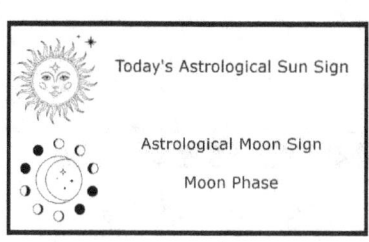

Today's Astrological Sun Sign

Astrological Moon Sign

Moon Phase

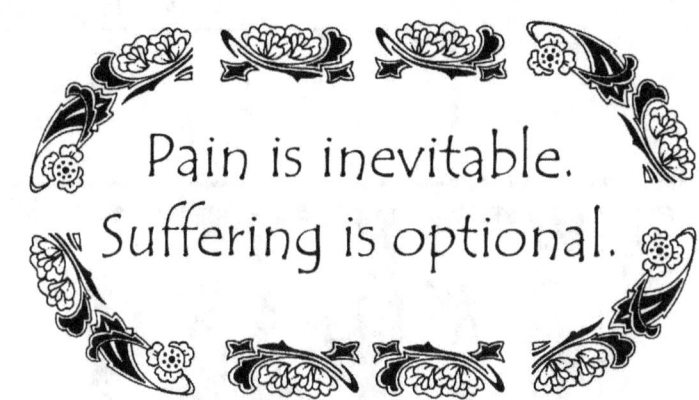

Pain is inevitable. Suffering is optional.

Notes

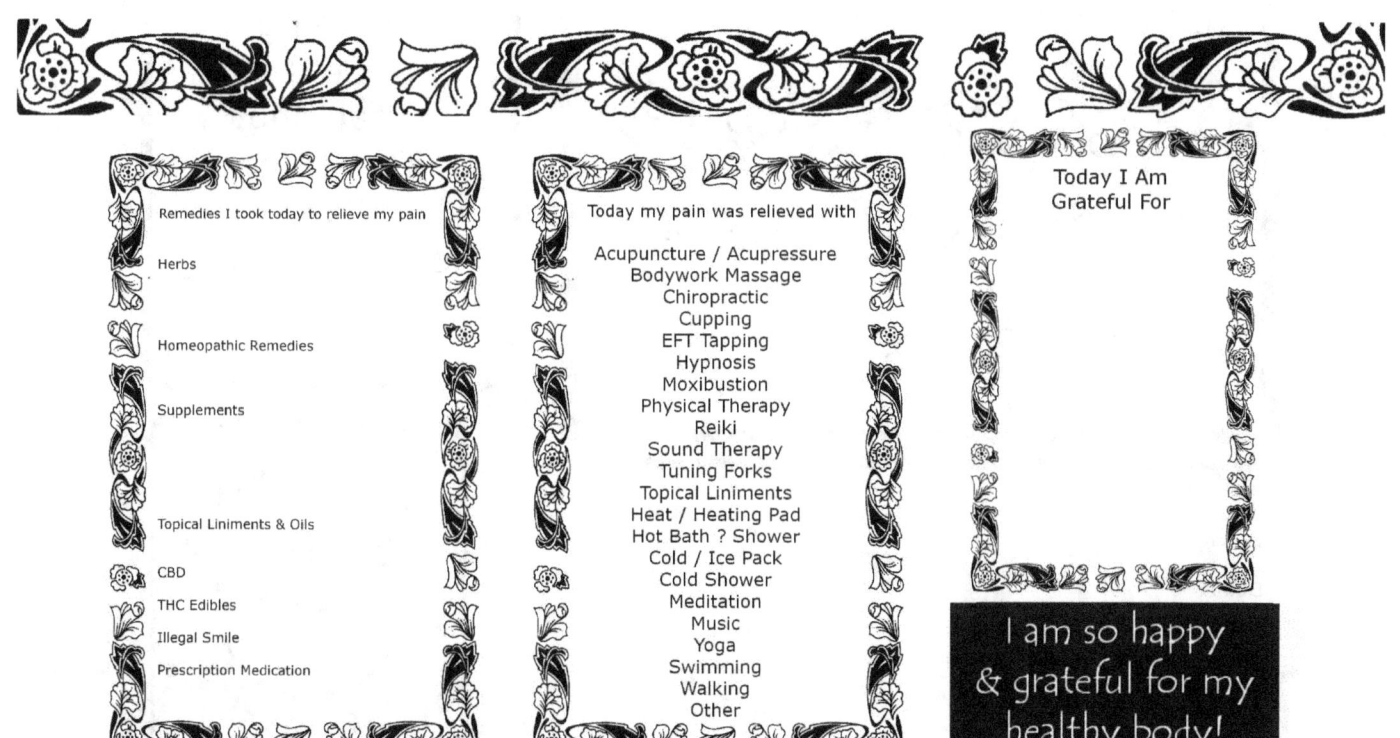

Remedies I took today to relieve my pain

Herbs

Homeopathic Remedies

Supplements

Topical Liniments & Oils

CBD

THC Edibles

Illegal Smile

Prescription Medication

Today my pain was relieved with

Acupuncture / Acupressure
Bodywork Massage
Chiropractic
Cupping
EFT Tapping
Hypnosis
Moxibustion
Physical Therapy
Reiki
Sound Therapy
Tuning Forks
Topical Liniments
Heat / Heating Pad
Hot Bath ? Shower
Cold / Ice Pack
Cold Shower
Meditation
Music
Yoga
Swimming
Walking
Other

Today I Am Grateful For

I am so happy & grateful for my healthy body!

Today's Day & Date

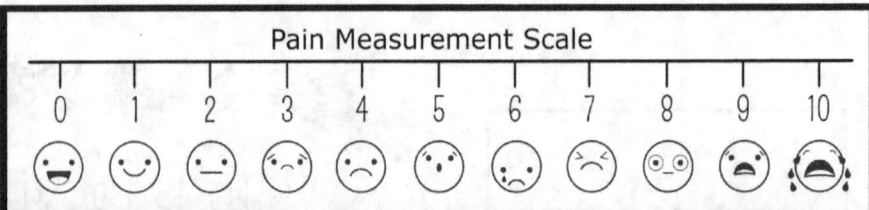

Highlight All Painful Areas

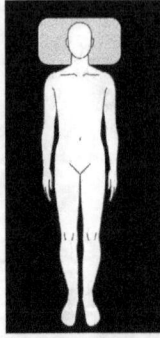 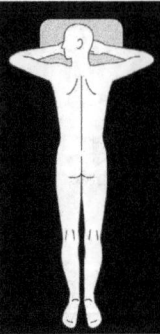 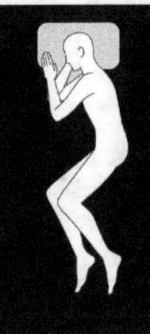 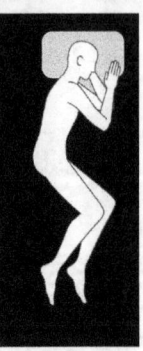

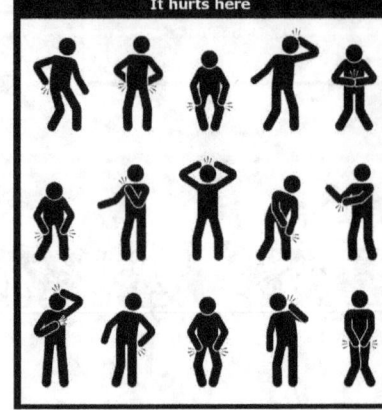

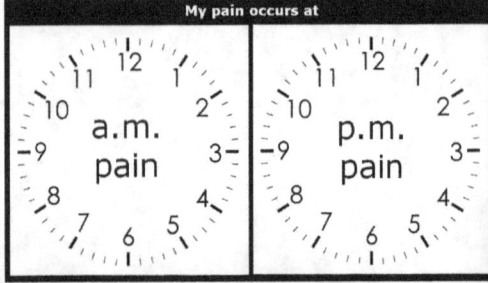

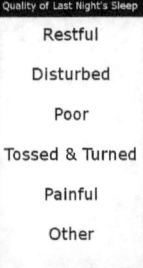

Quality of Last Night's Sleep
- Restful
- Disturbed
- Poor
- Tossed & Turned
- Painful
- Other

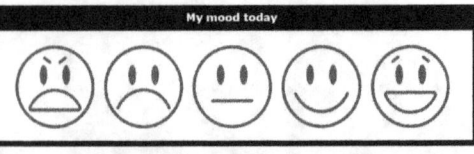

My pain is
Hot
Burning
Cold
Stabbing
Throbbing
Fixed
Moving Traveling
Constant
On & Off

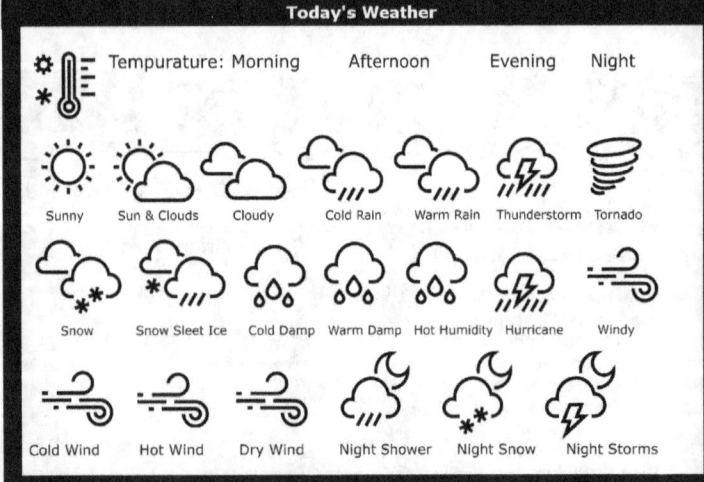

Breakfast

Lunch

Dinner

Snacks

Alcohol

Food Allergy Triggers

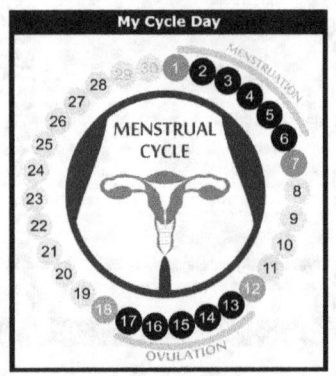

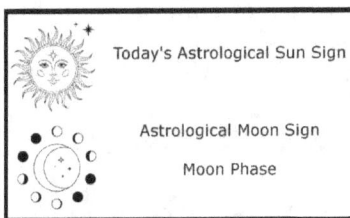

Today's Astrological Sun Sign

Astrological Moon Sign
Moon Phase

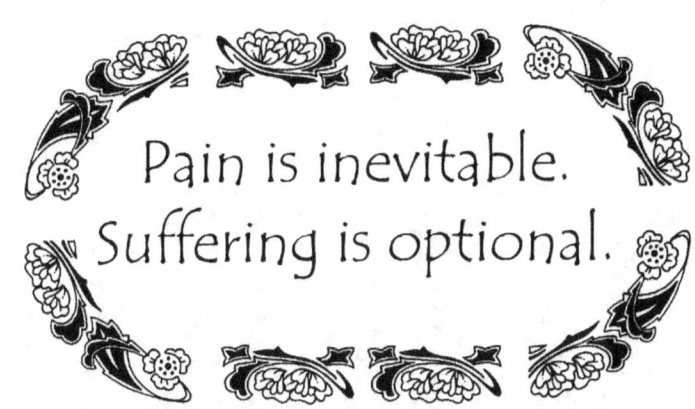

Pain is inevitable.
Suffering is optional.

Notes

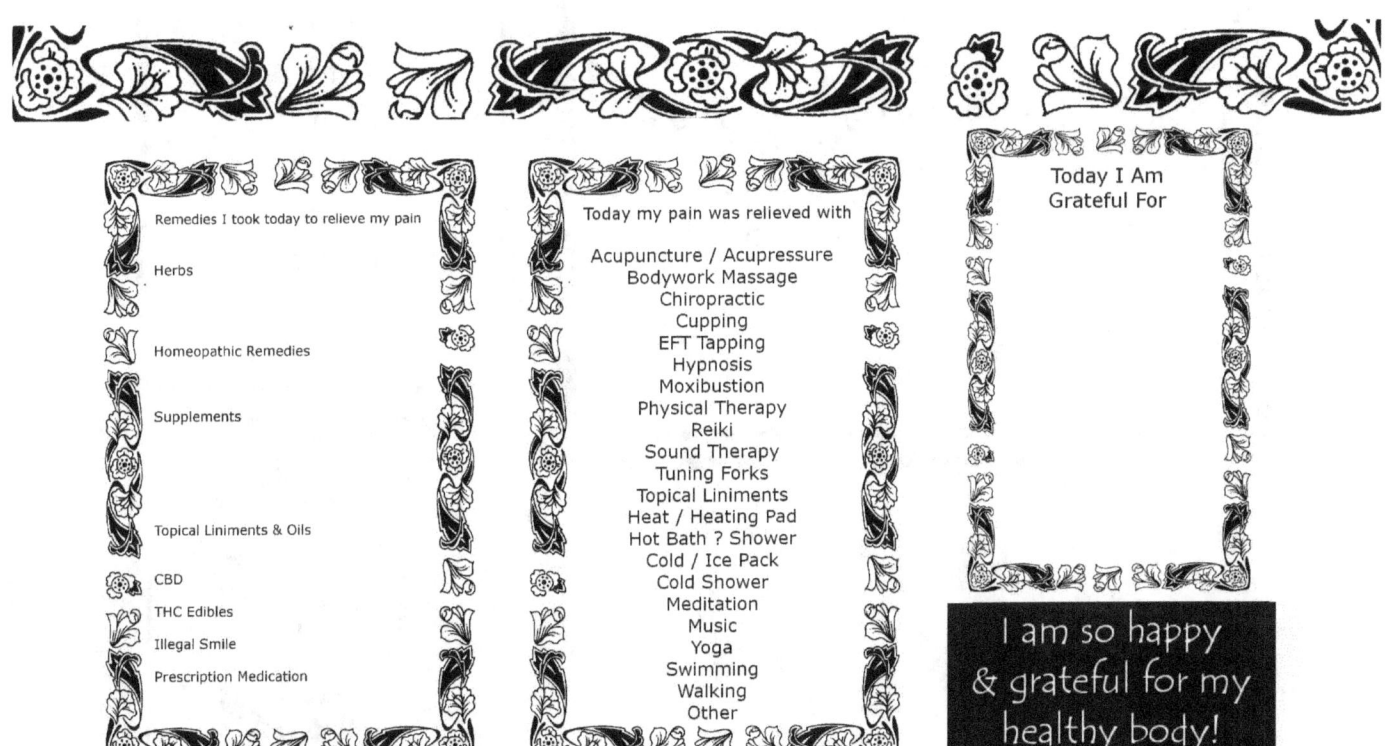

Remedies I took today to relieve my pain

Herbs

Homeopathic Remedies

Supplements

Topical Liniments & Oils

CBD
THC Edibles
Illegal Smile
Prescription Medication

Today my pain was relieved with

Acupuncture / Acupressure
Bodywork Massage
Chiropractic
Cupping
EFT Tapping
Hypnosis
Moxibustion
Physical Therapy
Reiki
Sound Therapy
Tuning Forks
Topical Liniments
Heat / Heating Pad
Hot Bath ? Shower
Cold / Ice Pack
Cold Shower
Meditation
Music
Yoga
Swimming
Walking
Other

Today I Am Grateful For

I am so happy & grateful for my healthy body!

Today's Day & Date

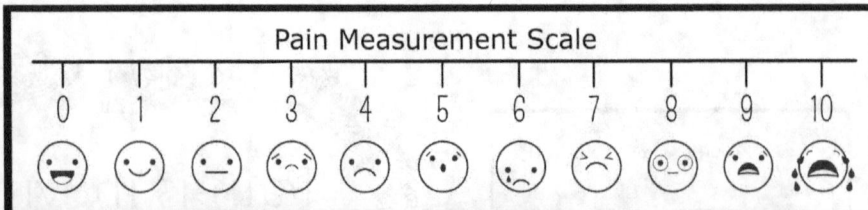

Highlight All Painful Areas

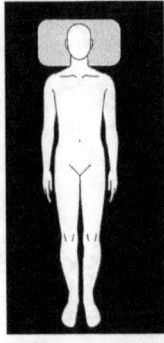 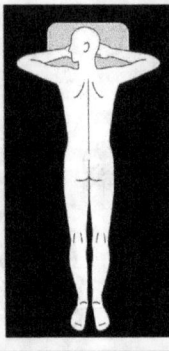 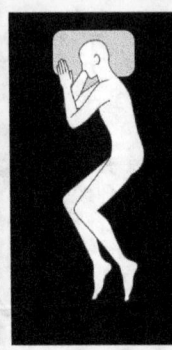 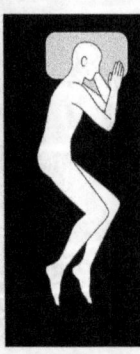

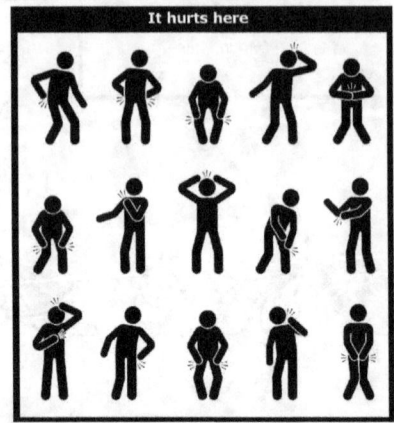
It hurts here

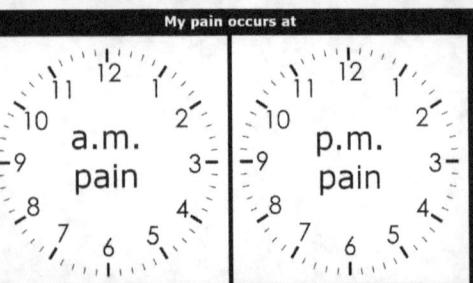
My pain occurs at — a.m. pain / p.m. pain

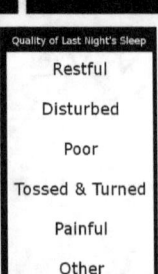
Quality of Last Night's Sleep
- Restful
- Disturbed
- Poor
- Tossed & Turned
- Painful
- Other

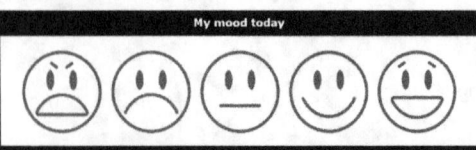
My mood today

My pain is
Hot
Burning
Cold
Stabbing
Throbbing
Fixed
Moving Traveling
Constant
On & Off

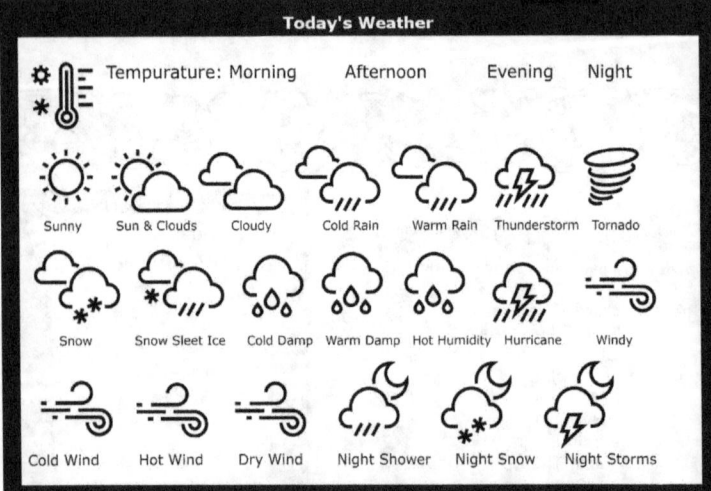
Today's Weather
Tempurature: Morning Afternoon Evening Night
Sunny | Sun & Clouds | Cloudy | Cold Rain | Warm Rain | Thunderstorm | Tornado
Snow | Snow Sleet Ice | Cold Damp | Warm Damp | Hot Humidity | Hurricane | Windy
Cold Wind | Hot Wind | Dry Wind | Night Shower | Night Snow | Night Storms

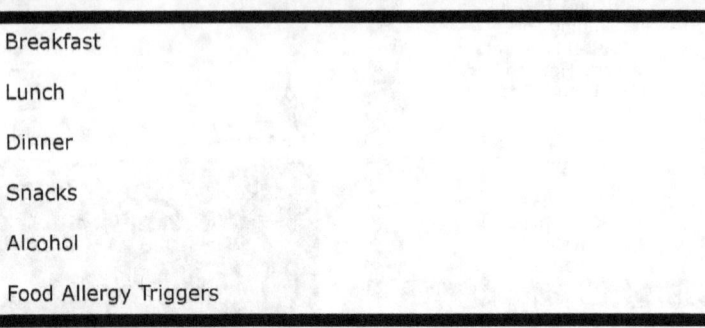

Breakfast

Lunch

Dinner

Snacks

Alcohol

Food Allergy Triggers

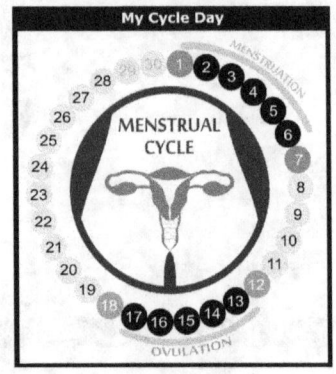
My Cycle Day

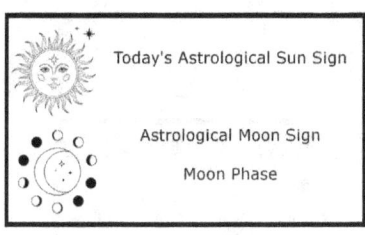

Today's Astrological Sun Sign

Astrological Moon Sign

Moon Phase

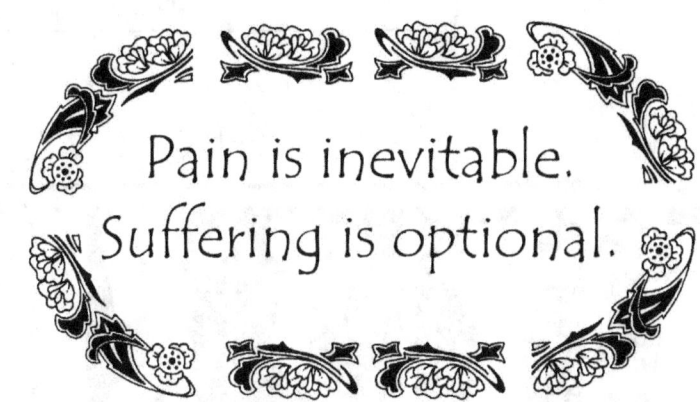

Pain is inevitable.
Suffering is optional.

Notes

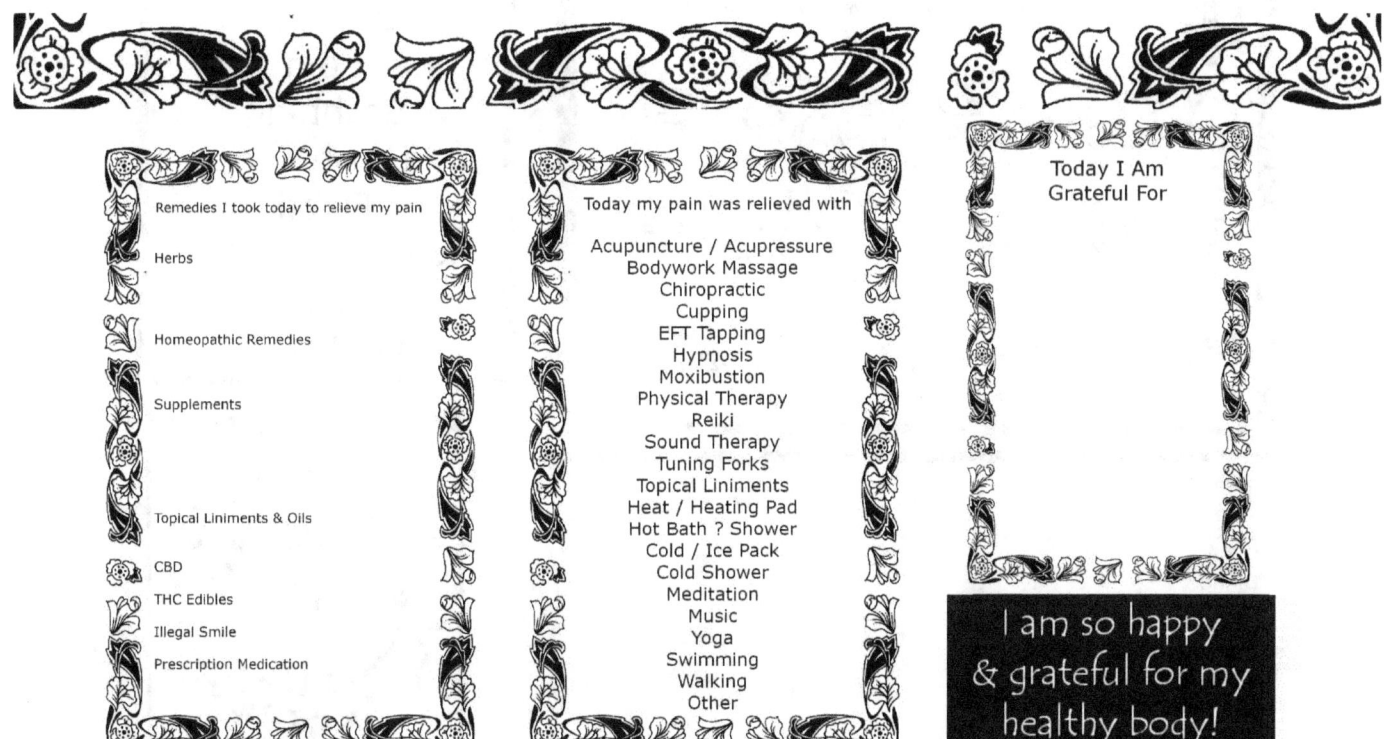

Remedies I took today to relieve my pain

Herbs

Homeopathic Remedies

Supplements

Topical Liniments & Oils

CBD

THC Edibles

Illegal Smile

Prescription Medication

Today my pain was relieved with

Acupuncture / Acupressure
Bodywork Massage
Chiropractic
Cupping
EFT Tapping
Hypnosis
Moxibustion
Physical Therapy
Reiki
Sound Therapy
Tuning Forks
Topical Liniments
Heat / Heating Pad
Hot Bath ? Shower
Cold / Ice Pack
Cold Shower
Meditation
Music
Yoga
Swimming
Walking
Other

Today I Am
Grateful For

I am so happy
& grateful for my
healthy body!

Today's Day & Date

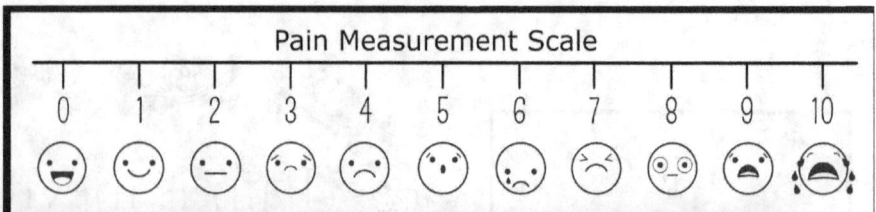

Pain Measurement Scale

Highlight All Painful Areas

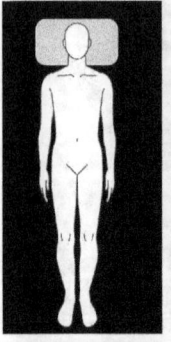 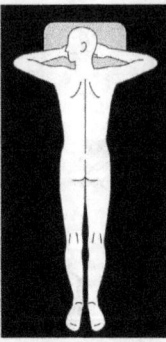 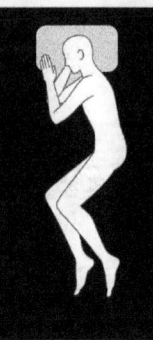 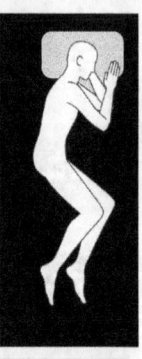

It hurts here

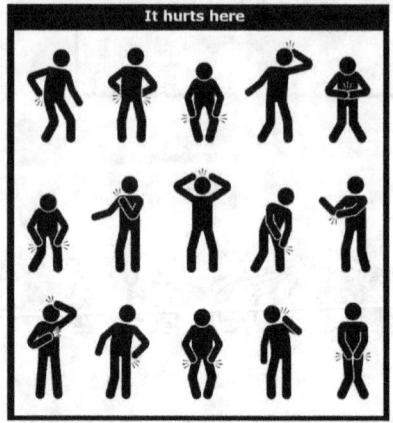

My pain occurs at

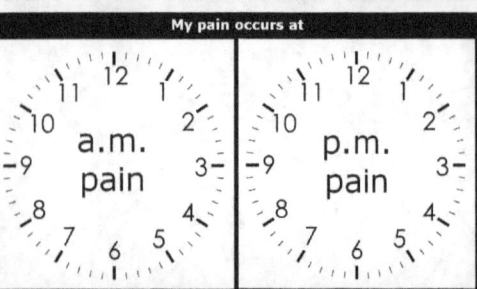
a.m. pain | p.m. pain

Quality of Last Night's Sleep
- Restful
- Disturbed
- Poor
- Tossed & Turned
- Painful
- Other

My mood today

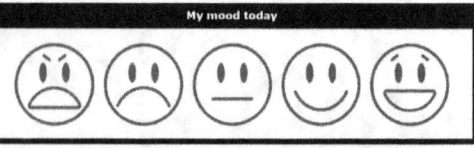

Today's Weather

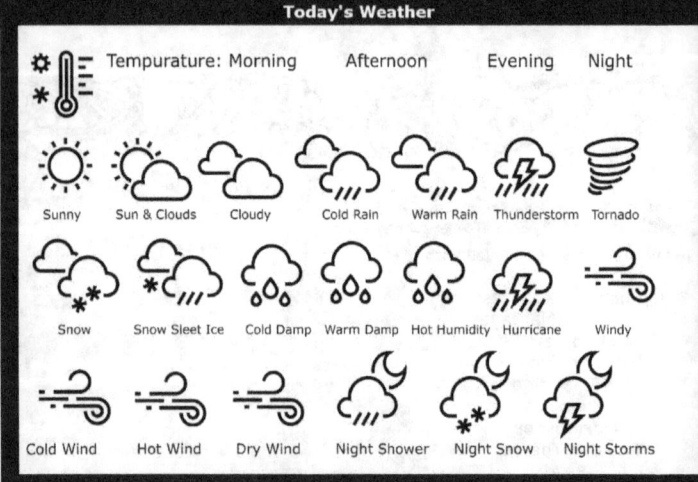

Temperature: Morning   Afternoon   Evening   Night

Sunny, Sun & Clouds, Cloudy, Cold Rain, Warm Rain, Thunderstorm, Tornado
Snow, Snow Sleet Ice, Cold Damp, Warm Damp, Hot Humidity, Hurricane, Windy
Cold Wind, Hot Wind, Dry Wind, Night Shower, Night Snow, Night Storms

My pain is

Hot
Burning
Cold
Stabbing
Throbbing
Fixed
Moving Traveling
Constant
On & Off

Breakfast

Lunch

Dinner

Snacks

Alcohol

Food Allergy Triggers

My Cycle Day

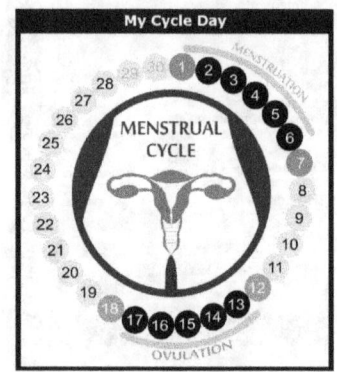

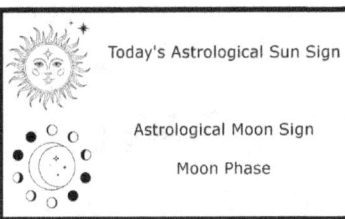

Today's Astrological Sun Sign

Astrological Moon Sign

Moon Phase

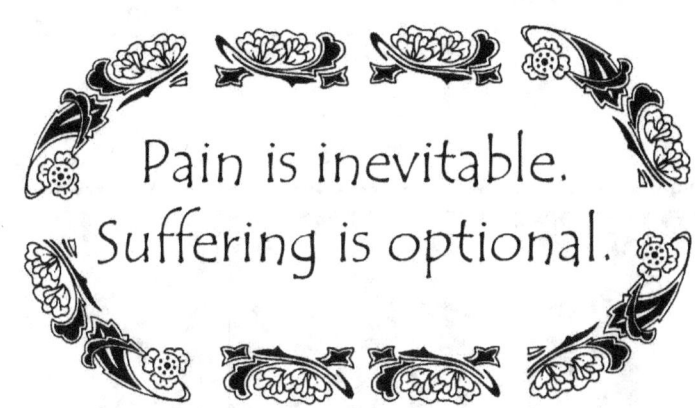

Pain is inevitable.
Suffering is optional.

Notes

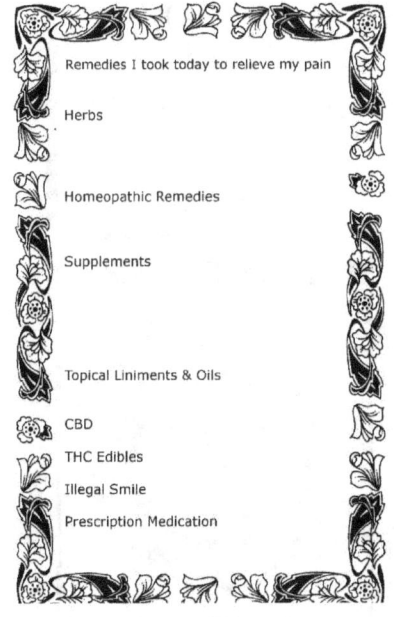

Remedies I took today to relieve my pain

Herbs

Homeopathic Remedies

Supplements

Topical Liniments & Oils

CBD

THC Edibles

Illegal Smile

Prescription Medication

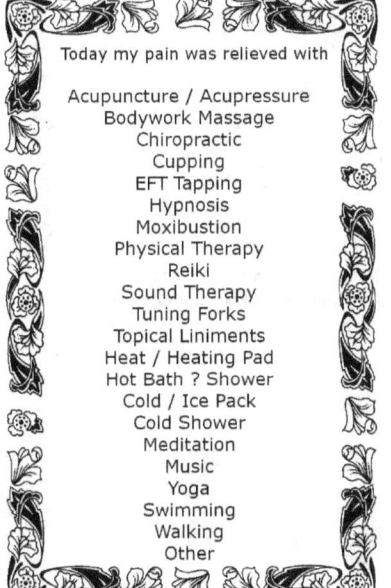

Today my pain was relieved with

Acupuncture / Acupressure
Bodywork Massage
Chiropractic
Cupping
EFT Tapping
Hypnosis
Moxibustion
Physical Therapy
Reiki
Sound Therapy
Tuning Forks
Topical Liniments
Heat / Heating Pad
Hot Bath ? Shower
Cold / Ice Pack
Cold Shower
Meditation
Music
Yoga
Swimming
Walking
Other

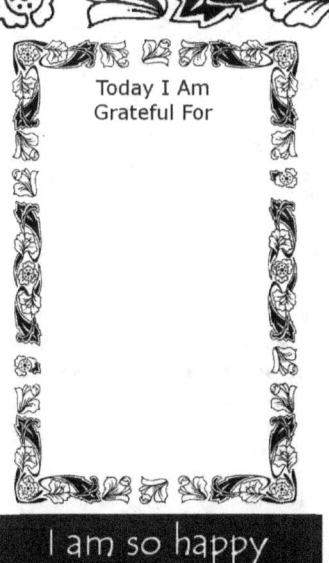

Today I Am
Grateful For

I am so happy
& grateful for my
healthy body!

Today's Day & Date

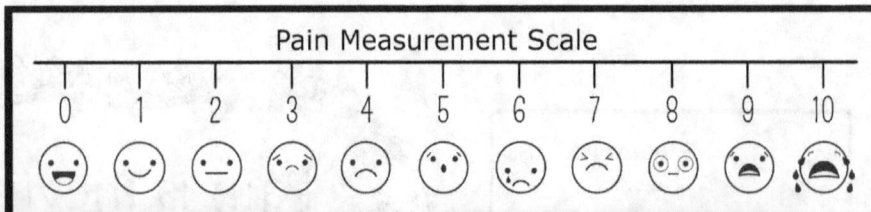

Highlight All Painful Areas

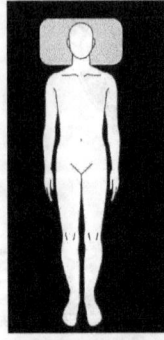 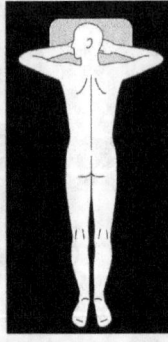 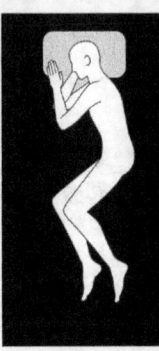 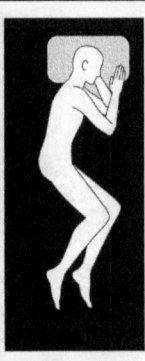

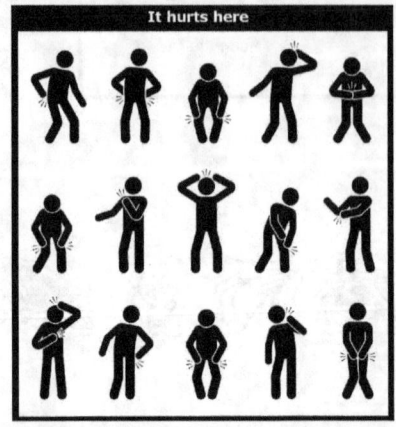

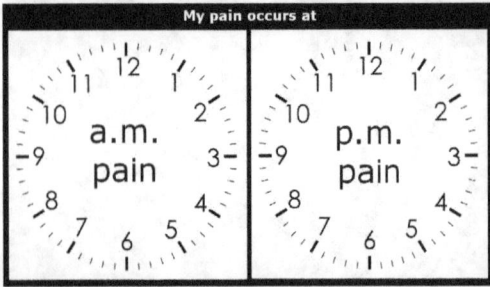

My pain occurs at — a.m. pain / p.m. pain

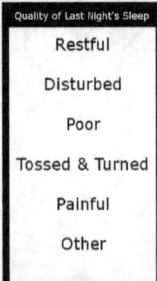

Quality of Last Night's Sleep
- Restful
- Disturbed
- Poor
- Tossed & Turned
- Painful
- Other

My mood today

My pain is
Hot
Burning
Cold
Stabbing
Throbbing
Fixed
Moving Traveling
Constant
On & Off

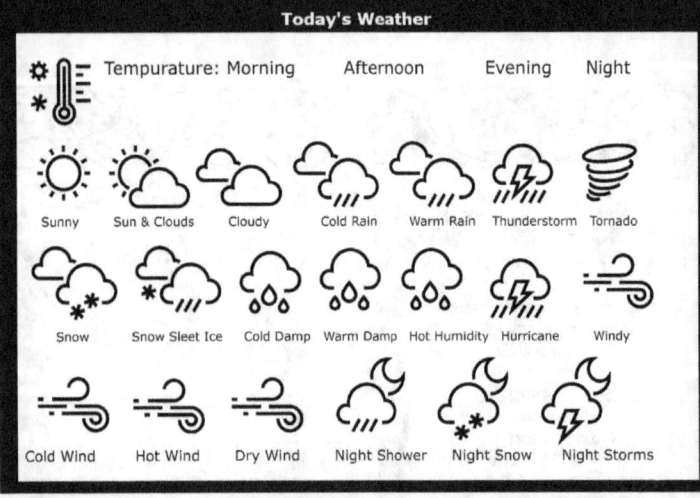

Today's Weather — Temperature: Morning, Afternoon, Evening, Night

Sunny, Sun & Clouds, Cloudy, Cold Rain, Warm Rain, Thunderstorm, Tornado
Snow, Snow Sleet Ice, Cold Damp, Warm Damp, Hot Humidity, Hurricane, Windy
Cold Wind, Hot Wind, Dry Wind, Night Shower, Night Snow, Night Storms

Breakfast

Lunch

Dinner

Snacks

Alcohol

Food Allergy Triggers

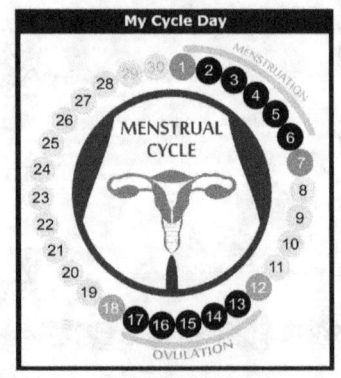

My Cycle Day

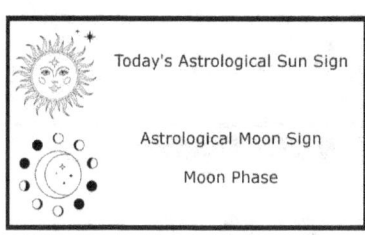

Today's Astrological Sun Sign

Astrological Moon Sign

Moon Phase

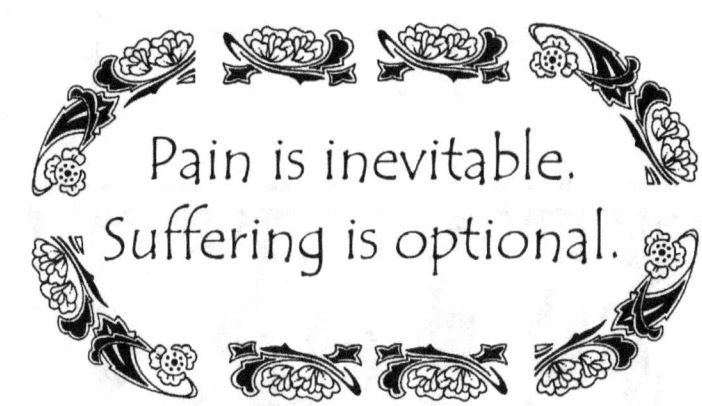

Pain is inevitable.
Suffering is optional.

Notes

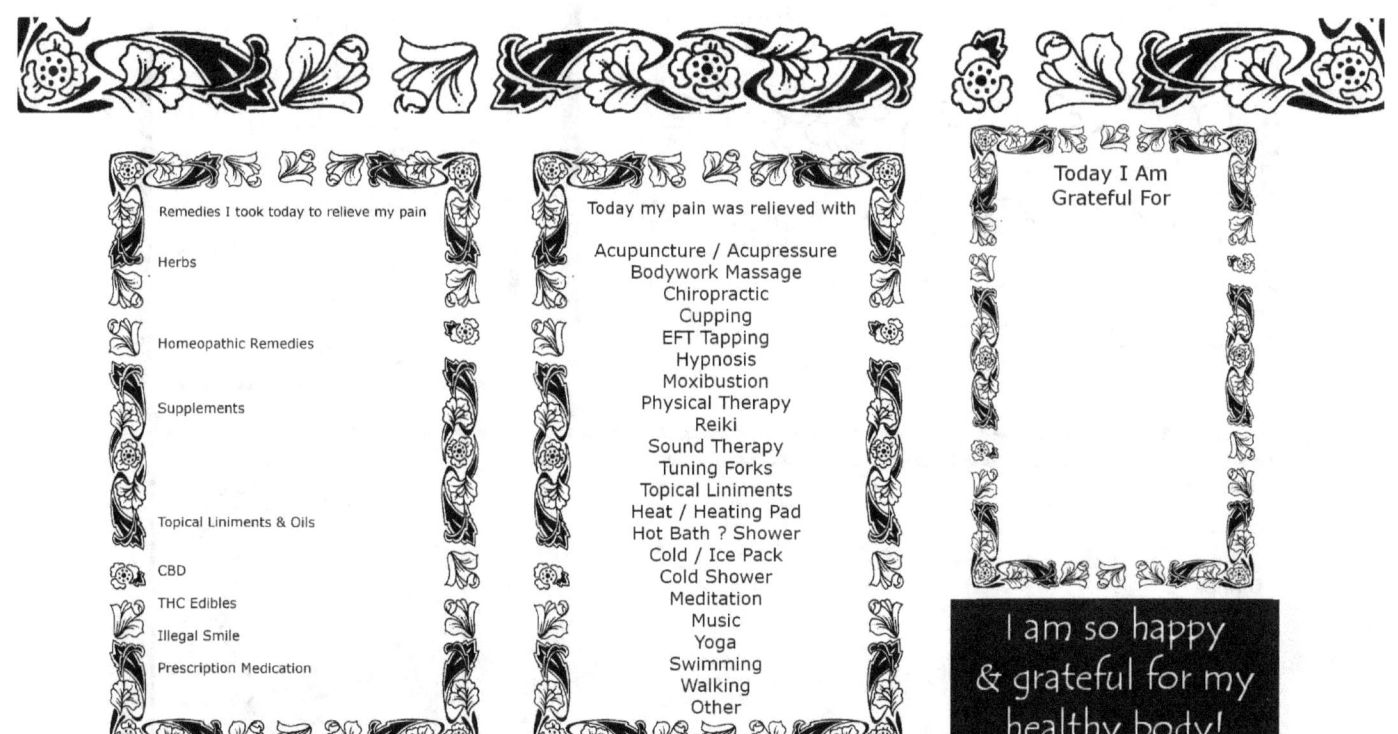

Remedies I took today to relieve my pain

Herbs

Homeopathic Remedies

Supplements

Topical Liniments & Oils

CBD

THC Edibles

Illegal Smile

Prescription Medication

Today my pain was relieved with

Acupuncture / Acupressure
Bodywork Massage
Chiropractic
Cupping
EFT Tapping
Hypnosis
Moxibustion
Physical Therapy
Reiki
Sound Therapy
Tuning Forks
Topical Liniments
Heat / Heating Pad
Hot Bath ? Shower
Cold / Ice Pack
Cold Shower
Meditation
Music
Yoga
Swimming
Walking
Other

Today I Am Grateful For

I am so happy & grateful for my healthy body!

Today's Day & Date

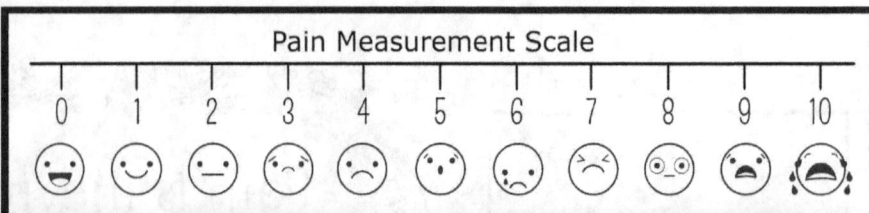

Highlight All Painful Areas

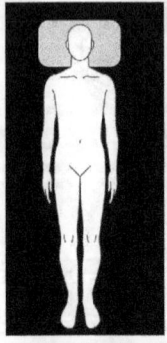 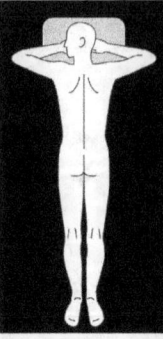 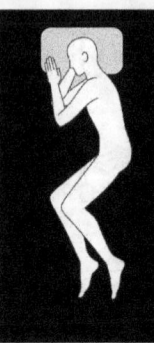 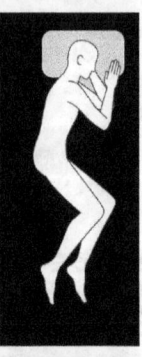

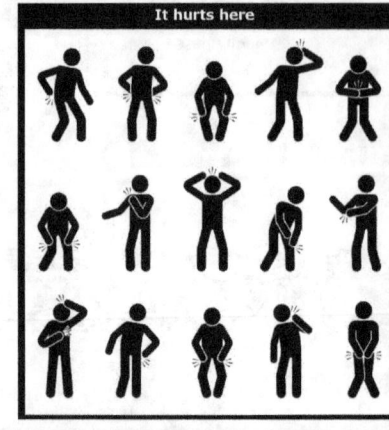
It hurts here

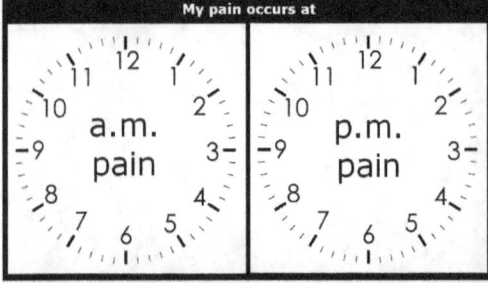
My pain occurs at — a.m. pain / p.m. pain

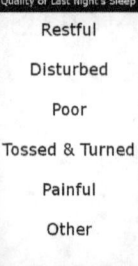
Quality of Last Night's Sleep
- Restful
- Disturbed
- Poor
- Tossed & Turned
- Painful
- Other

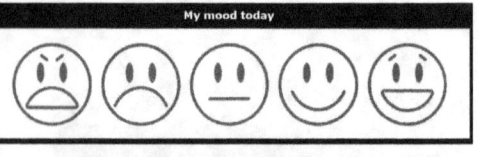
My mood today

My pain is
Hot
Burning
Cold
Stabbing
Throbbing
Fixed
Moving Traveling
Constant
On & Off

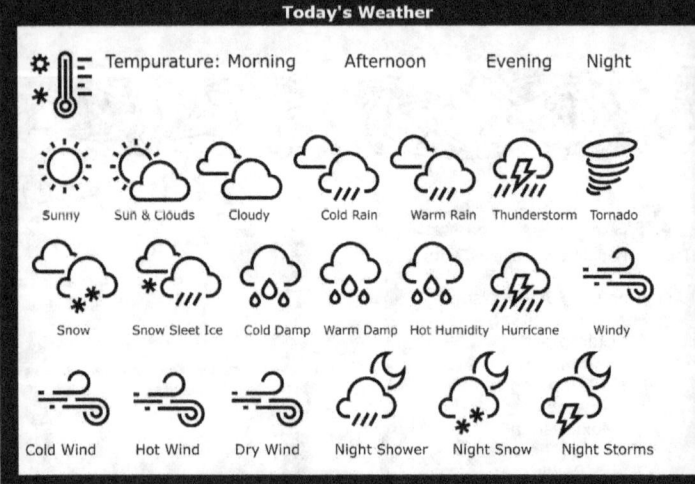
Today's Weather

Breakfast

Lunch

Dinner

Snacks

Alcohol

Food Allergy Triggers

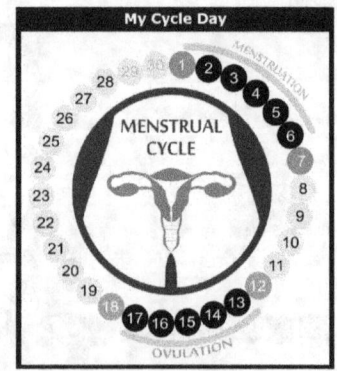
My Cycle Day

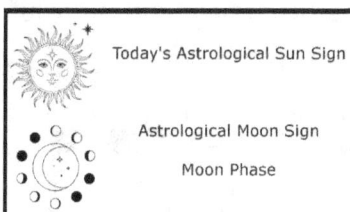

Today's Astrological Sun Sign

Astrological Moon Sign

Moon Phase

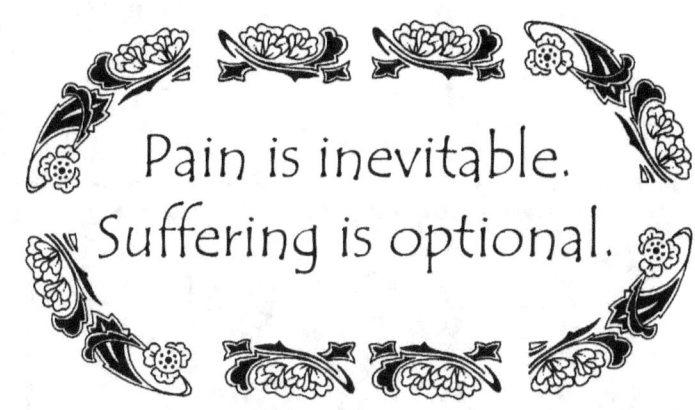

Pain is inevitable.
Suffering is optional.

Notes

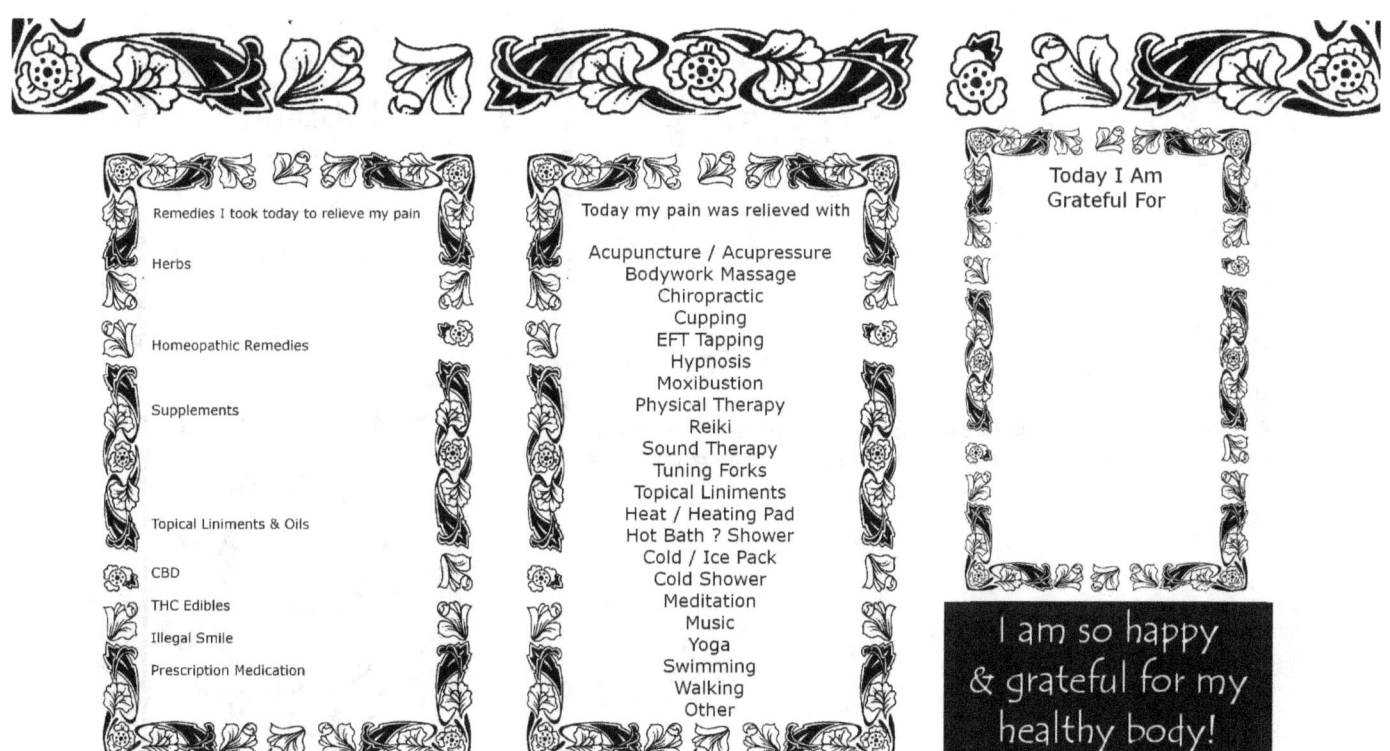

Remedies I took today to relieve my pain

Herbs

Homeopathic Remedies

Supplements

Topical Liniments & Oils

CBD

THC Edibles

Illegal Smile

Prescription Medication

Today my pain was relieved with

Acupuncture / Acupressure
Bodywork Massage
Chiropractic
Cupping
EFT Tapping
Hypnosis
Moxibustion
Physical Therapy
Reiki
Sound Therapy
Tuning Forks
Topical Liniments
Heat / Heating Pad
Hot Bath ? Shower
Cold / Ice Pack
Cold Shower
Meditation
Music
Yoga
Swimming
Walking
Other

Today I Am Grateful For

I am so happy & grateful for my healthy body!

Today's Day & Date

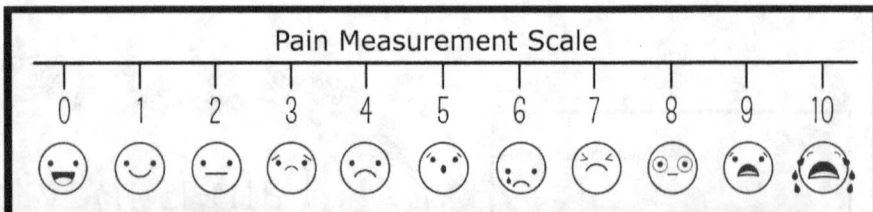

Highlight All Painful Areas

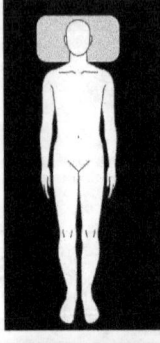 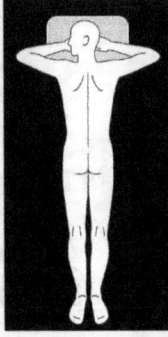 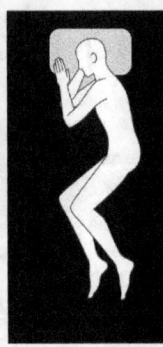 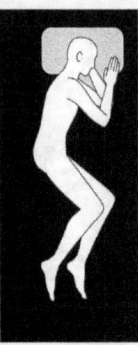

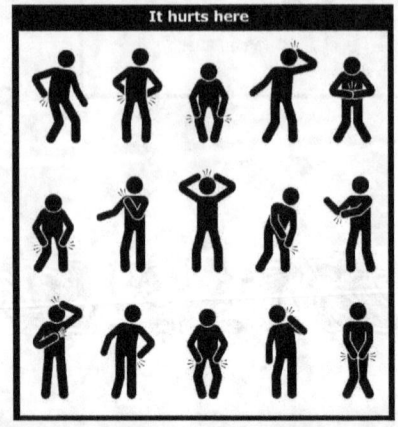
It hurts here

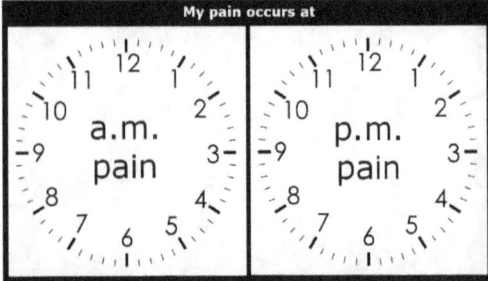
My pain occurs at — a.m. pain / p.m. pain

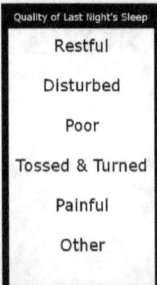

Quality of Last Night's Sleep
- Restful
- Disturbed
- Poor
- Tossed & Turned
- Painful
- Other

My mood today

My pain is
Hot
Burning
Cold
Stabbing
Throbbing
Fixed
Moving Traveling
Constant
On & Off

Today's Weather

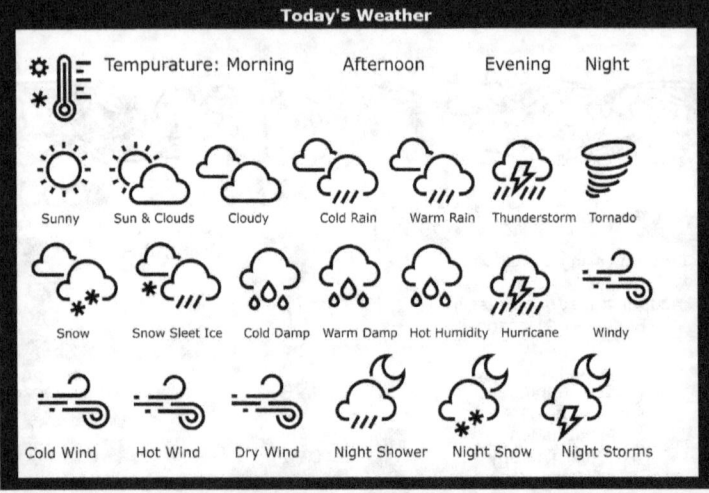

Tempurature: Morning   Afternoon   Evening   Night

Sunny, Sun & Clouds, Cloudy, Cold Rain, Warm Rain, Thunderstorm, Tornado
Snow, Snow Sleet Ice, Cold Damp, Warm Damp, Hot Humidity, Hurricane, Windy
Cold Wind, Hot Wind, Dry Wind, Night Shower, Night Snow, Night Storms

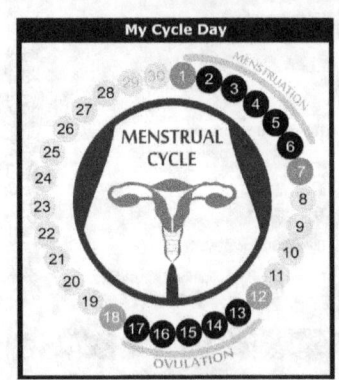
My Cycle Day

Breakfast

Lunch

Dinner

Snacks

Alcohol

Food Allergy Triggers

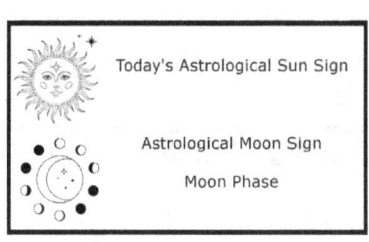

Today's Astrological Sun Sign

Astrological Moon Sign

Moon Phase

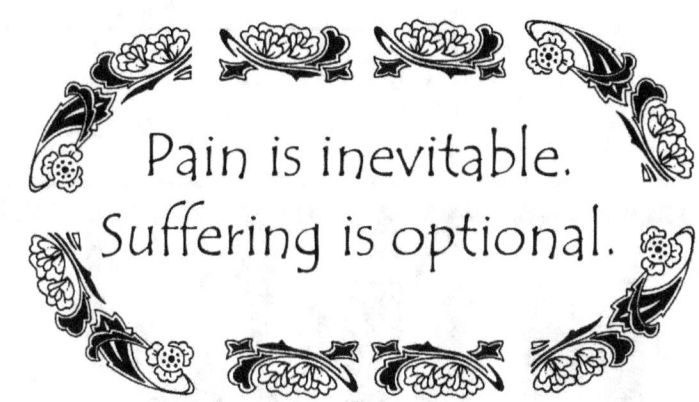

Pain is inevitable.
Suffering is optional.

Notes

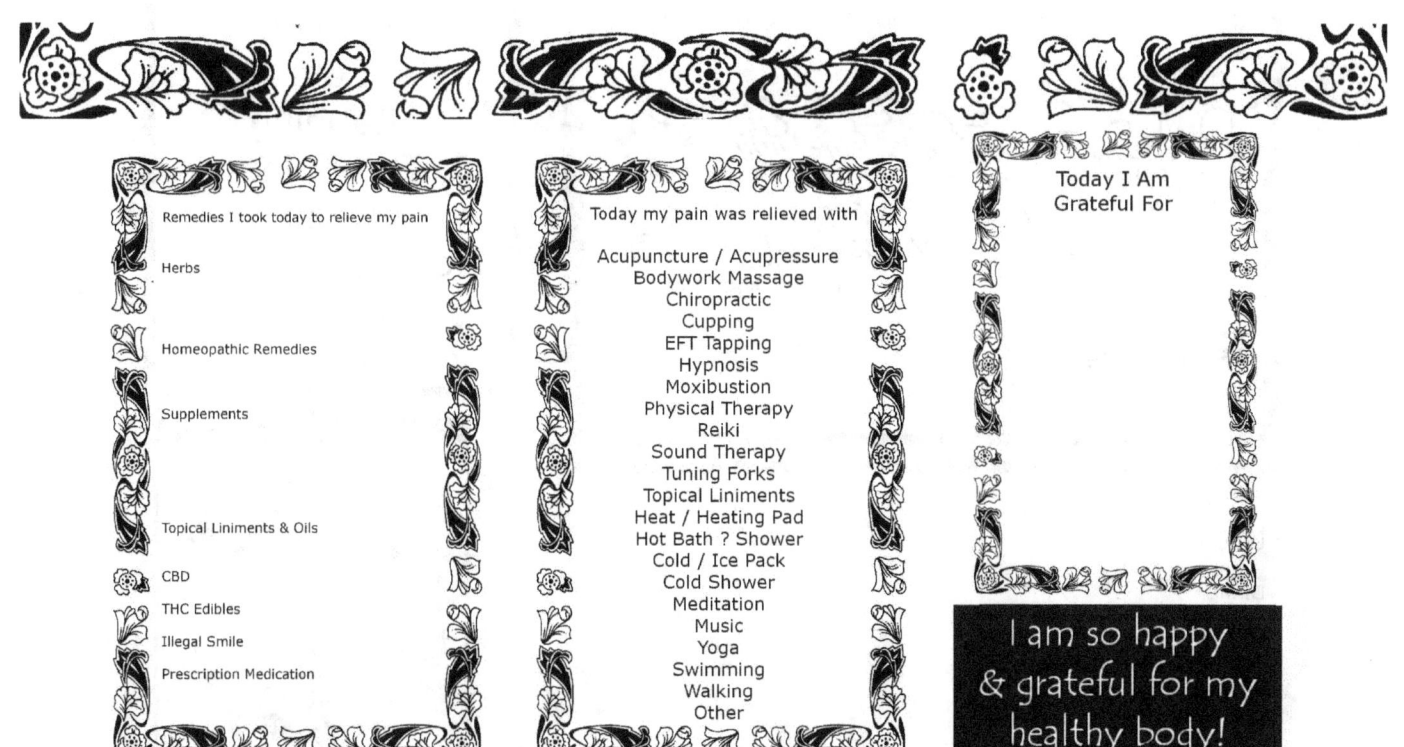

Remedies I took today to relieve my pain

Herbs

Homeopathic Remedies

Supplements

Topical Liniments & Oils

CBD

THC Edibles

Illegal Smile

Prescription Medication

Today my pain was relieved with

Acupuncture / Acupressure
Bodywork Massage
Chiropractic
Cupping
EFT Tapping
Hypnosis
Moxibustion
Physical Therapy
Reiki
Sound Therapy
Tuning Forks
Topical Liniments
Heat / Heating Pad
Hot Bath ? Shower
Cold / Ice Pack
Cold Shower
Meditation
Music
Yoga
Swimming
Walking
Other

Today I Am Grateful For

I am so happy & grateful for my healthy body!

Today's Day & Date

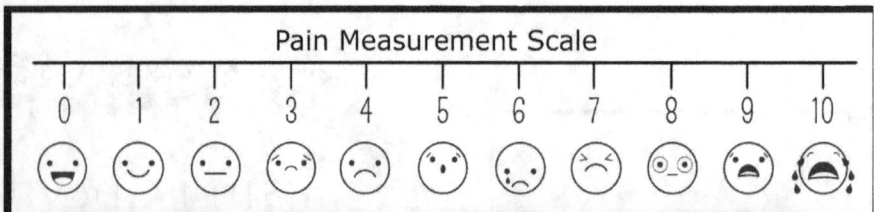

Highlight All Painful Areas

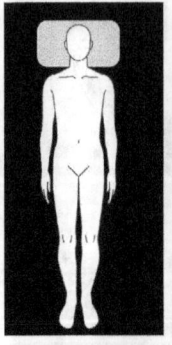 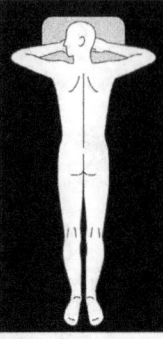 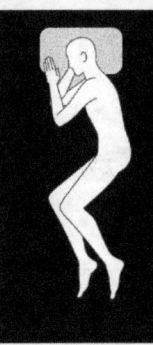 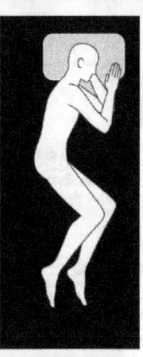

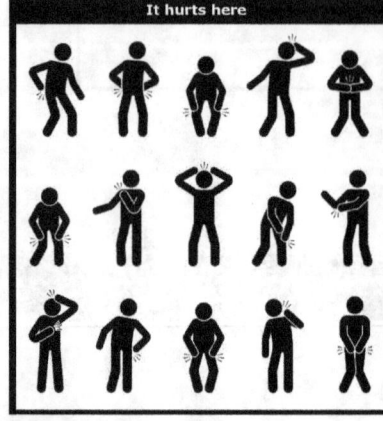

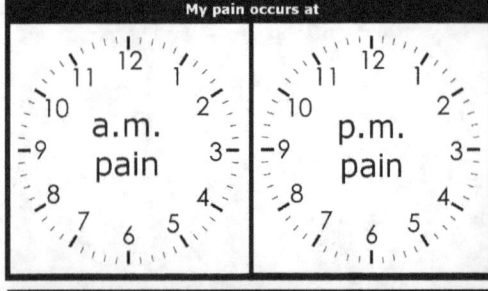

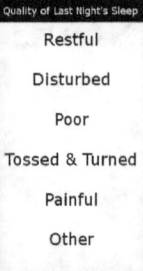

Quality of Last Night's Sleep
- Restful
- Disturbed
- Poor
- Tossed & Turned
- Painful
- Other

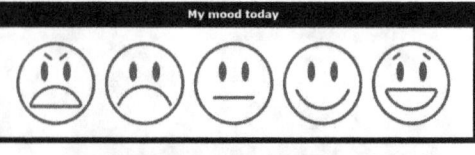

My pain is
Hot
Burning
Cold
Stabbing
Throbbing
Fixed
Moving Traveling
Constant
On & Off

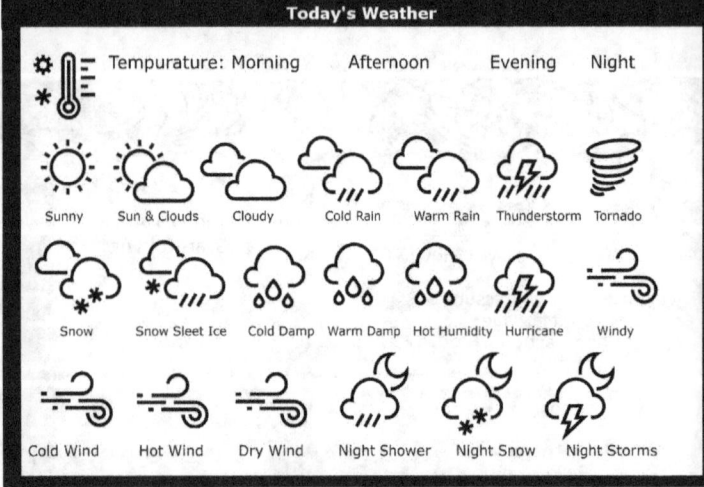

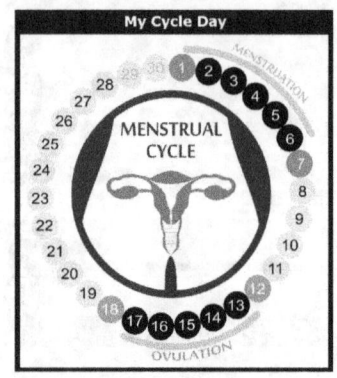

Breakfast

Lunch

Dinner

Snacks

Alcohol

Food Allergy Triggers

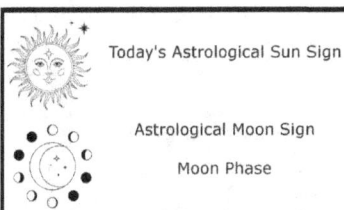

Today's Astrological Sun Sign

Astrological Moon Sign

Moon Phase

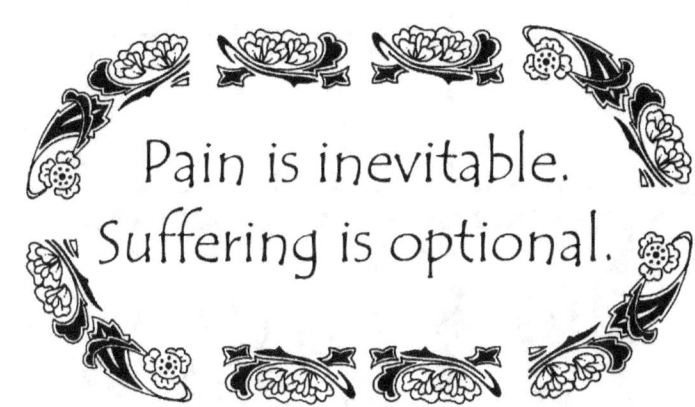

Pain is inevitable.
Suffering is optional.

Notes

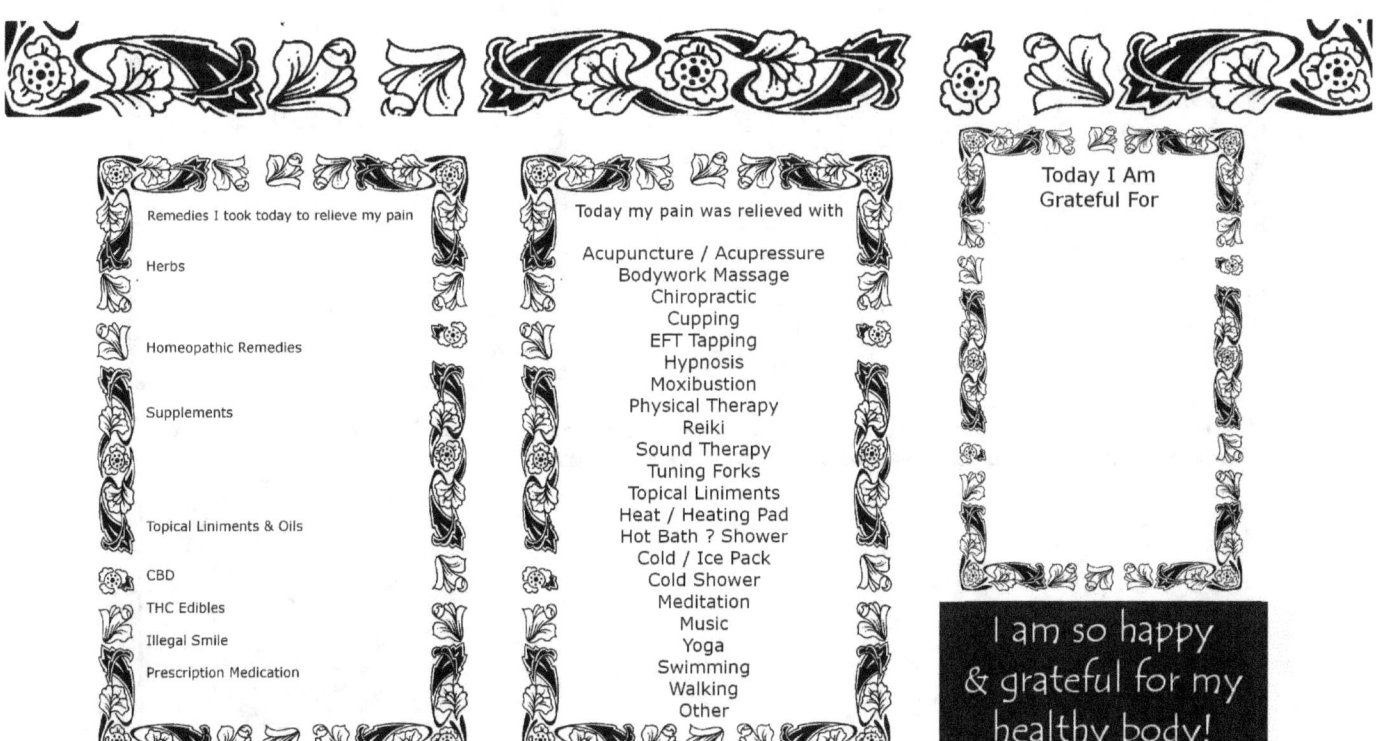

Remedies I took today to relieve my pain

Herbs

Homeopathic Remedies

Supplements

Topical Liniments & Oils

CBD

THC Edibles

Illegal Smile

Prescription Medication

Today my pain was relieved with

Acupuncture / Acupressure
Bodywork Massage
Chiropractic
Cupping
EFT Tapping
Hypnosis
Moxibustion
Physical Therapy
Reiki
Sound Therapy
Tuning Forks
Topical Liniments
Heat / Heating Pad
Hot Bath ? Shower
Cold / Ice Pack
Cold Shower
Meditation
Music
Yoga
Swimming
Walking
Other

Today I Am Grateful For

I am so happy & grateful for my healthy body!

Today's Day & Date

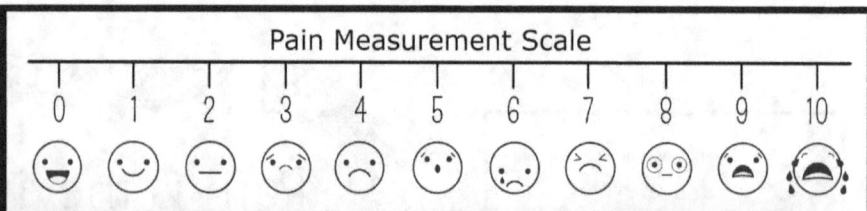

Highlight All Painful Areas

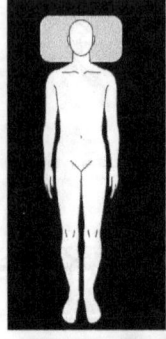 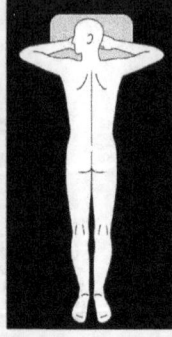 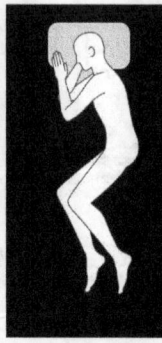 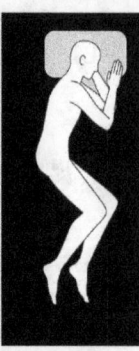

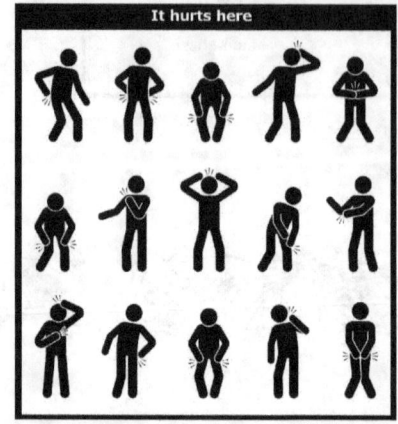

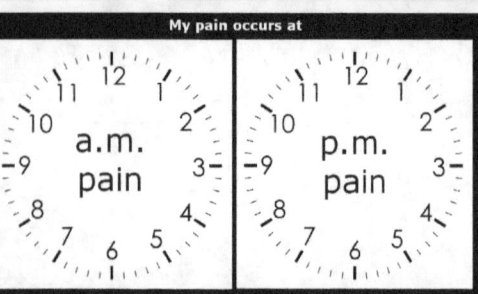

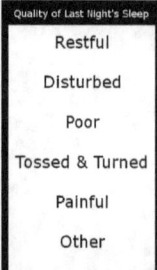

Quality of Last Night's Sleep
- Restful
- Disturbed
- Poor
- Tossed & Turned
- Painful
- Other

Today's Weather

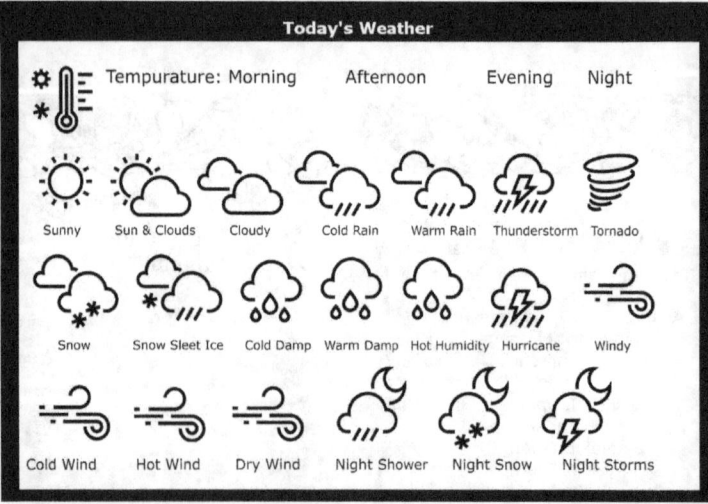

My pain is

Hot
Burning
Cold
Stabbing
Throbbing
Fixed
Moving Traveling
Constant
On & Off

Breakfast

Lunch

Dinner

Snacks

Alcohol

Food Allergy Triggers

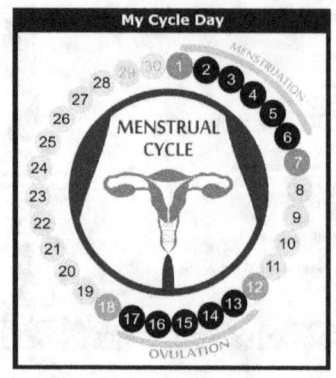

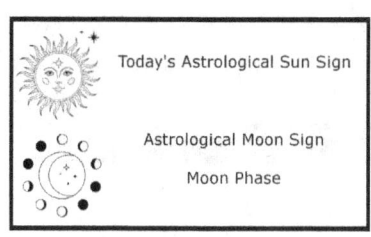

Today's Astrological Sun Sign

Astrological Moon Sign

Moon Phase

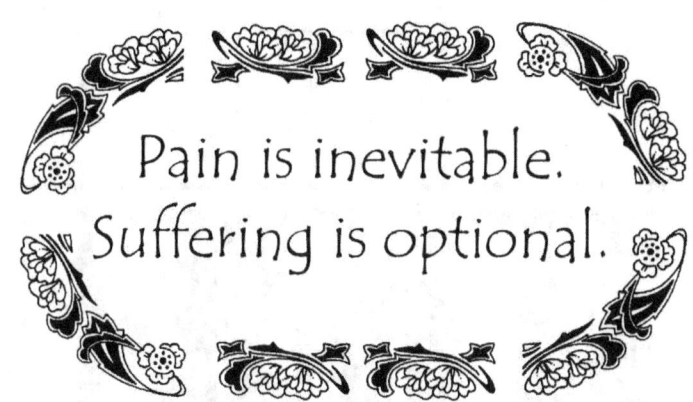

Pain is inevitable.
Suffering is optional.

Notes

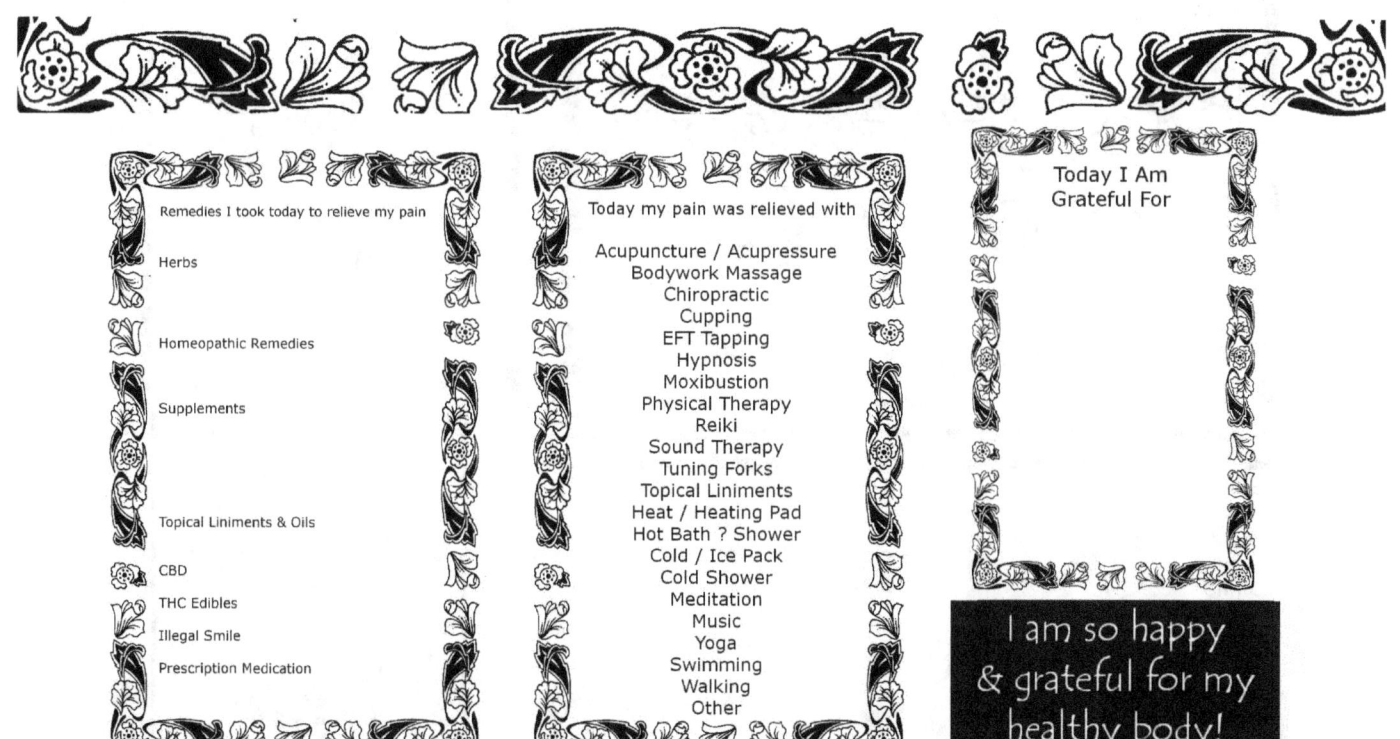

Remedies I took today to relieve my pain

Herbs

Homeopathic Remedies

Supplements

Topical Liniments & Oils

CBD

THC Edibles

Illegal Smile

Prescription Medication

Today my pain was relieved with

Acupuncture / Acupressure
Bodywork Massage
Chiropractic
Cupping
EFT Tapping
Hypnosis
Moxibustion
Physical Therapy
Reiki
Sound Therapy
Tuning Forks
Topical Liniments
Heat / Heating Pad
Hot Bath ? Shower
Cold / Ice Pack
Cold Shower
Meditation
Music
Yoga
Swimming
Walking
Other

Today I Am Grateful For

I am so happy & grateful for my healthy body!

Today's Day & Date

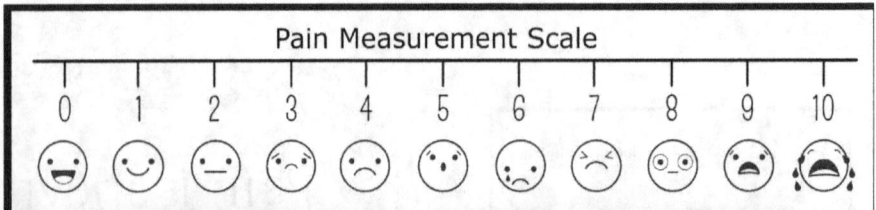

Highlight All Painful Areas

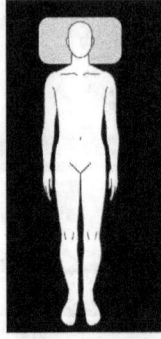 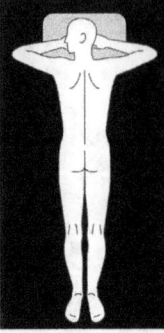 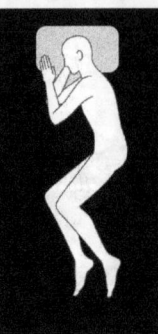 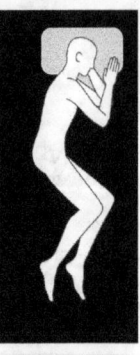

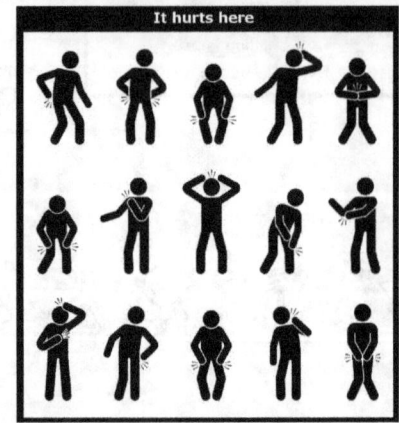
It hurts here

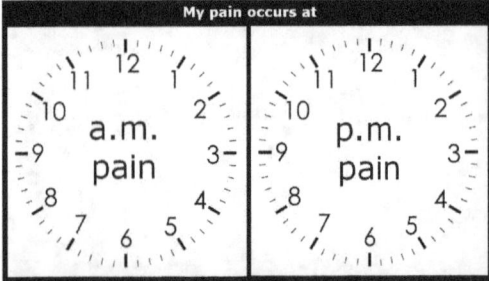
My pain occurs at — a.m. pain / p.m. pain

Quality of Last Night's Sleep
- Restful
- Disturbed
- Poor
- Tossed & Turned
- Painful
- Other

My mood today

My pain is
Hot
Burning
Cold
Stabbing
Throbbing
Fixed
Moving Traveling
Constant
On & Off

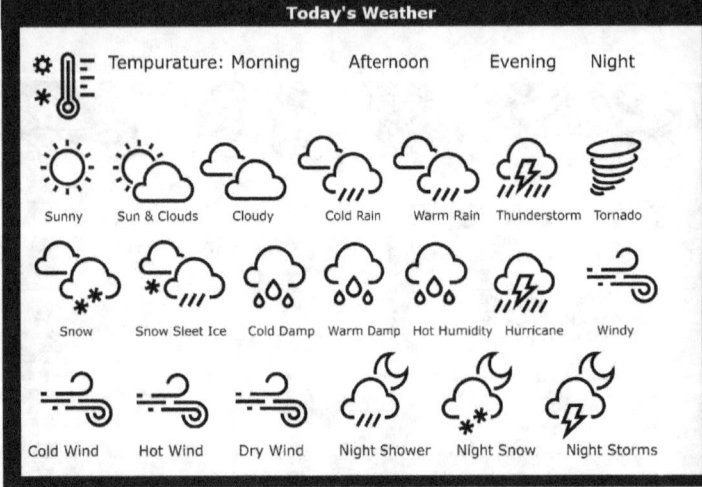
Today's Weather — Temperature: Morning, Afternoon, Evening, Night
Sunny, Sun & Clouds, Cloudy, Cold Rain, Warm Rain, Thunderstorm, Tornado
Snow, Snow Sleet Ice, Cold Damp, Warm Damp, Hot Humidity, Hurricane, Windy
Cold Wind, Hot Wind, Dry Wind, Night Shower, Night Snow, Night Storms

Breakfast

Lunch

Dinner

Snacks

Alcohol

Food Allergy Triggers

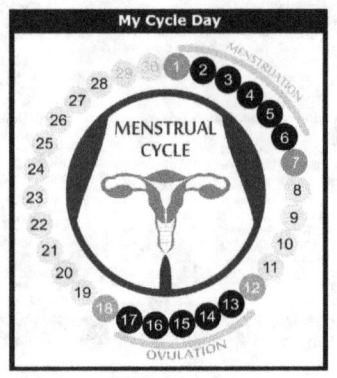
My Cycle Day

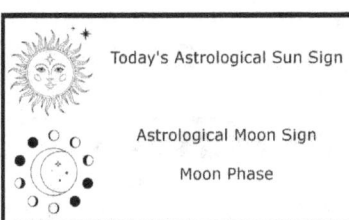

Today's Astrological Sun Sign

Astrological Moon Sign

Moon Phase

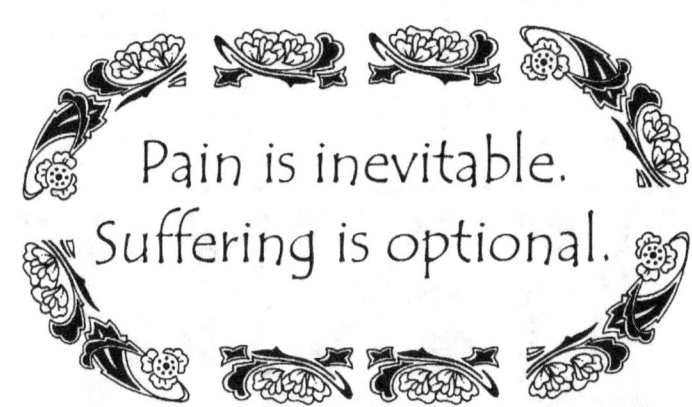

Pain is inevitable.
Suffering is optional.

Notes

Remedies I took today to relieve my pain

Herbs

Homeopathic Remedies

Supplements

Topical Liniments & Oils

CBD

THC Edibles

Illegal Smile

Prescription Medication

Today my pain was relieved with

Acupuncture / Acupressure
Bodywork Massage
Chiropractic
Cupping
EFT Tapping
Hypnosis
Moxibustion
Physical Therapy
Reiki
Sound Therapy
Tuning Forks
Topical Liniments
Heat / Heating Pad
Hot Bath ? Shower
Cold / Ice Pack
Cold Shower
Meditation
Music
Yoga
Swimming
Walking
Other

Today I Am Grateful For

I am so happy & grateful for my healthy body!

Today's Day & Date

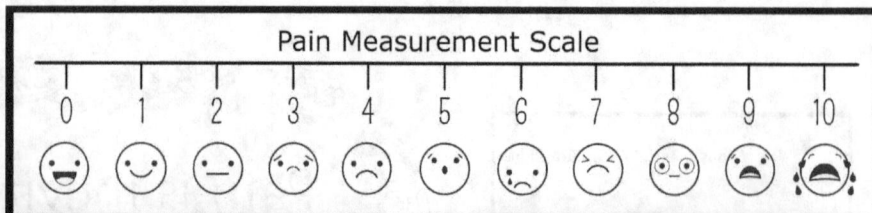

Highlight All Painful Areas

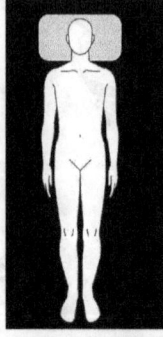 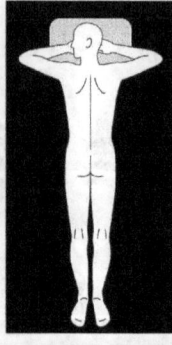 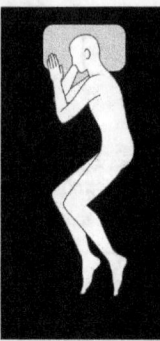 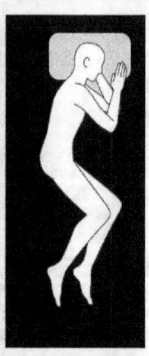

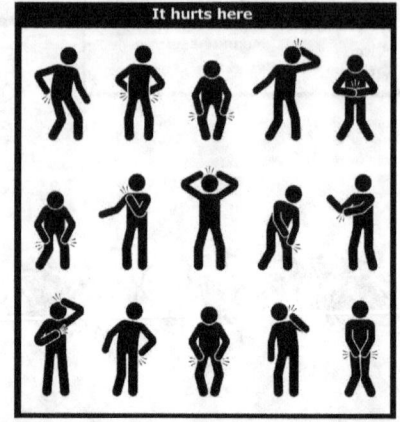
It hurts here

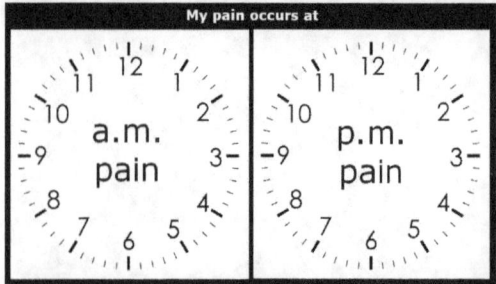
My pain occurs at — a.m. pain / p.m. pain

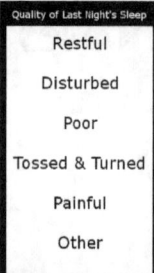

Quality of Last Night's Sleep
- Restful
- Disturbed
- Poor
- Tossed & Turned
- Painful
- Other

My mood today

My pain is

Hot
Burning
Cold
Stabbing
Throbbing
Fixed
Moving Traveling
Constant
On & Off

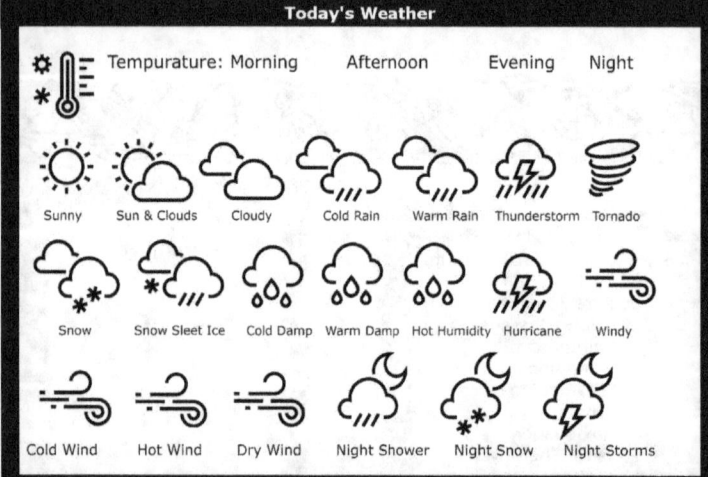
Today's Weather — Temperature: Morning, Afternoon, Evening, Night

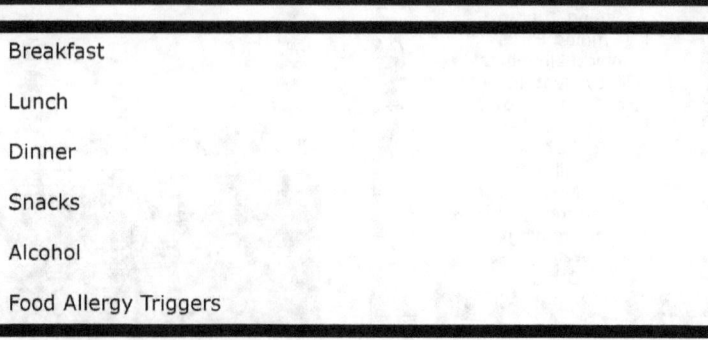

Breakfast

Lunch

Dinner

Snacks

Alcohol

Food Allergy Triggers

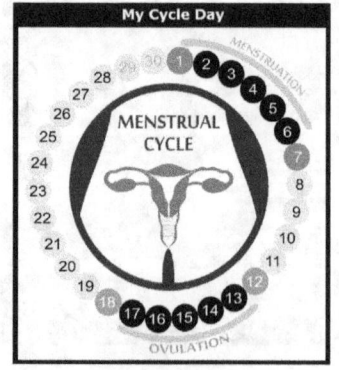
My Cycle Day

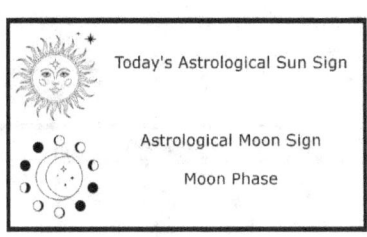

Today's Astrological Sun Sign

Astrological Moon Sign

Moon Phase

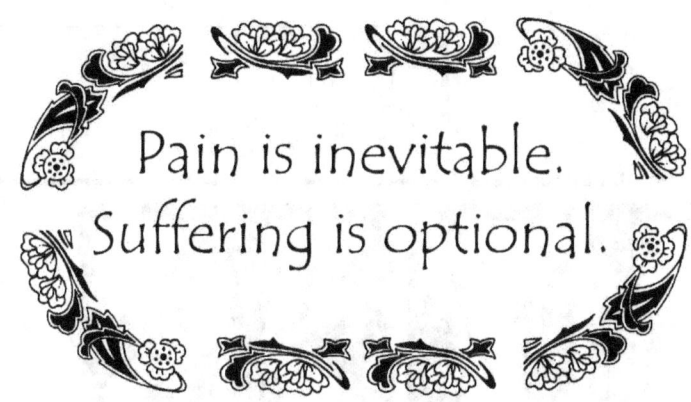

Pain is inevitable.
Suffering is optional.

Notes

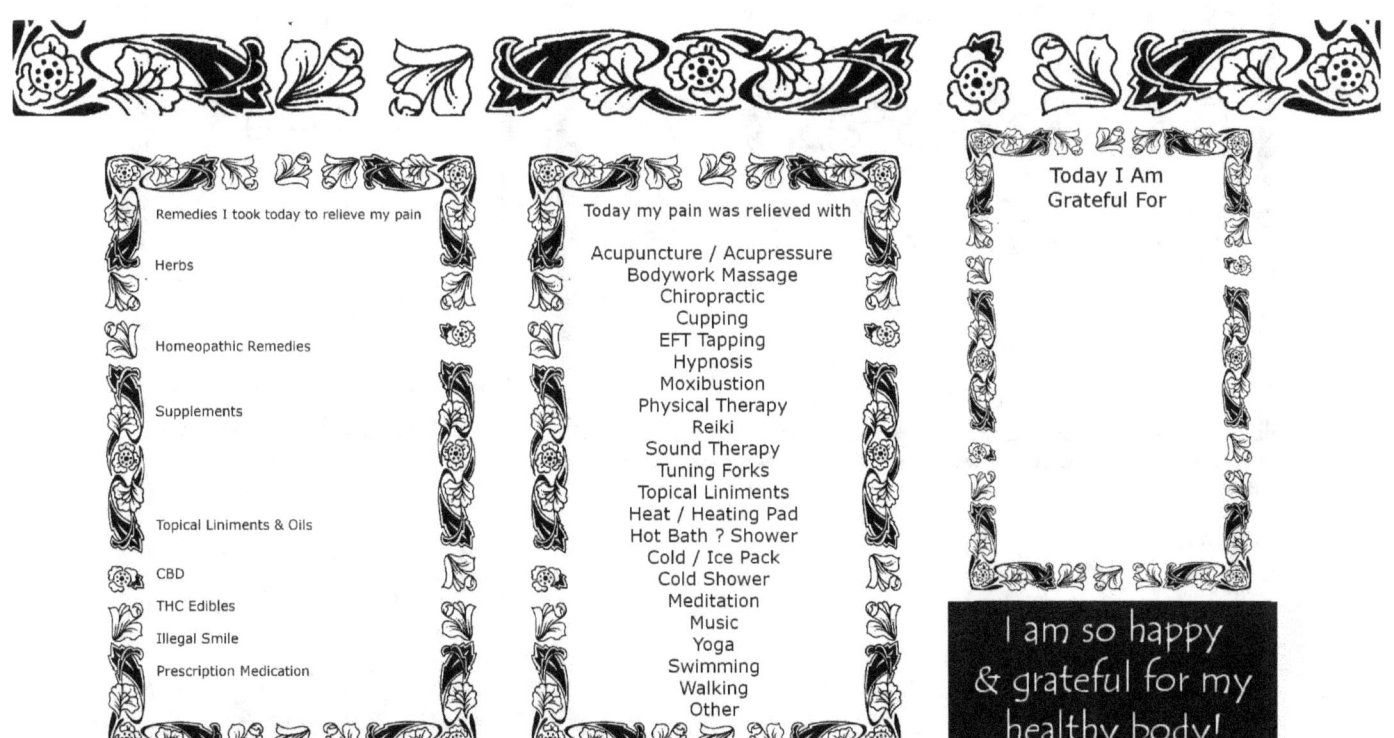

Remedies I took today to relieve my pain

Herbs

Homeopathic Remedies

Supplements

Topical Liniments & Oils

CBD

THC Edibles

Illegal Smile

Prescription Medication

Today my pain was relieved with

Acupuncture / Acupressure
Bodywork Massage
Chiropractic
Cupping
EFT Tapping
Hypnosis
Moxibustion
Physical Therapy
Reiki
Sound Therapy
Tuning Forks
Topical Liniments
Heat / Heating Pad
Hot Bath ? Shower
Cold / Ice Pack
Cold Shower
Meditation
Music
Yoga
Swimming
Walking
Other

Today I Am Grateful For

I am so happy & grateful for my healthy body!

Today's Day & Date

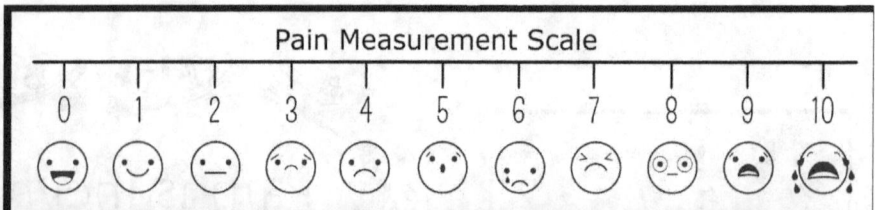

Highlight All Painful Areas

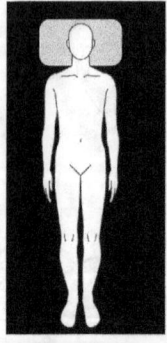 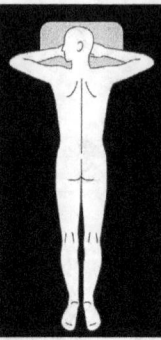 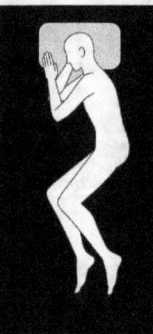 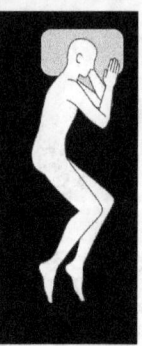

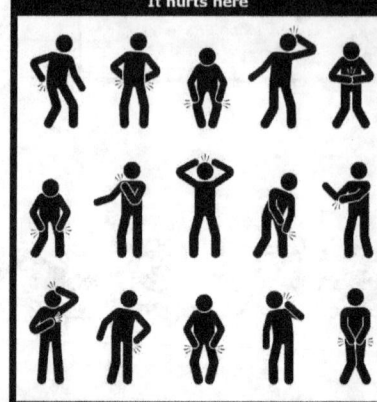

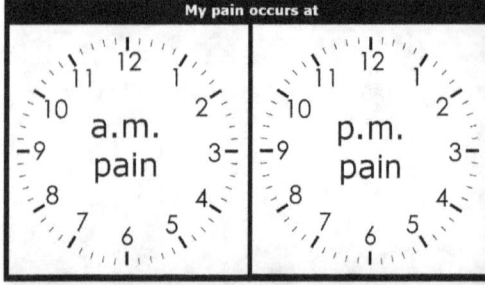

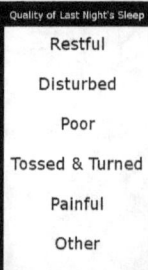

Quality of Last Night's Sleep
- Restful
- Disturbed
- Poor
- Tossed & Turned
- Painful
- Other

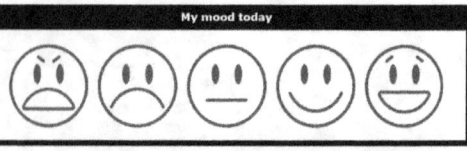

My pain is
Hot
Burning
Cold
Stabbing
Throbbing
Fixed
Moving Traveling
Constant
On & Off

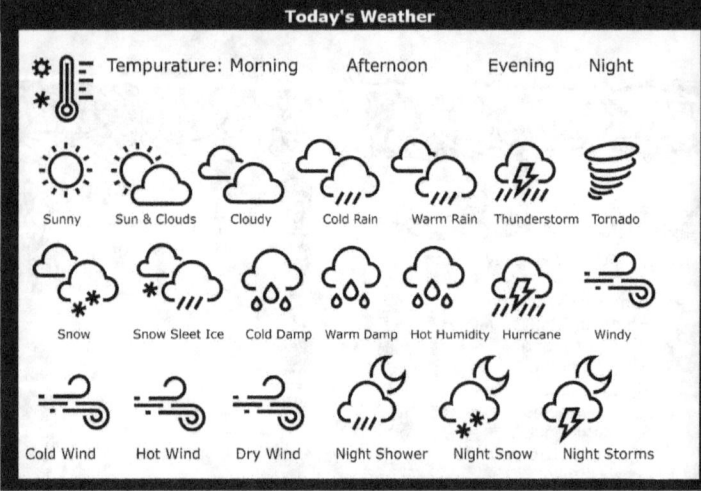

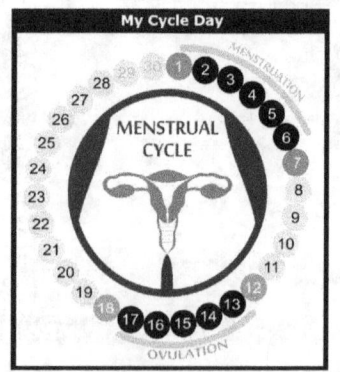

Breakfast

Lunch

Dinner

Snacks

Alcohol

Food Allergy Triggers

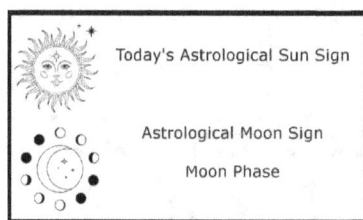

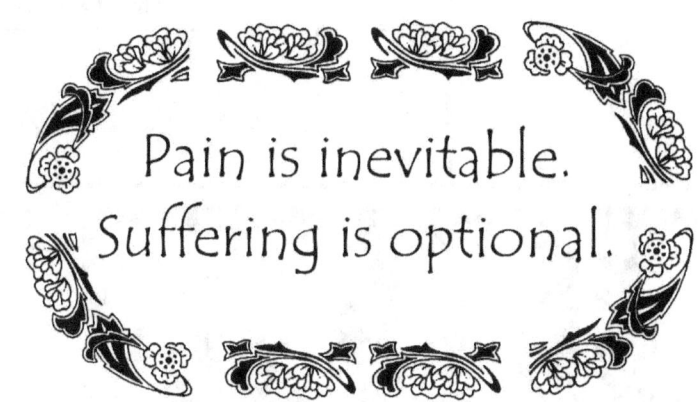

Notes

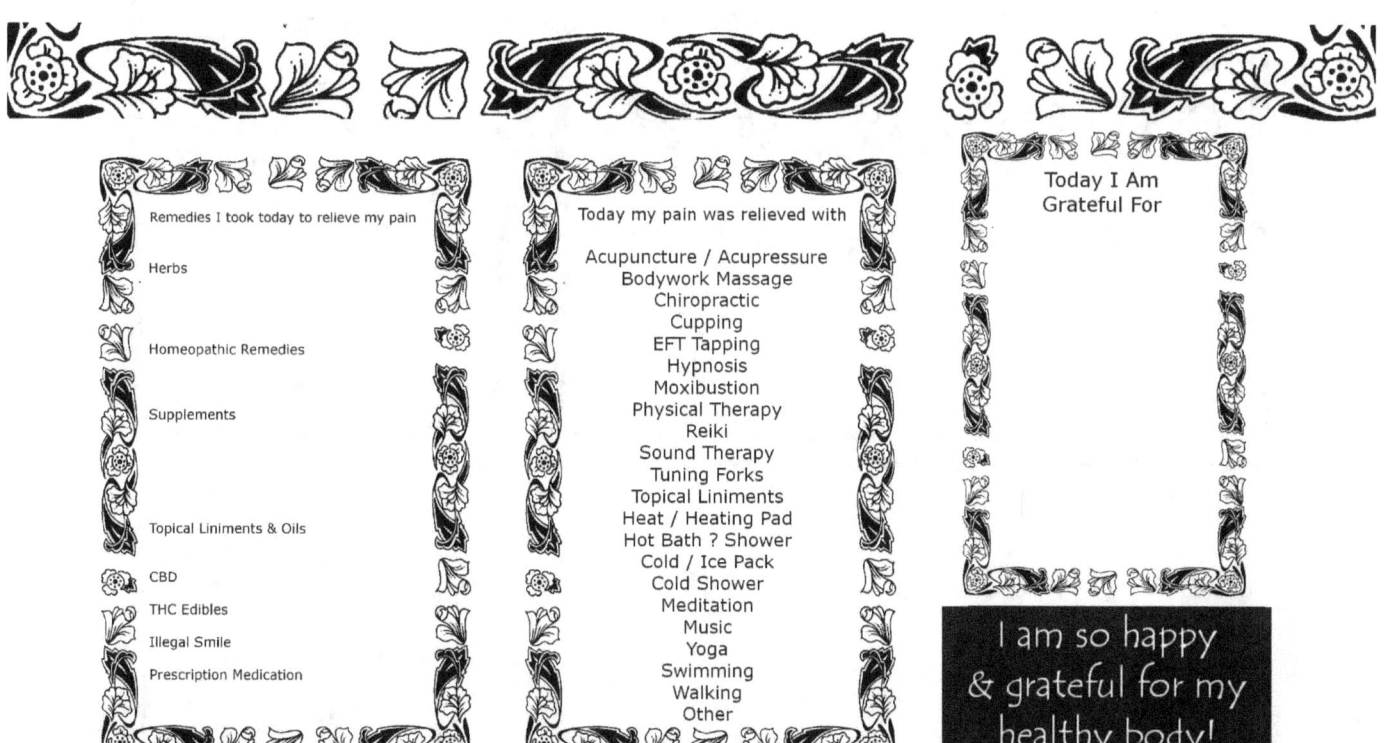

Remedies I took today to relieve my pain

Herbs

Homeopathic Remedies

Supplements

Topical Liniments & Oils

CBD

THC Edibles

Illegal Smile

Prescription Medication

Today my pain was relieved with

Acupuncture / Acupressure
Bodywork Massage
Chiropractic
Cupping
EFT Tapping
Hypnosis
Moxibustion
Physical Therapy
Reiki
Sound Therapy
Tuning Forks
Topical Liniments
Heat / Heating Pad
Hot Bath ? Shower
Cold / Ice Pack
Cold Shower
Meditation
Music
Yoga
Swimming
Walking
Other

Today I Am Grateful For

I am so happy & grateful for my healthy body!

Today's Day & Date

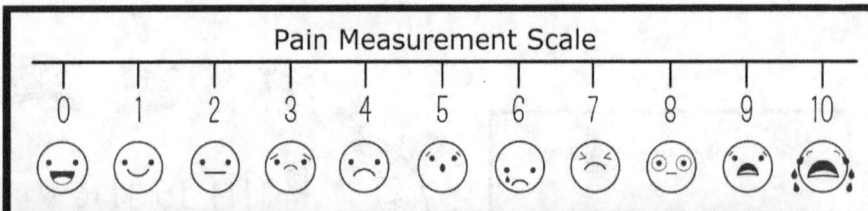

Highlight All Painful Areas

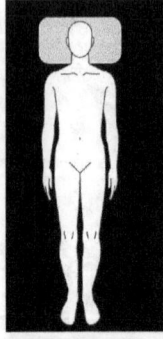 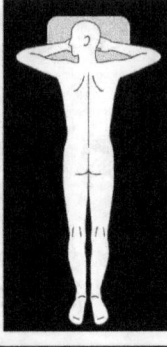 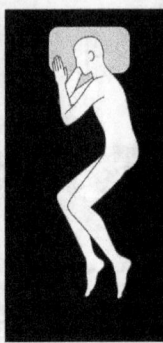 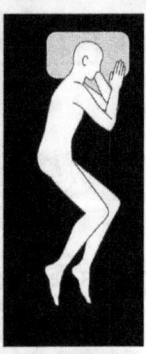

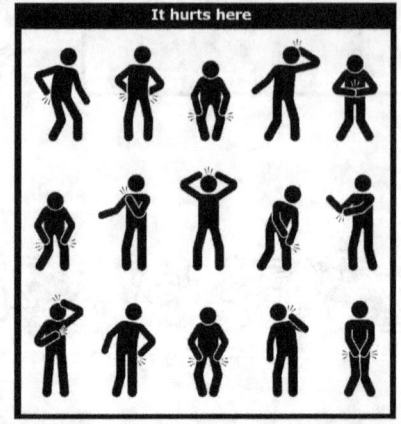

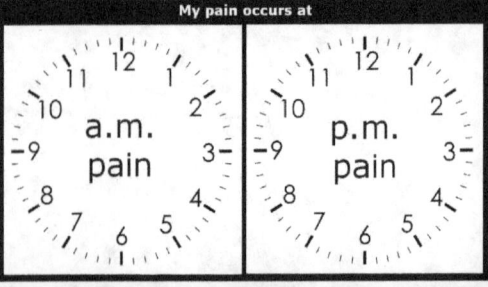

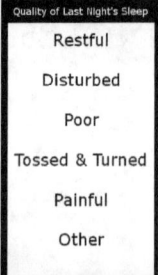

Quality of Last Night's Sleep
- Restful
- Disturbed
- Poor
- Tossed & Turned
- Painful
- Other

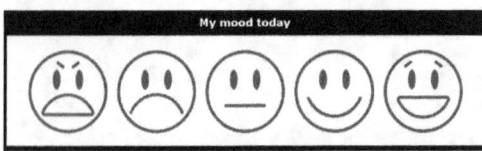

My mood today

My pain is
Hot
Burning
Cold
Stabbing
Throbbing
Fixed
Moving Traveling
Constant
On & Off

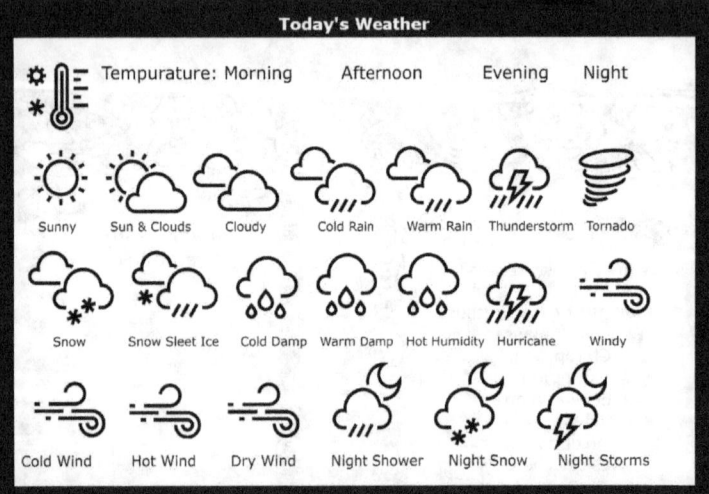

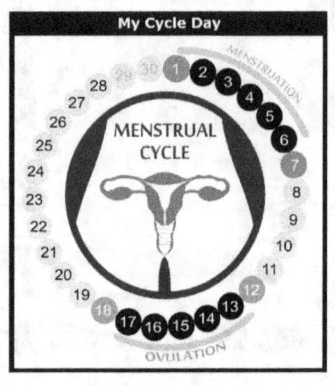

Breakfast

Lunch

Dinner

Snacks

Alcohol

Food Allergy Triggers

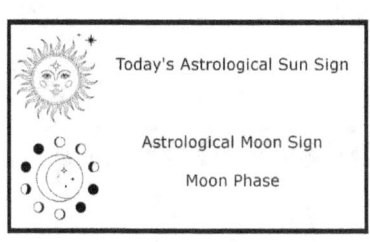

Today's Astrological Sun Sign

Astrological Moon Sign

Moon Phase

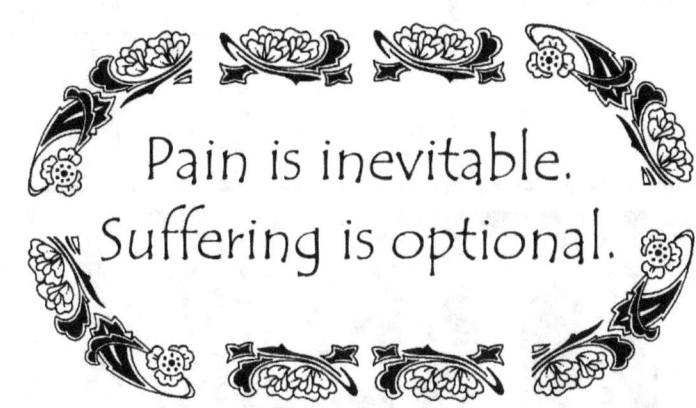

Pain is inevitable. Suffering is optional.

Notes

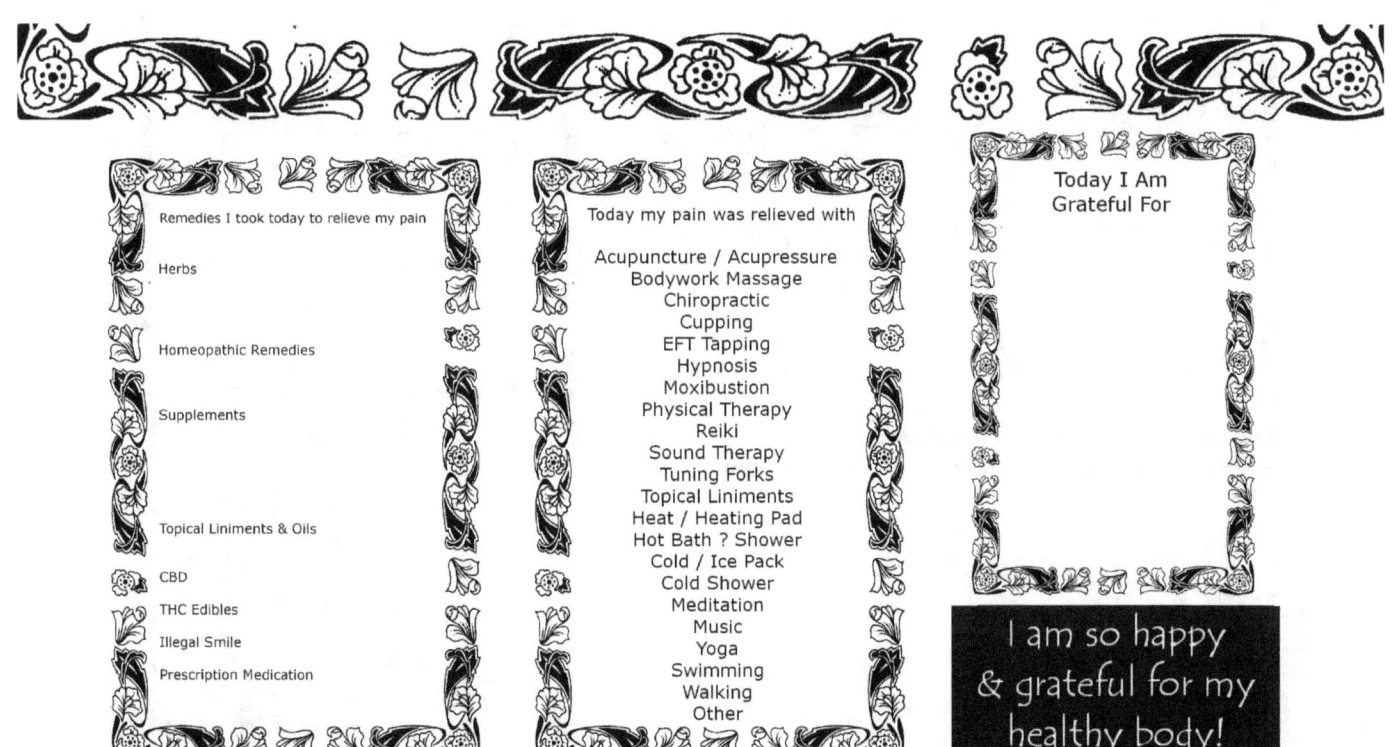

Remedies I took today to relieve my pain

Herbs

Homeopathic Remedies

Supplements

Topical Liniments & Oils

CBD

THC Edibles

Illegal Smile

Prescription Medication

Today my pain was relieved with

Acupuncture / Acupressure
Bodywork Massage
Chiropractic
Cupping
EFT Tapping
Hypnosis
Moxibustion
Physical Therapy
Reiki
Sound Therapy
Tuning Forks
Topical Liniments
Heat / Heating Pad
Hot Bath ? Shower
Cold / Ice Pack
Cold Shower
Meditation
Music
Yoga
Swimming
Walking
Other

Today I Am Grateful For

I am so happy & grateful for my healthy body!

Today's Day & Date

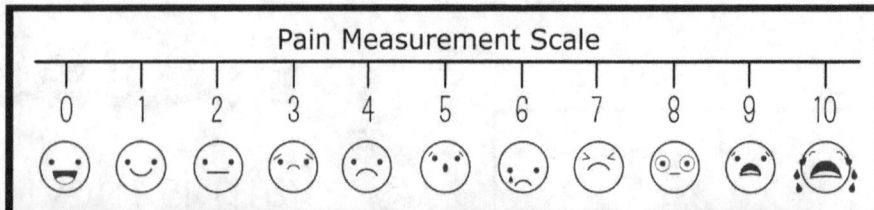

Highlight All Painful Areas

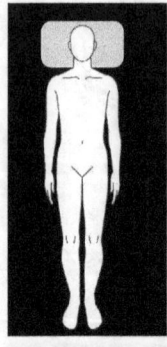 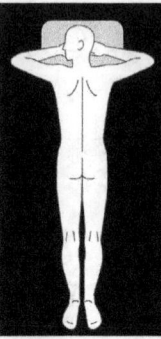 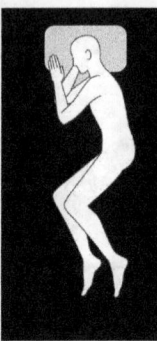 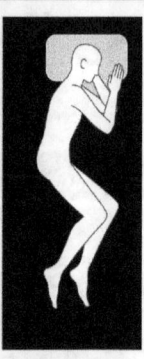

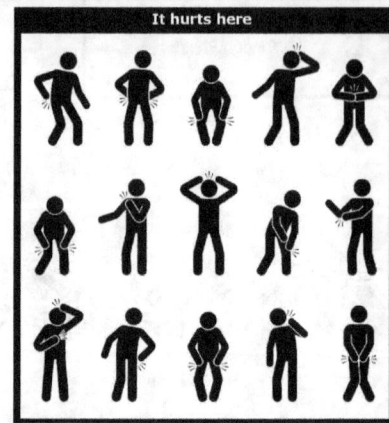
It hurts here

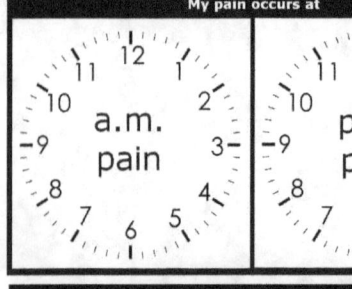
My pain occurs at — a.m. pain / p.m. pain

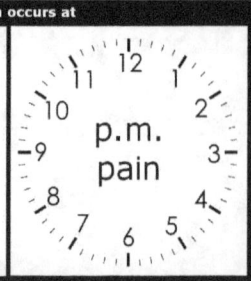
Quality of Last Night's Sleep
- Restful
- Disturbed
- Poor
- Tossed & Turned
- Painful
- Other

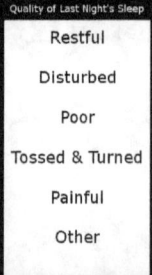
My mood today

My pain is
Hot
Burning
Cold
Stabbing
Throbbing
Fixed
Moving Traveling
Constant
On & Off

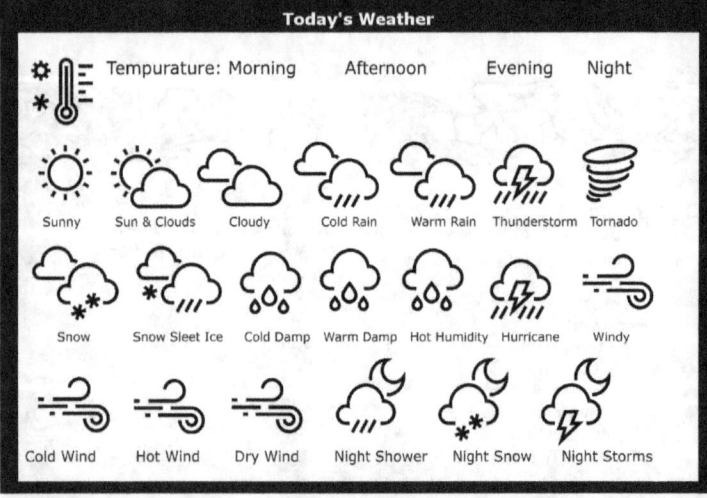
Today's Weather

Tempurature: Morning Afternoon Evening Night

Sunny, Sun & Clouds, Cloudy, Cold Rain, Warm Rain, Thunderstorm, Tornado
Snow, Snow Sleet Ice, Cold Damp, Warm Damp, Hot Humidity, Hurricane, Windy
Cold Wind, Hot Wind, Dry Wind, Night Shower, Night Snow, Night Storms

Breakfast

Lunch

Dinner

Snacks

Alcohol

Food Allergy Triggers

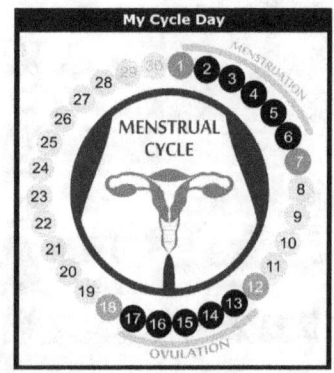
My Cycle Day

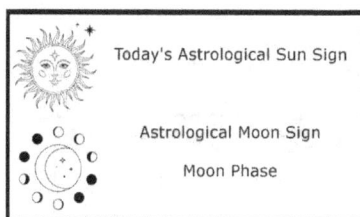

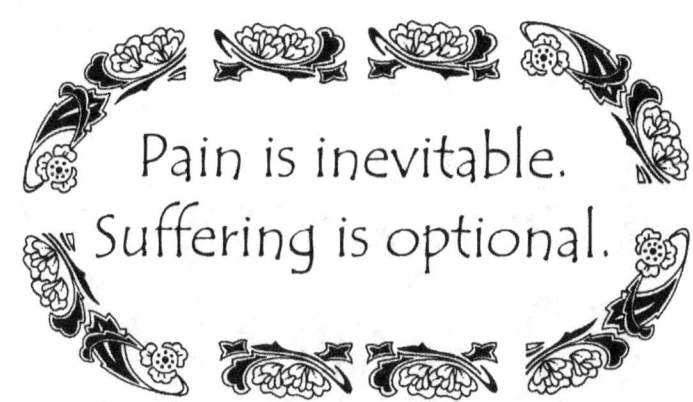

Pain is inevitable. Suffering is optional.

Notes

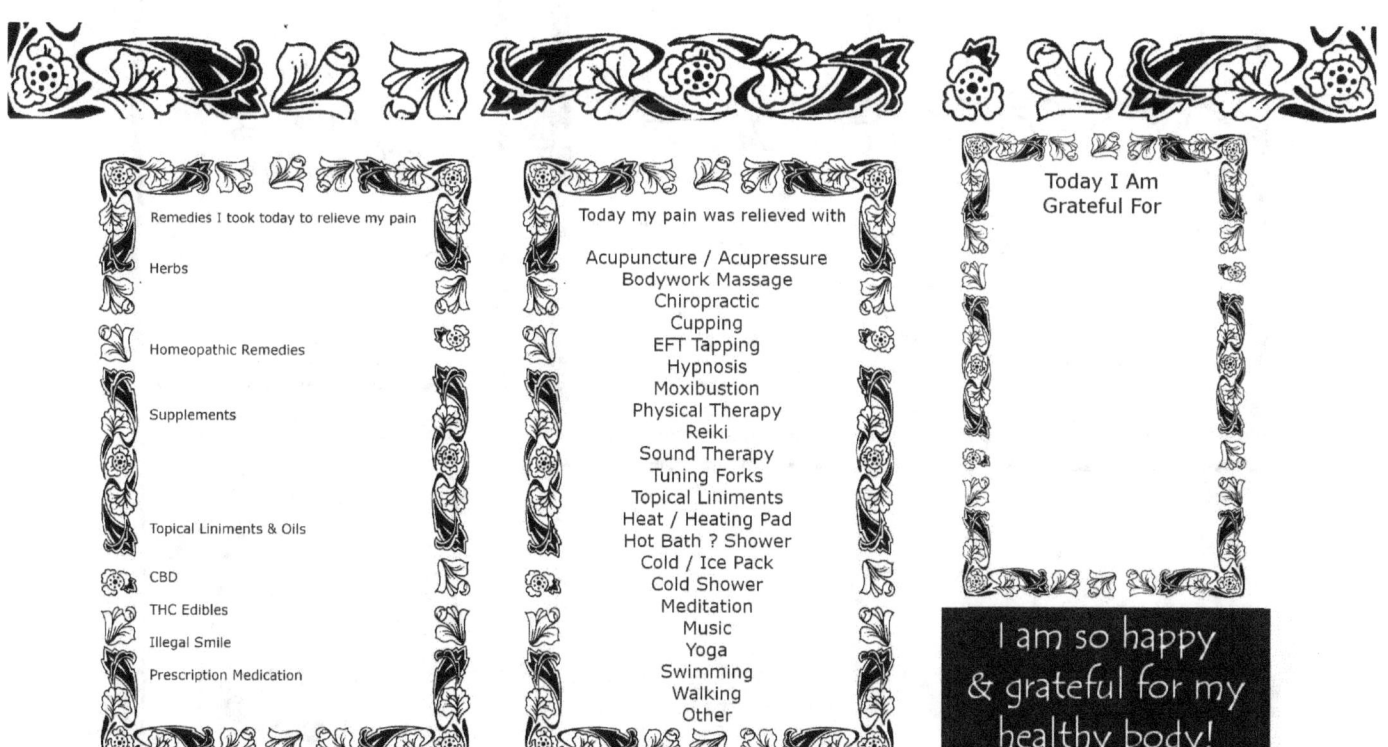

Remedies I took today to relieve my pain

Herbs

Homeopathic Remedies

Supplements

Topical Liniments & Oils

CBD

THC Edibles

Illegal Smile

Prescription Medication

Today my pain was relieved with

Acupuncture / Acupressure
Bodywork Massage
Chiropractic
Cupping
EFT Tapping
Hypnosis
Moxibustion
Physical Therapy
Reiki
Sound Therapy
Tuning Forks
Topical Liniments
Heat / Heating Pad
Hot Bath ? Shower
Cold / Ice Pack
Cold Shower
Meditation
Music
Yoga
Swimming
Walking
Other

Today I Am Grateful For

I am so happy & grateful for my healthy body!

Today's Day & Date

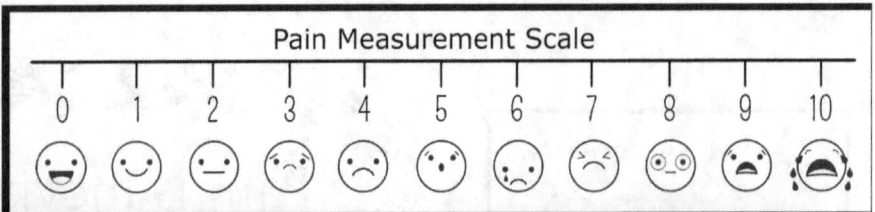

Highlight All Painful Areas

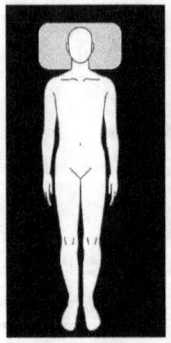 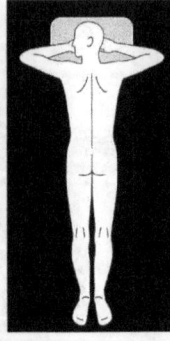 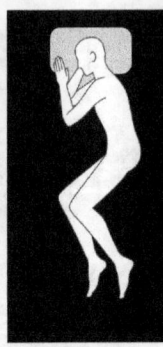 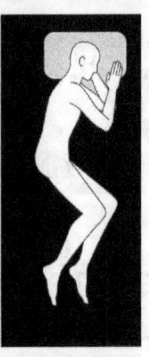

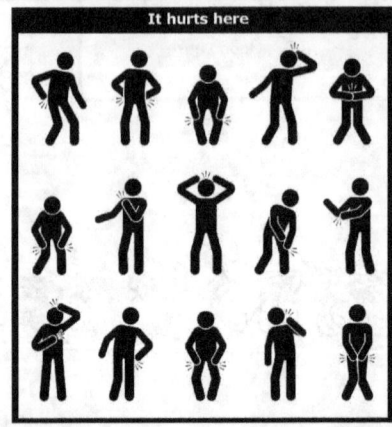
It hurts here

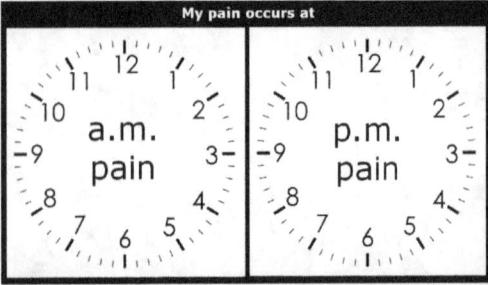
My pain occurs at — a.m. pain / p.m. pain

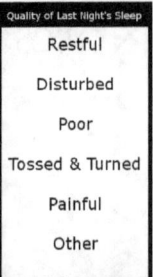

Quality of Last Night's Sleep
- Restful
- Disturbed
- Poor
- Tossed & Turned
- Painful
- Other

My mood today

My pain is
Hot
Burning
Cold
Stabbing
Throbbing
Fixed
Moving Traveling
Constant
On & Off

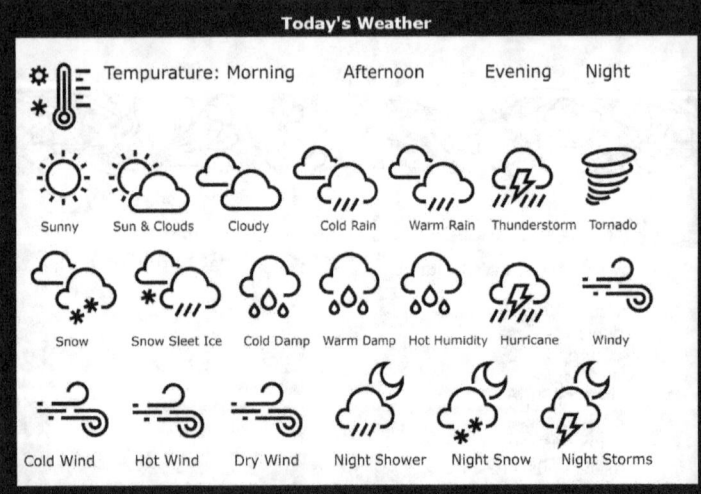
Today's Weather — Temperature: Morning, Afternoon, Evening, Night

Breakfast

Lunch

Dinner

Snacks

Alcohol

Food Allergy Triggers

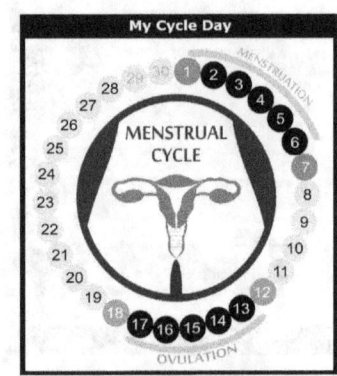
My Cycle Day

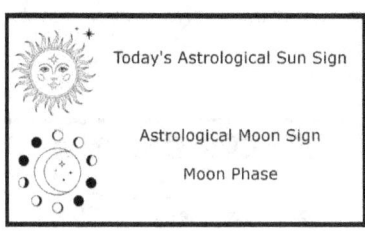

Today's Astrological Sun Sign

Astrological Moon Sign

Moon Phase

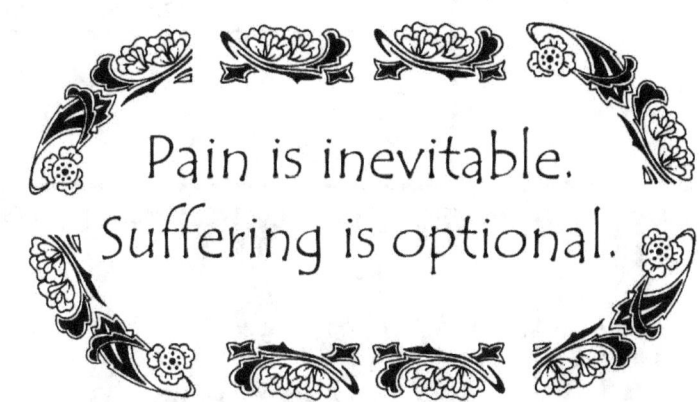

Pain is inevitable.
Suffering is optional.

Notes

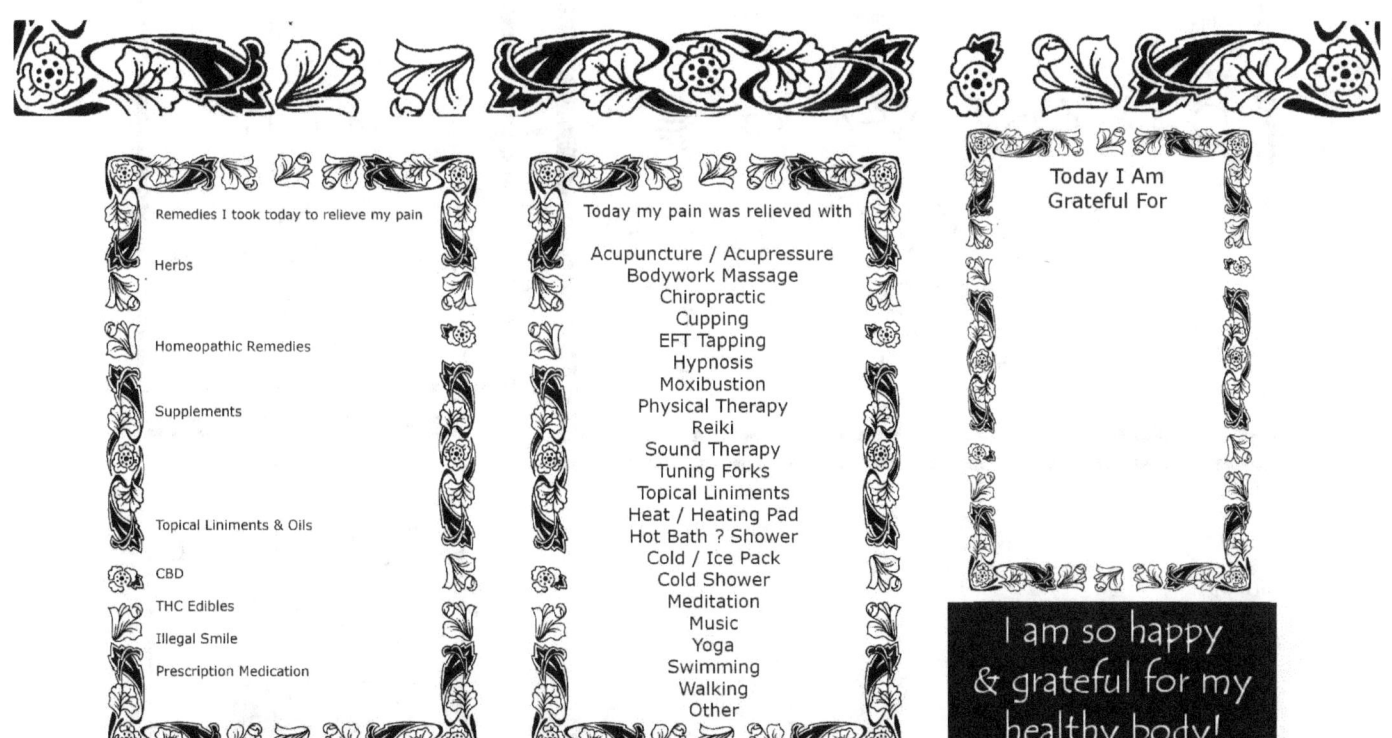

Remedies I took today to relieve my pain

Herbs

Homeopathic Remedies

Supplements

Topical Liniments & Oils

CBD

THC Edibles

Illegal Smile

Prescription Medication

Today my pain was relieved with

Acupuncture / Acupressure
Bodywork Massage
Chiropractic
Cupping
EFT Tapping
Hypnosis
Moxibustion
Physical Therapy
Reiki
Sound Therapy
Tuning Forks
Topical Liniments
Heat / Heating Pad
Hot Bath ? Shower
Cold / Ice Pack
Cold Shower
Meditation
Music
Yoga
Swimming
Walking
Other

Today I Am
Grateful For

I am so happy & grateful for my healthy body!

Today's Day & Date

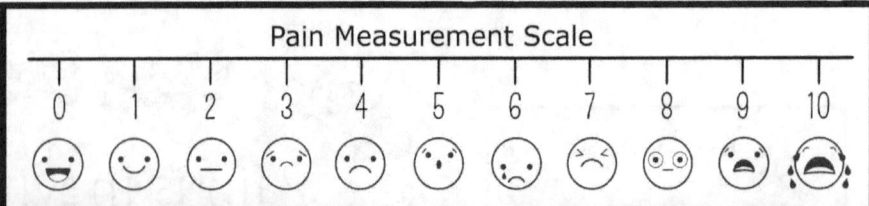

Highlight All Painful Areas

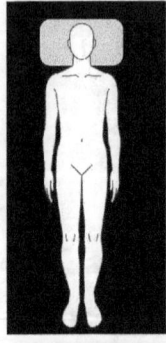 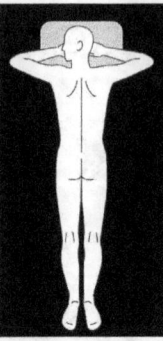 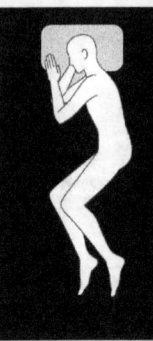 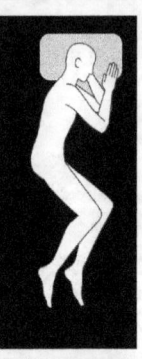

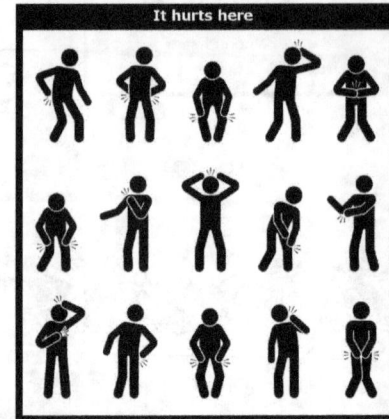
It hurts here

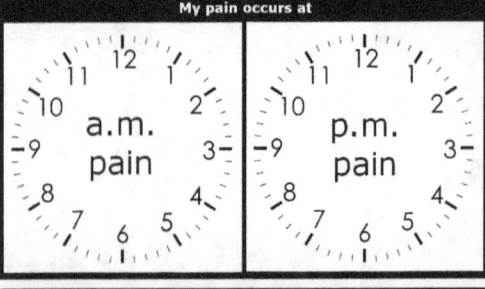
My pain occurs at — a.m. pain / p.m. pain

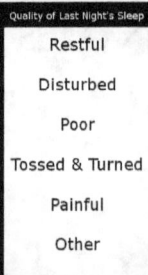
Quality of Last Night's Sleep
- Restful
- Disturbed
- Poor
- Tossed & Turned
- Painful
- Other

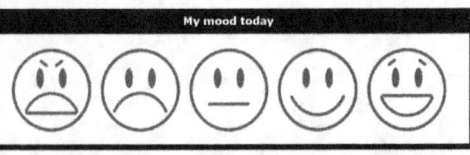
My mood today

My pain is
Hot
Burning
Cold
Stabbing
Throbbing
Fixed
Moving Traveling
Constant
On & Off

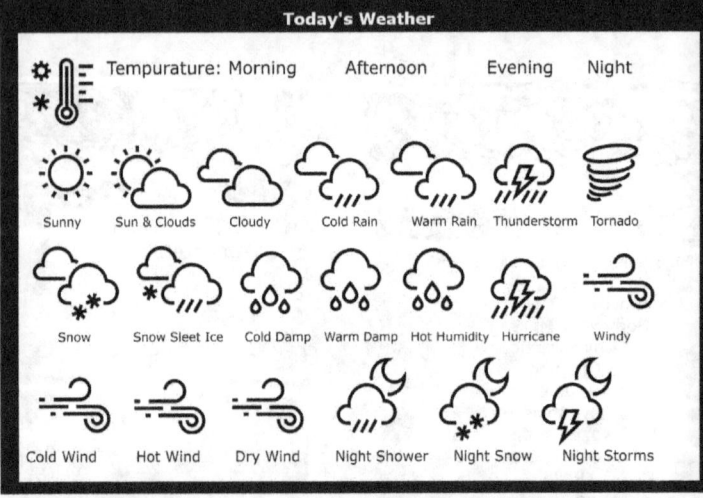
Today's Weather — Temperature: Morning, Afternoon, Evening, Night

Sunny, Sun & Clouds, Cloudy, Cold Rain, Warm Rain, Thunderstorm, Tornado
Snow, Snow Sleet Ice, Cold Damp, Warm Damp, Hot Humidity, Hurricane, Windy
Cold Wind, Hot Wind, Dry Wind, Night Shower, Night Snow, Night Storms

Breakfast

Lunch

Dinner

Snacks

Alcohol

Food Allergy Triggers

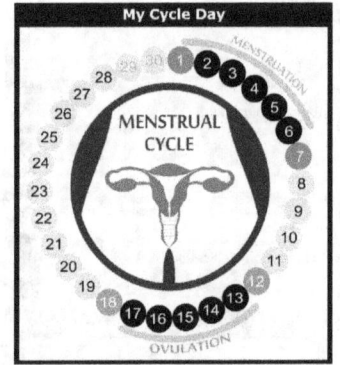
My Cycle Day

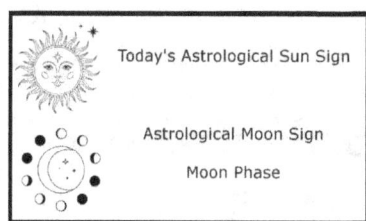

Today's Astrological Sun Sign

Astrological Moon Sign

Moon Phase

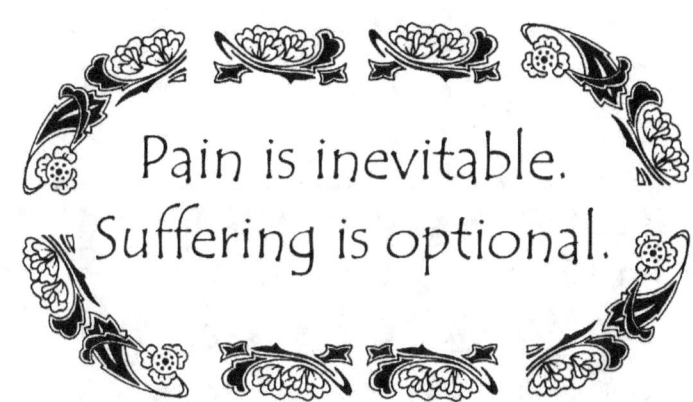

Pain is inevitable.
Suffering is optional.

Notes

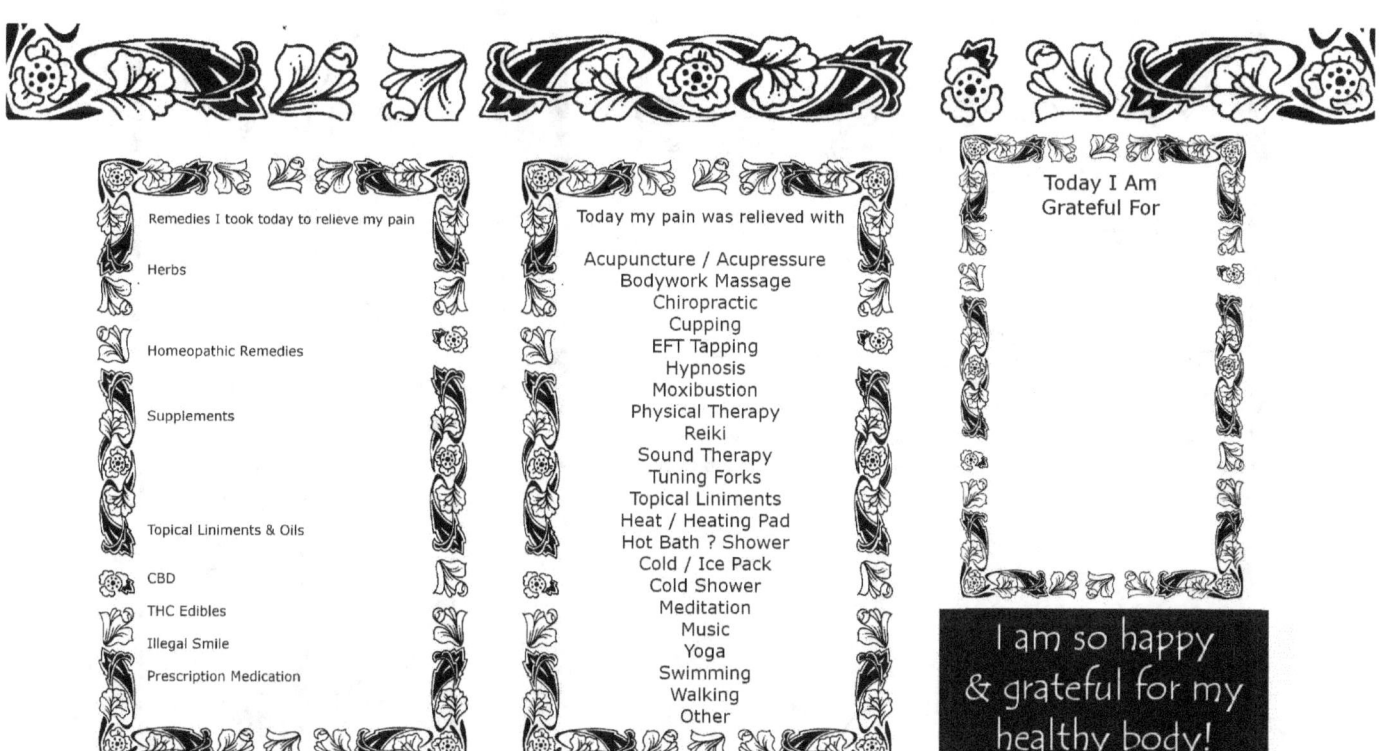

Remedies I took today to relieve my pain

Herbs

Homeopathic Remedies

Supplements

Topical Liniments & Oils

CBD
THC Edibles
Illegal Smile
Prescription Medication

Today my pain was relieved with

Acupuncture / Acupressure
Bodywork Massage
Chiropractic
Cupping
EFT Tapping
Hypnosis
Moxibustion
Physical Therapy
Reiki
Sound Therapy
Tuning Forks
Topical Liniments
Heat / Heating Pad
Hot Bath ? Shower
Cold / Ice Pack
Cold Shower
Meditation
Music
Yoga
Swimming
Walking
Other

Today I Am Grateful For

I am so happy & grateful for my healthy body!

Today's Day & Date

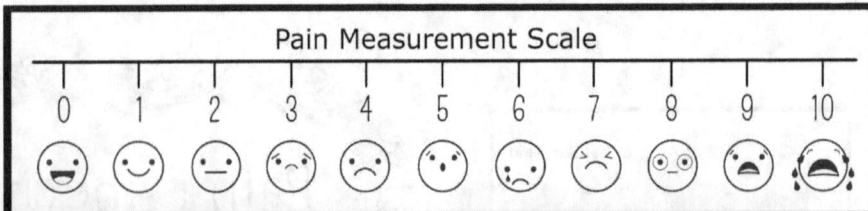

Highlight All Painful Areas

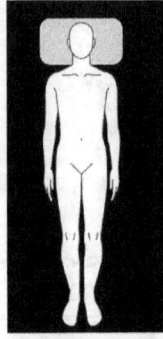 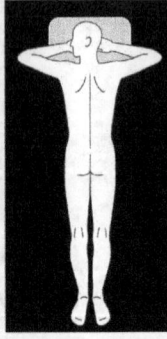 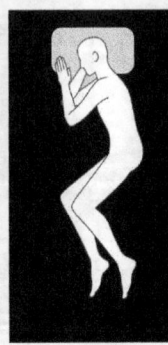 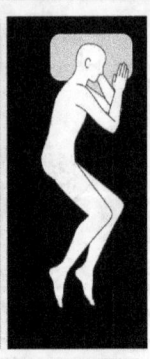

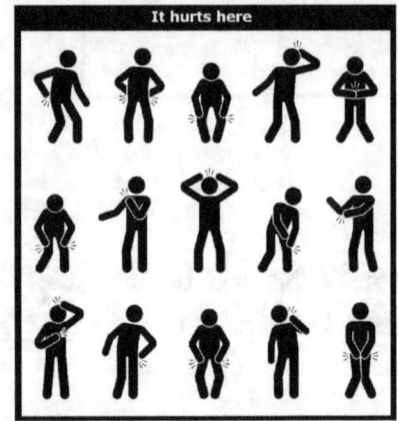
It hurts here

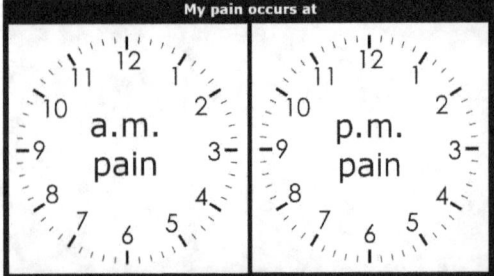
My pain occurs at — a.m. pain / p.m. pain

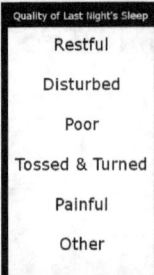

Quality of Last Night's Sleep
- Restful
- Disturbed
- Poor
- Tossed & Turned
- Painful
- Other

My mood today

My pain is
Hot
Burning
Cold
Stabbing
Throbbing
Fixed
Moving Traveling
Constant
On & Off

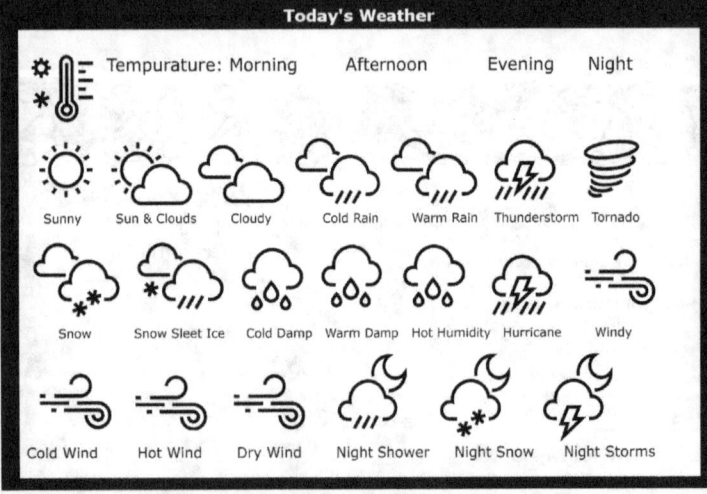
Today's Weather — Temperature: Morning, Afternoon, Evening, Night

Breakfast

Lunch

Dinner

Snacks

Alcohol

Food Allergy Triggers

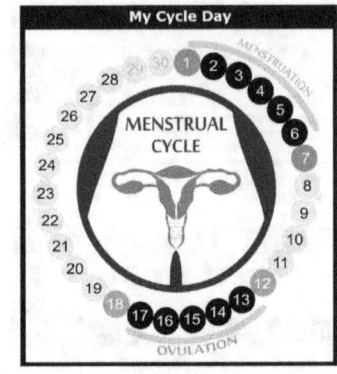
My Cycle Day

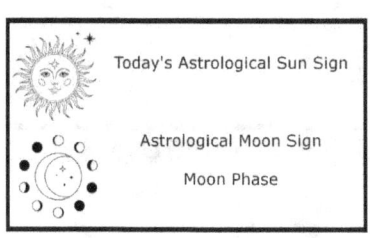

Today's Astrological Sun Sign

Astrological Moon Sign

Moon Phase

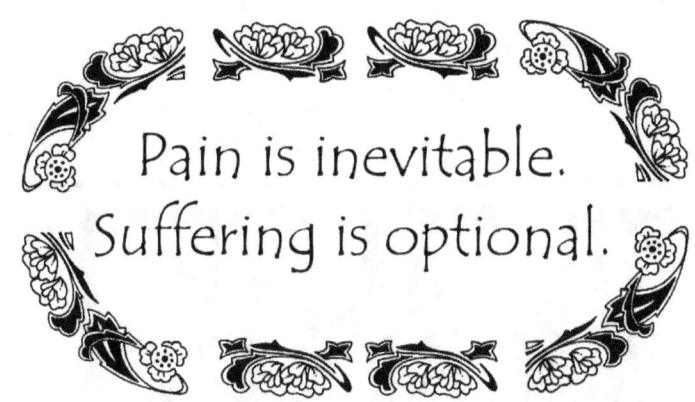

Pain is inevitable. Suffering is optional.

Notes

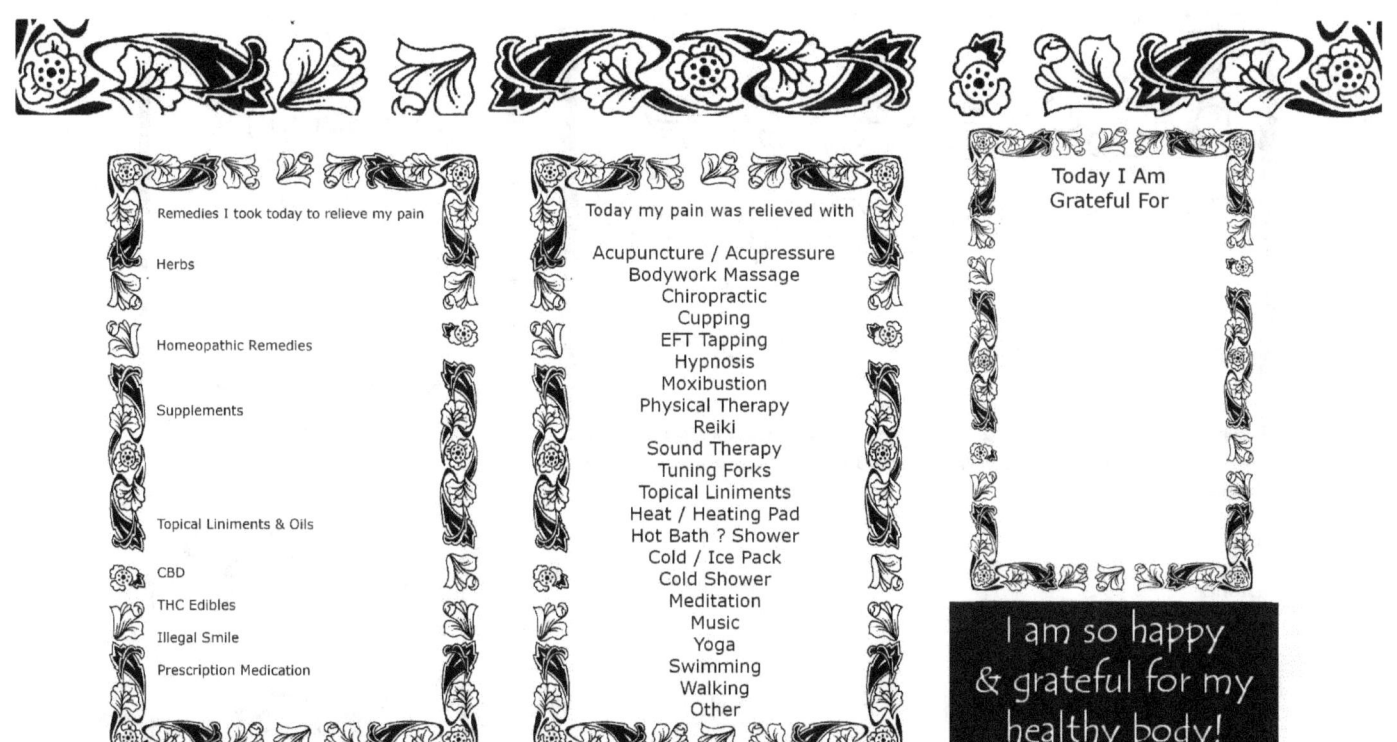

Remedies I took today to relieve my pain

Herbs

Homeopathic Remedies

Supplements

Topical Liniments & Oils

CBD
THC Edibles
Illegal Smile
Prescription Medication

Today my pain was relieved with

Acupuncture / Acupressure
Bodywork Massage
Chiropractic
Cupping
EFT Tapping
Hypnosis
Moxibustion
Physical Therapy
Reiki
Sound Therapy
Tuning Forks
Topical Liniments
Heat / Heating Pad
Hot Bath ? Shower
Cold / Ice Pack
Cold Shower
Meditation
Music
Yoga
Swimming
Walking
Other

Today I Am Grateful For

I am so happy & grateful for my healthy body!

Today's Day & Date

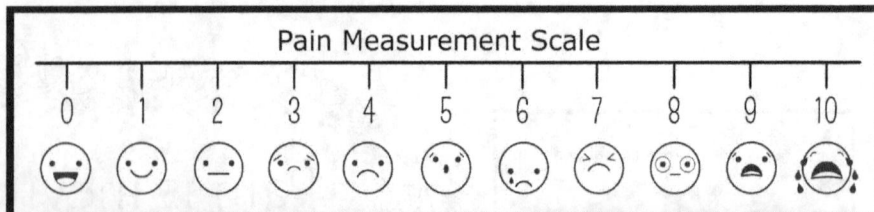

Pain Measurement Scale
0 1 2 3 4 5 6 7 8 9 10

Highlight All Painful Areas

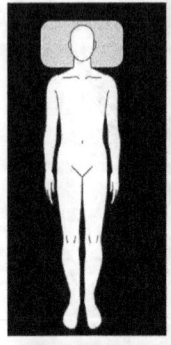 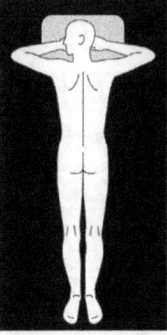 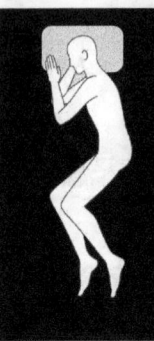 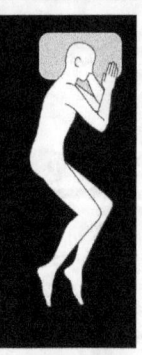

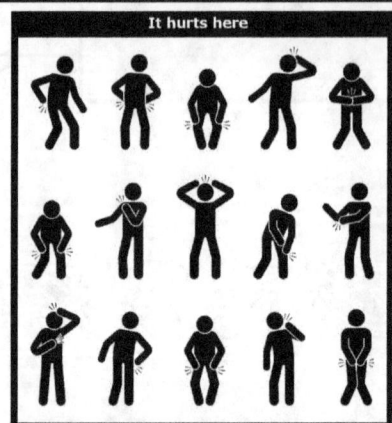
It hurts here

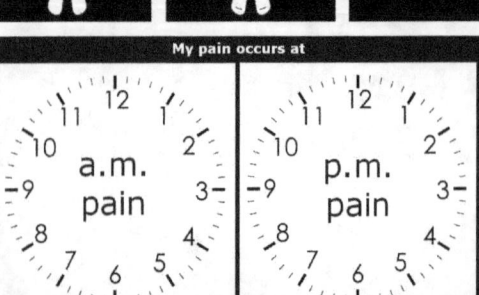
My pain occurs at — a.m. pain / p.m. pain

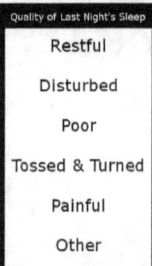
Quality of Last Night's Sleep
- Restful
- Disturbed
- Poor
- Tossed & Turned
- Painful
- Other

My mood today

My pain is
Hot
Burning
Cold
Stabbing
Throbbing
Fixed
Moving Traveling
Constant
On & Off

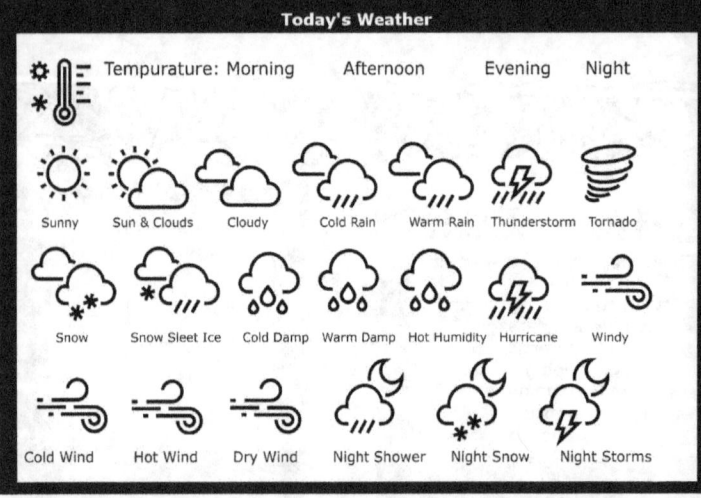
Today's Weather
Tempurature: Morning Afternoon Evening Night

Sunny, Sun & Clouds, Cloudy, Cold Rain, Warm Rain, Thunderstorm, Tornado
Snow, Snow Sleet Ice, Cold Damp, Warm Damp, Hot Humidity, Hurricane, Windy
Cold Wind, Hot Wind, Dry Wind, Night Shower, Night Snow, Night Storms

Breakfast

Lunch

Dinner

Snacks

Alcohol

Food Allergy Triggers

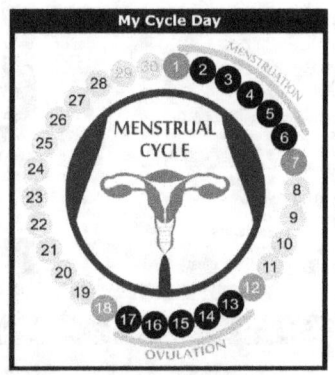
My Cycle Day

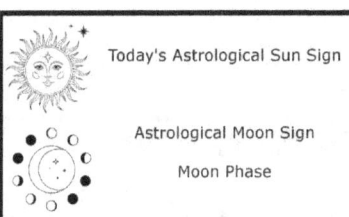

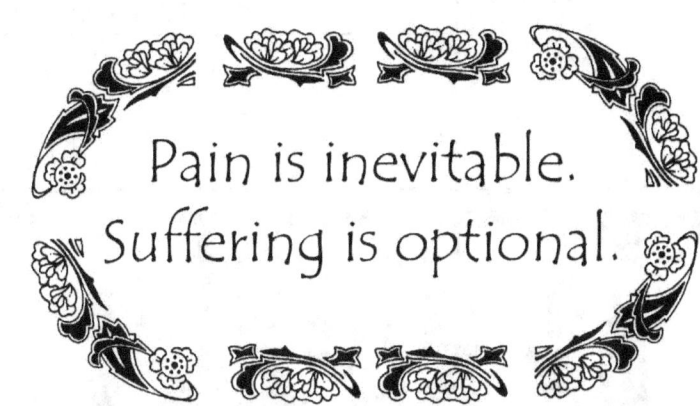

Notes

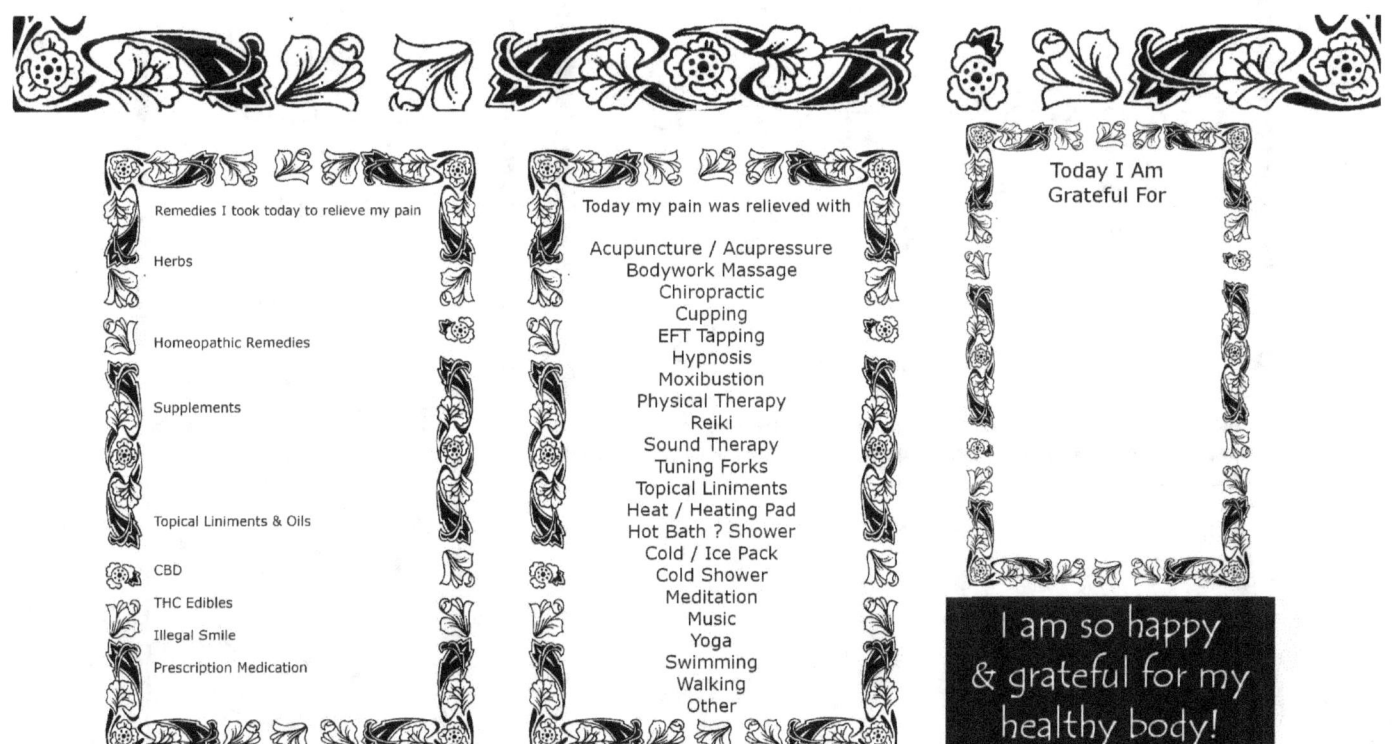

Remedies I took today to relieve my pain

Herbs

Homeopathic Remedies

Supplements

Topical Liniments & Oils

CBD

THC Edibles

Illegal Smile

Prescription Medication

Today my pain was relieved with

Acupuncture / Acupressure
Bodywork Massage
Chiropractic
Cupping
EFT Tapping
Hypnosis
Moxibustion
Physical Therapy
Reiki
Sound Therapy
Tuning Forks
Topical Liniments
Heat / Heating Pad
Hot Bath ? Shower
Cold / Ice Pack
Cold Shower
Meditation
Music
Yoga
Swimming
Walking
Other

Today I Am Grateful For

I am so happy & grateful for my healthy body!

Today's Day & Date

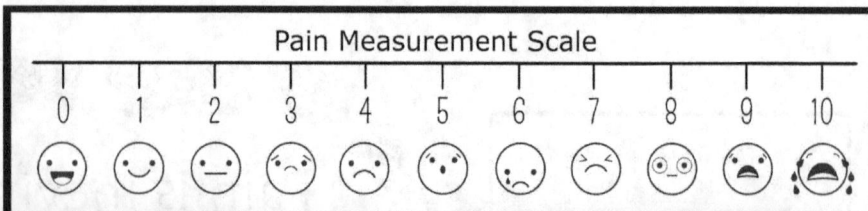

Highlight All Painful Areas

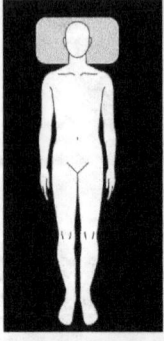 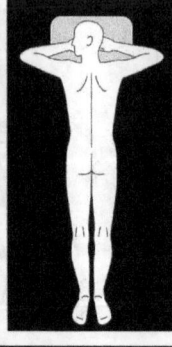 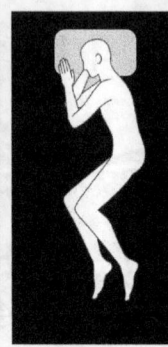 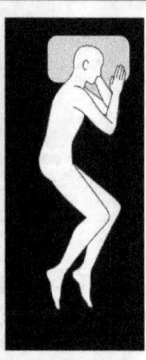

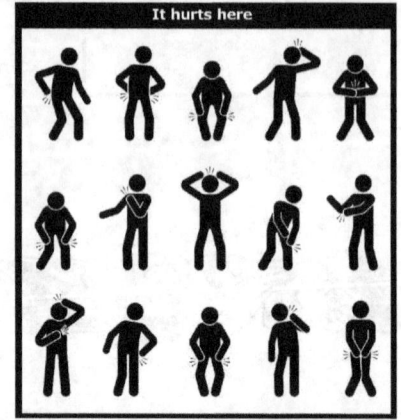

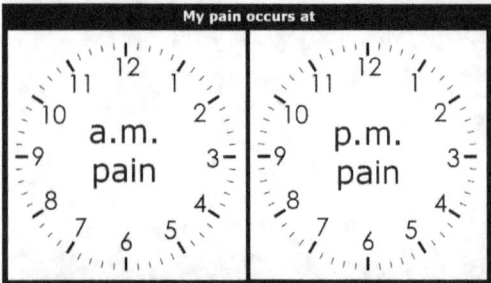

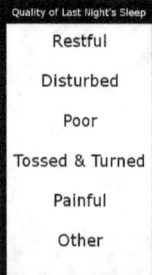

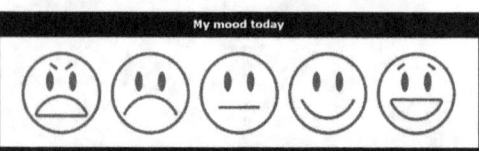

My pain is
Hot
Burning
Cold
Stabbing
Throbbing
Fixed
Moving Traveling
Constant
On & Off

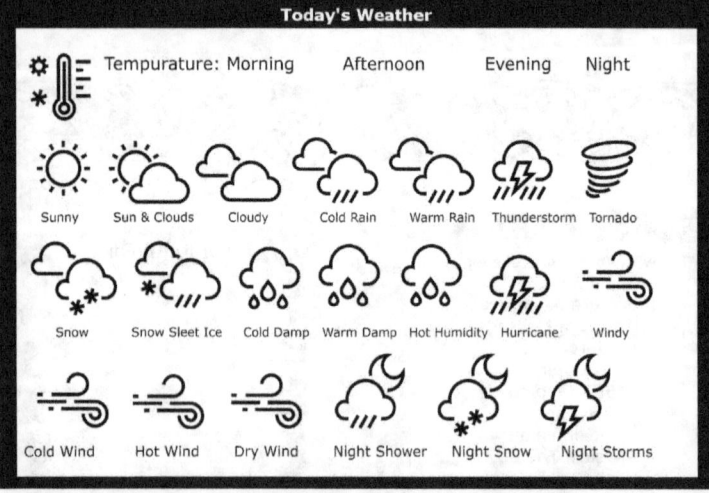

Breakfast

Lunch

Dinner

Snacks

Alcohol

Food Allergy Triggers

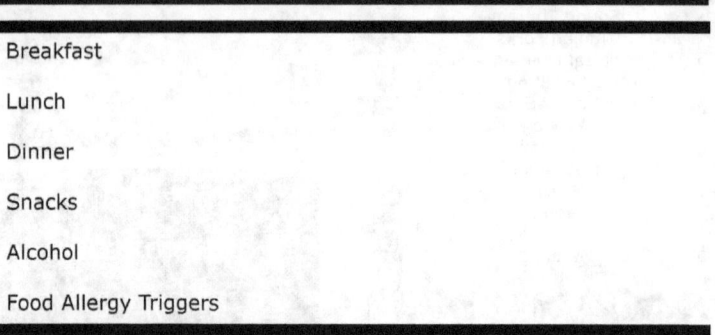

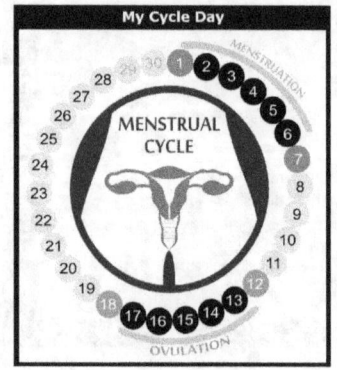

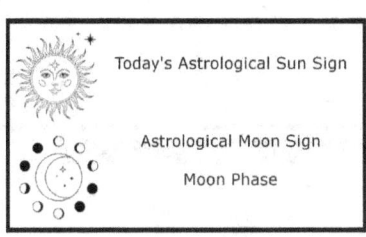

Today's Astrological Sun Sign

Astrological Moon Sign

Moon Phase

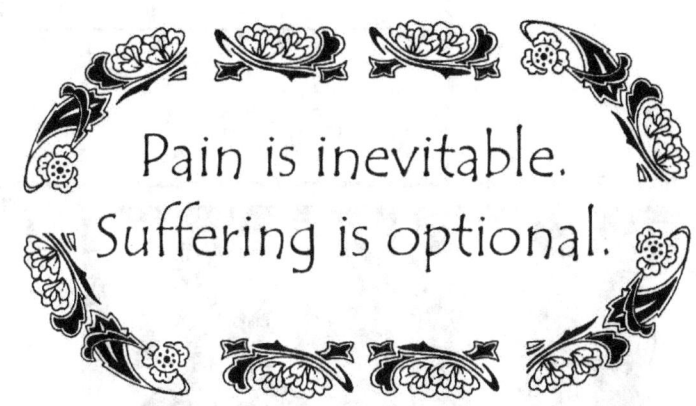

Pain is inevitable.
Suffering is optional.

Notes

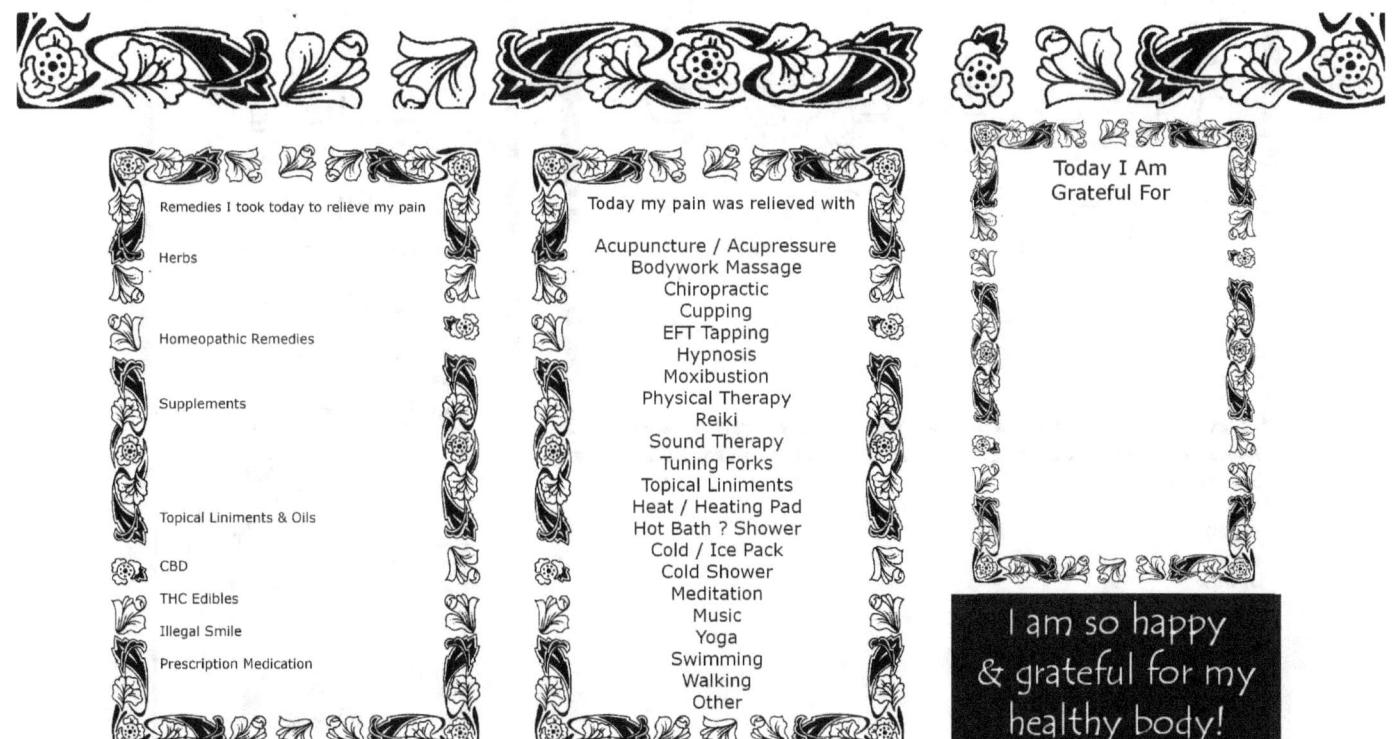

Remedies I took today to relieve my pain

Herbs

Homeopathic Remedies

Supplements

Topical Liniments & Oils

CBD
THC Edibles
Illegal Smile
Prescription Medication

Today my pain was relieved with

Acupuncture / Acupressure
Bodywork Massage
Chiropractic
Cupping
EFT Tapping
Hypnosis
Moxibustion
Physical Therapy
Reiki
Sound Therapy
Tuning Forks
Topical Liniments
Heat / Heating Pad
Hot Bath ? Shower
Cold / Ice Pack
Cold Shower
Meditation
Music
Yoga
Swimming
Walking
Other

Today I Am Grateful For

I am so happy & grateful for my healthy body!

Today's Day & Date

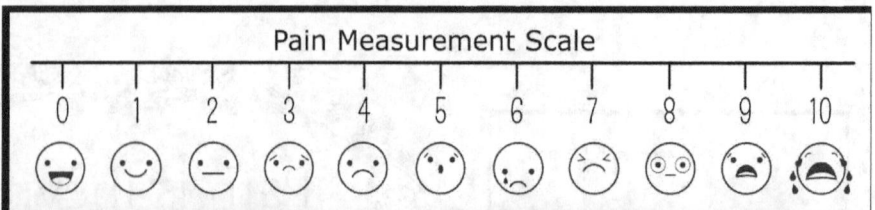

Highlight All Painful Areas

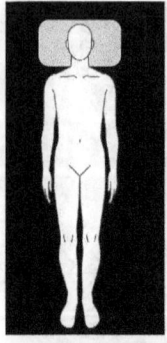 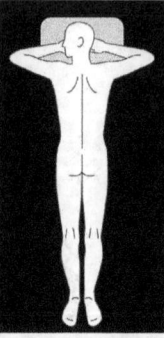 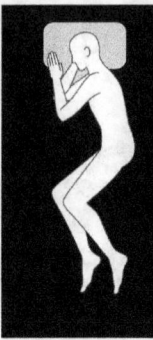 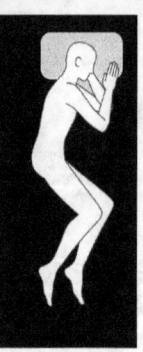

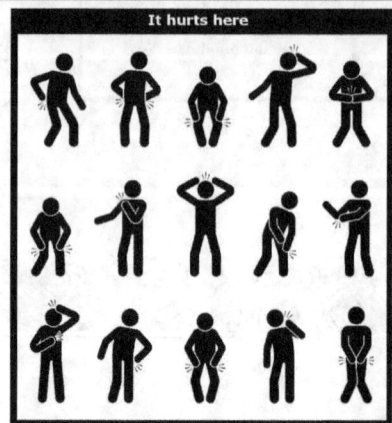

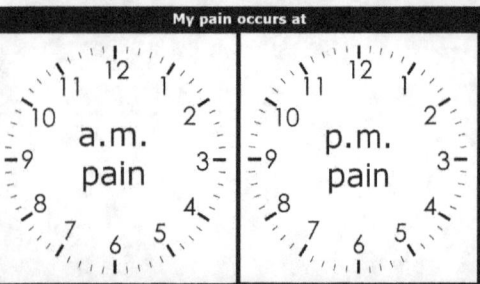

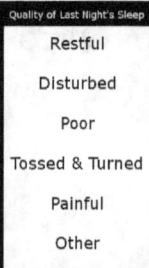

Quality of Last Night's Sleep
- Restful
- Disturbed
- Poor
- Tossed & Turned
- Painful
- Other

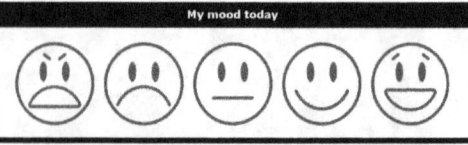

My pain is
Hot
Burning
Cold
Stabbing
Throbbing
Fixed
Moving Traveling
Constant
On & Off

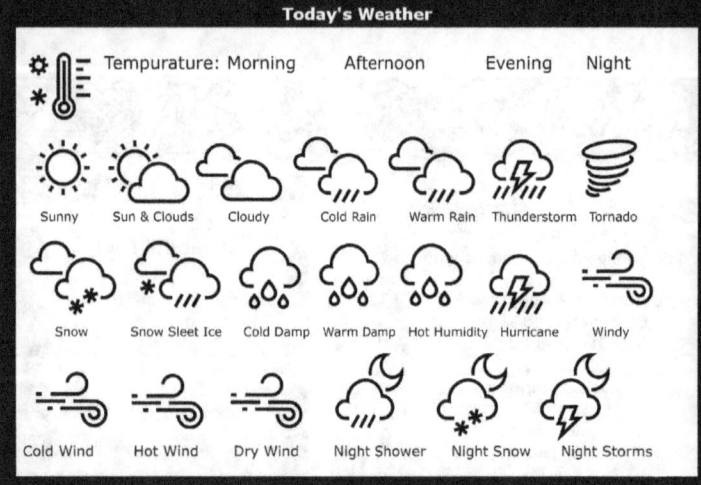

Breakfast

Lunch

Dinner

Snacks

Alcohol

Food Allergy Triggers

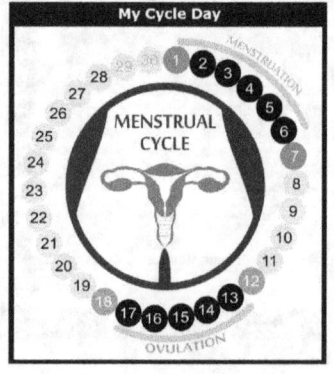

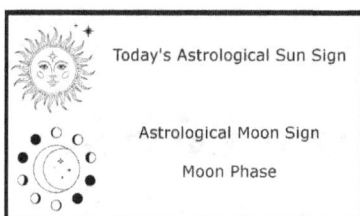

Today's Astrological Sun Sign

Astrological Moon Sign

Moon Phase

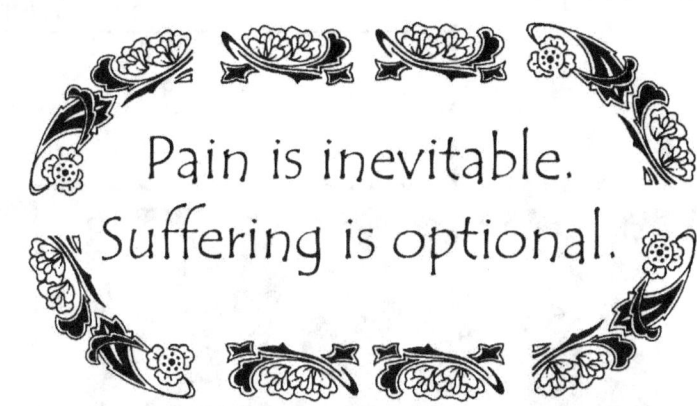

Pain is inevitable.
Suffering is optional.

Notes

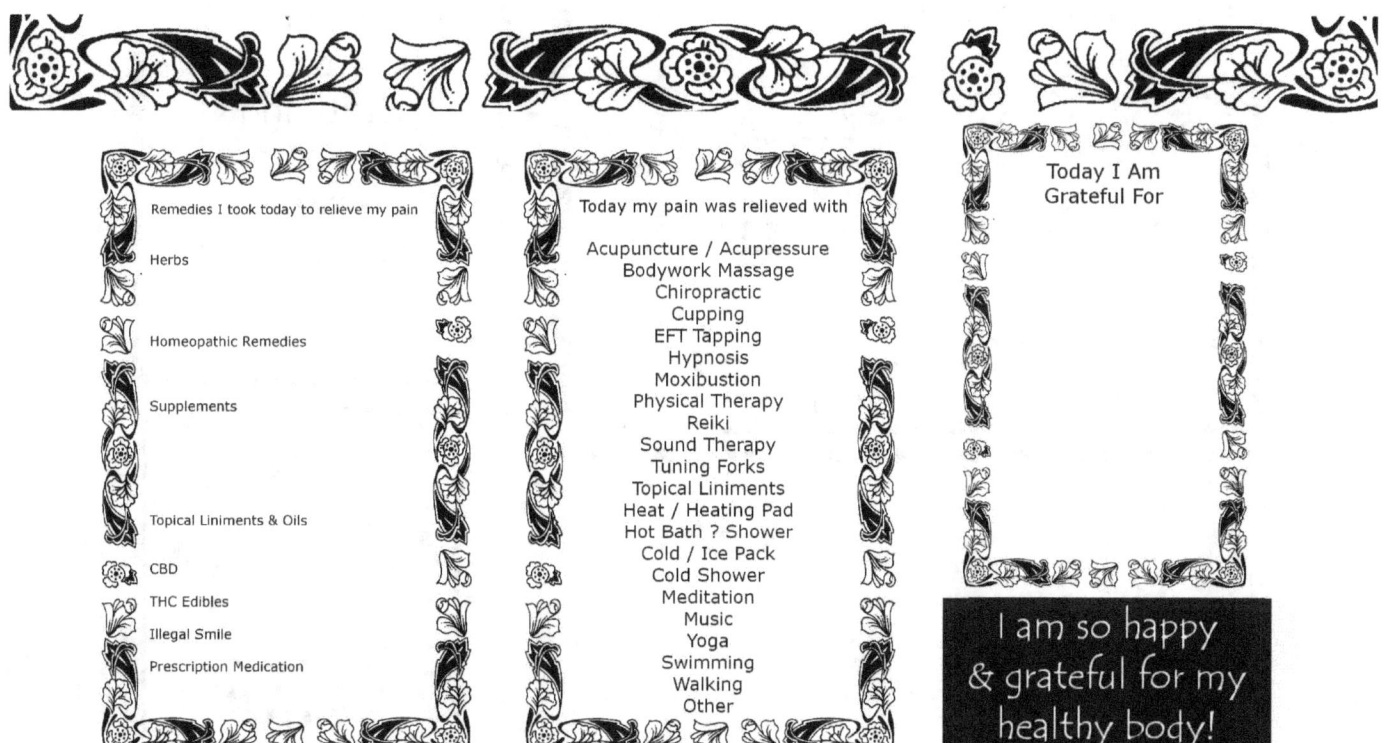

Remedies I took today to relieve my pain

Herbs

Homeopathic Remedies

Supplements

Topical Liniments & Oils

CBD

THC Edibles

Illegal Smile

Prescription Medication

Today my pain was relieved with

Acupuncture / Acupressure
Bodywork Massage
Chiropractic
Cupping
EFT Tapping
Hypnosis
Moxibustion
Physical Therapy
Reiki
Sound Therapy
Tuning Forks
Topical Liniments
Heat / Heating Pad
Hot Bath ? Shower
Cold / Ice Pack
Cold Shower
Meditation
Music
Yoga
Swimming
Walking
Other

Today I Am Grateful For

I am so happy & grateful for my healthy body!

Today's Day & Date

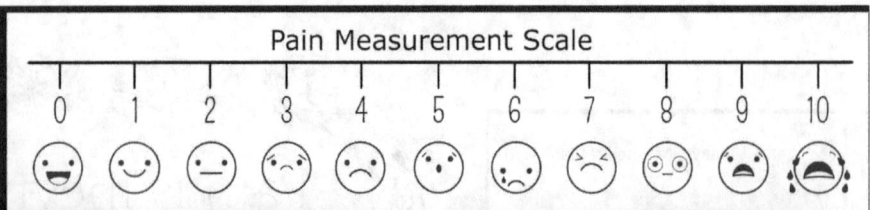

Highlight All Painful Areas

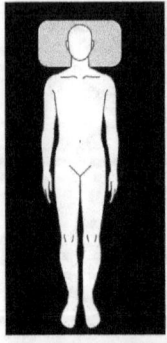 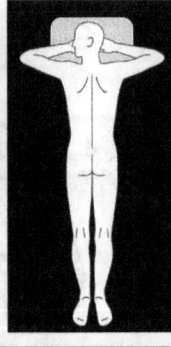 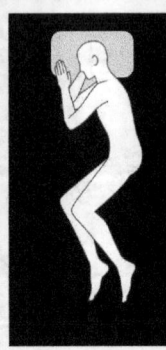 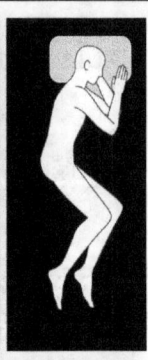

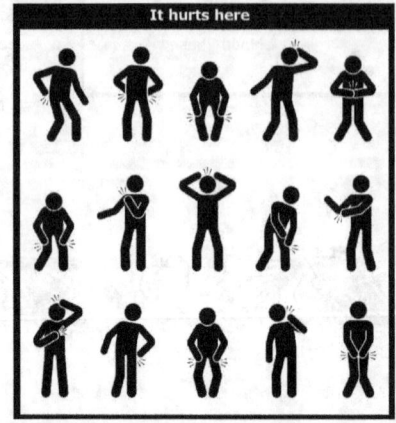

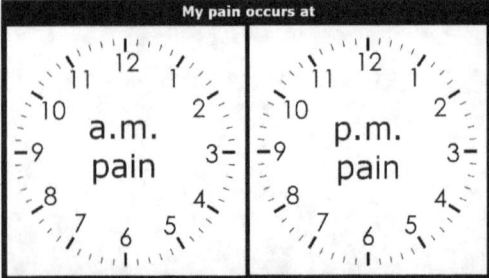

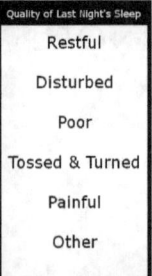

Quality of Last Night's Sleep
Restful
Disturbed
Poor
Tossed & Turned
Painful
Other

My pain is
Hot
Burning
Cold
Stabbing
Throbbing
Fixed
Moving Traveling
Constant
On & Off

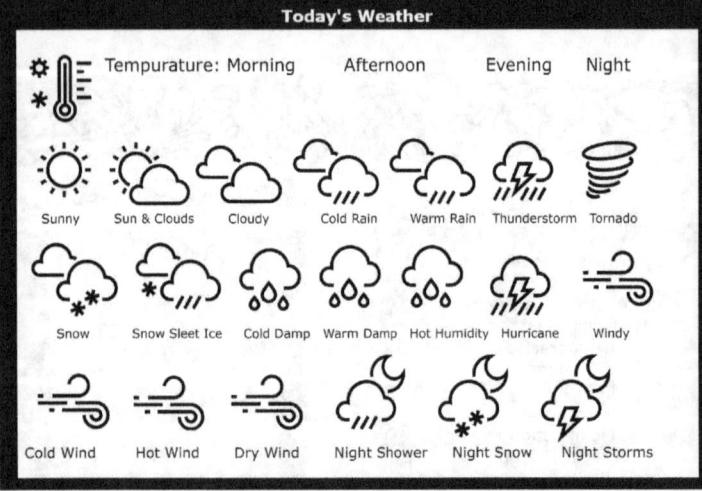

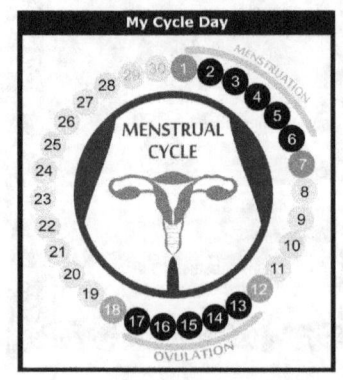

Breakfast

Lunch

Dinner

Snacks

Alcohol

Food Allergy Triggers

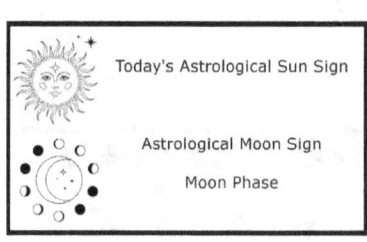

Today's Astrological Sun Sign

Astrological Moon Sign

Moon Phase

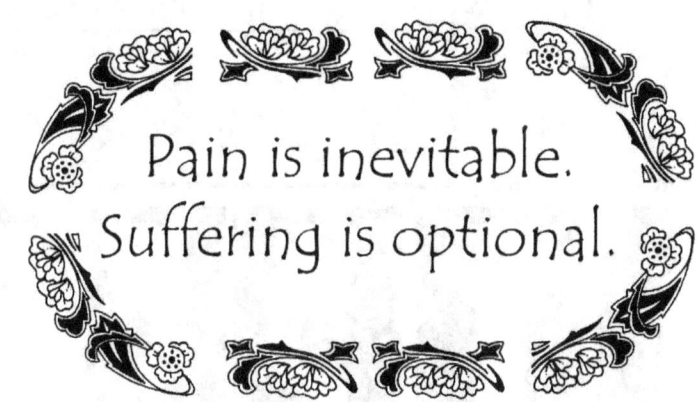

Pain is inevitable.
Suffering is optional.

Notes

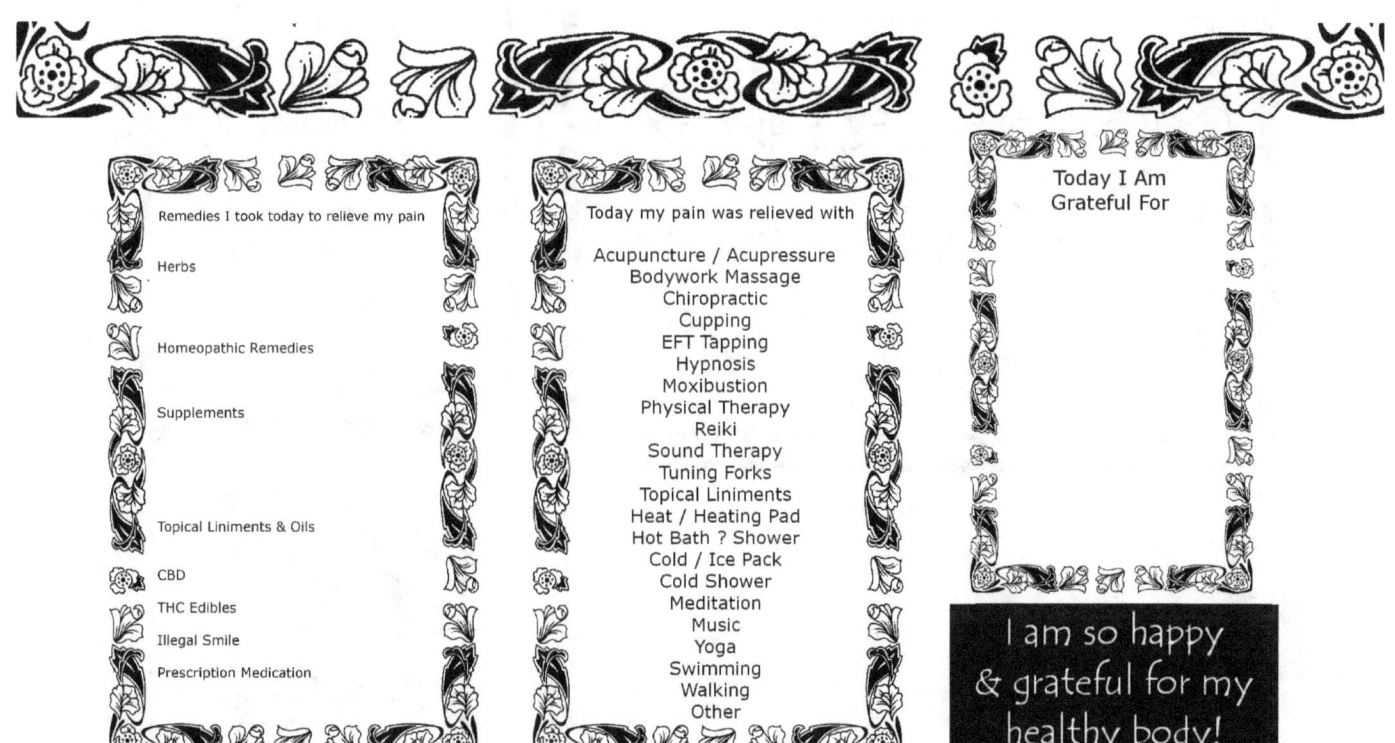

Remedies I took today to relieve my pain

Herbs

Homeopathic Remedies

Supplements

Topical Liniments & Oils

CBD

THC Edibles

Illegal Smile

Prescription Medication

Today my pain was relieved with

Acupuncture / Acupressure
Bodywork Massage
Chiropractic
Cupping
EFT Tapping
Hypnosis
Moxibustion
Physical Therapy
Reiki
Sound Therapy
Tuning Forks
Topical Liniments
Heat / Heating Pad
Hot Bath ? Shower
Cold / Ice Pack
Cold Shower
Meditation
Music
Yoga
Swimming
Walking
Other

Today I Am Grateful For

I am so happy & grateful for my healthy body!

Today's Day & Date

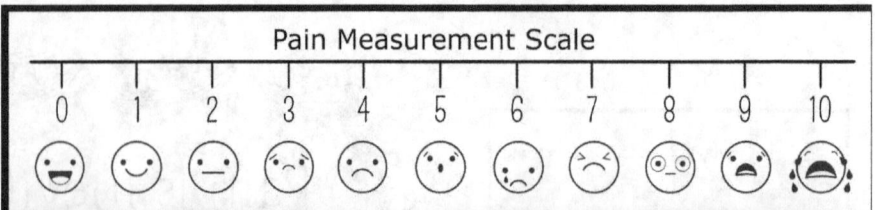

Highlight All Painful Areas

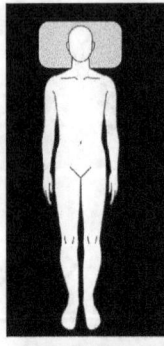 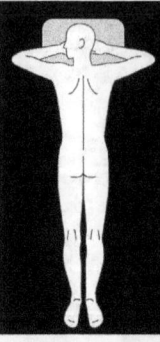 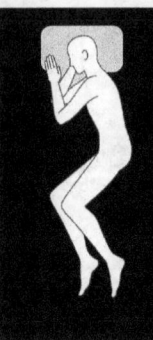 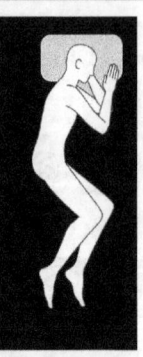 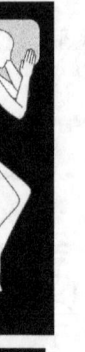

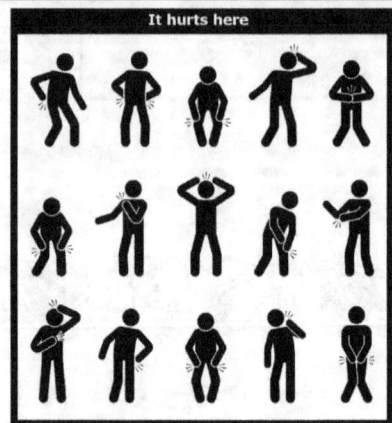

It hurts here

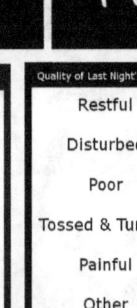

My pain occurs at — a.m. pain / p.m. pain

Quality of Last Night's Sleep
- Restful
- Disturbed
- Poor
- Tossed & Turned
- Painful
- Other

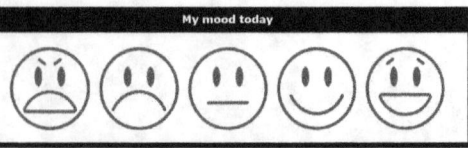

My mood today

My pain is
Hot
Burning
Cold
Stabbing
Throbbing
Fixed
Moving Traveling
Constant
On & Off

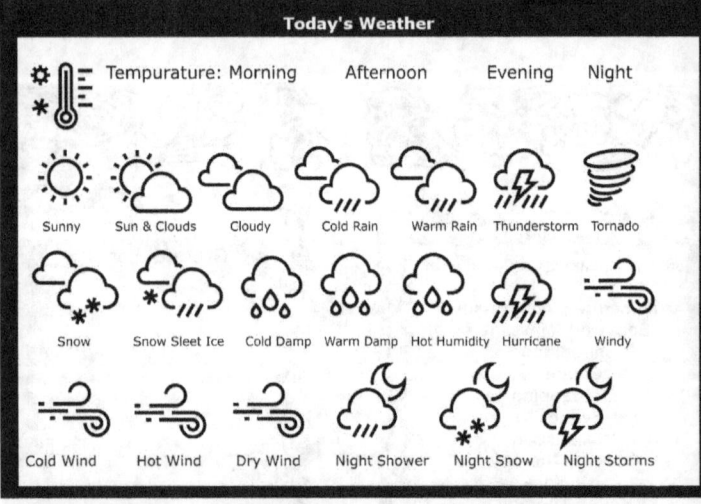

Breakfast

Lunch

Dinner

Snacks

Alcohol

Food Allergy Triggers

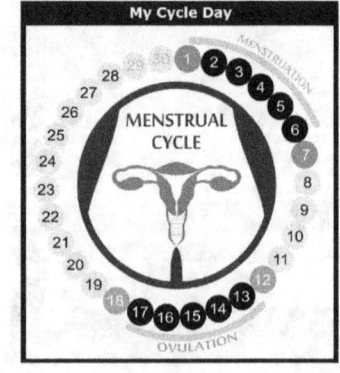

My Cycle Day

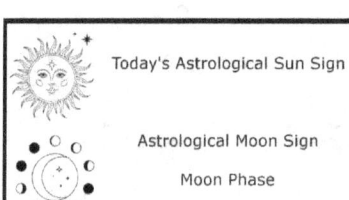

Today's Astrological Sun Sign

Astrological Moon Sign

Moon Phase

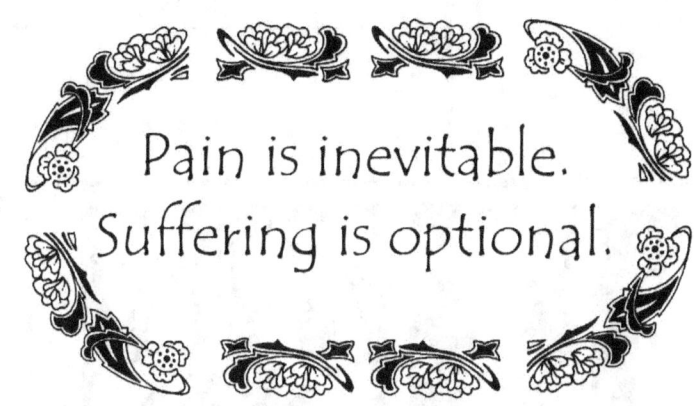

Pain is inevitable.
Suffering is optional.

Notes

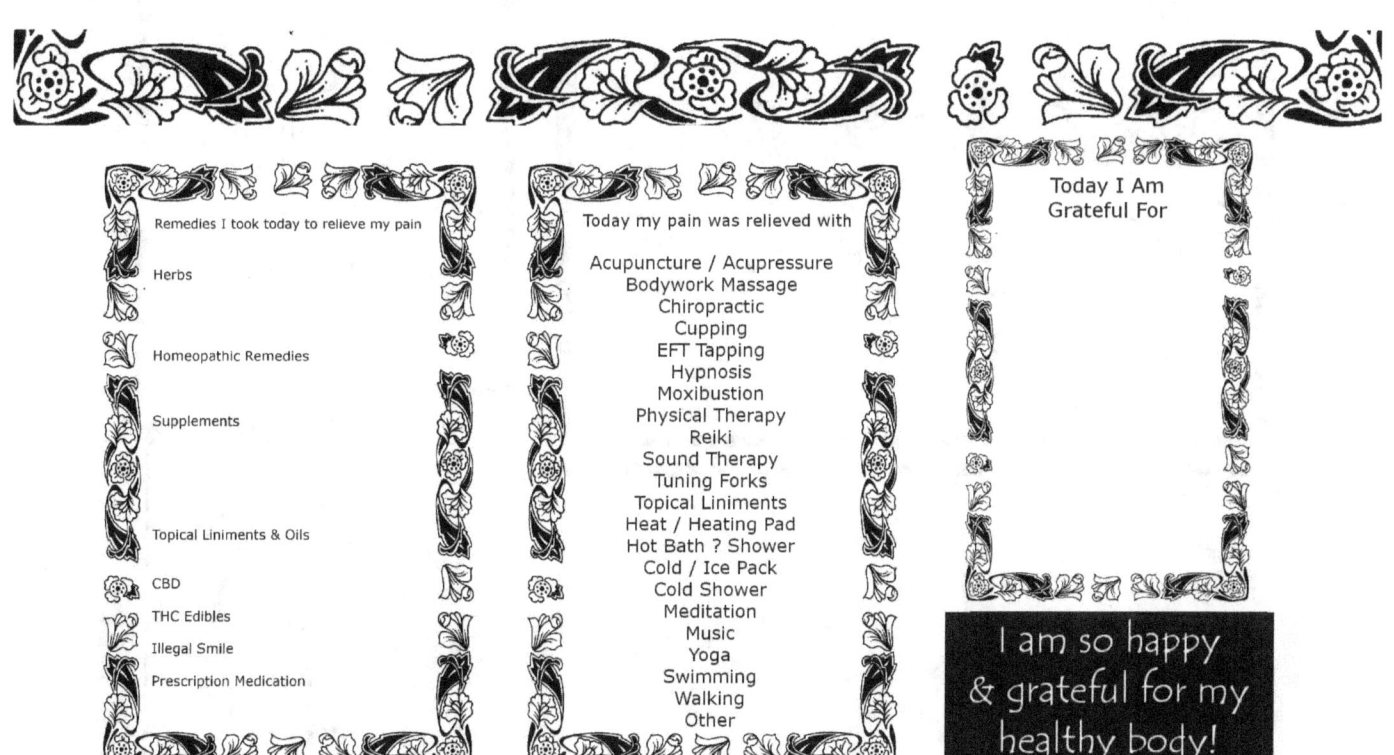

Remedies I took today to relieve my pain

Herbs

Homeopathic Remedies

Supplements

Topical Liniments & Oils

CBD
THC Edibles
Illegal Smile
Prescription Medication

Today my pain was relieved with

Acupuncture / Acupressure
Bodywork Massage
Chiropractic
Cupping
EFT Tapping
Hypnosis
Moxibustion
Physical Therapy
Reiki
Sound Therapy
Tuning Forks
Topical Liniments
Heat / Heating Pad
Hot Bath ? Shower
Cold / Ice Pack
Cold Shower
Meditation
Music
Yoga
Swimming
Walking
Other

Today I Am Grateful For

I am so happy & grateful for my healthy body!

Today's Day & Date

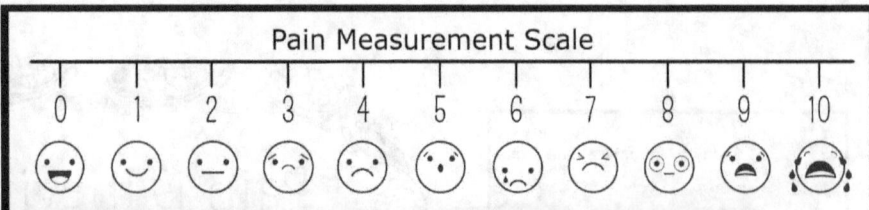

Highlight All Painful Areas

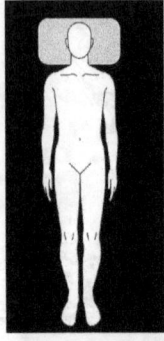 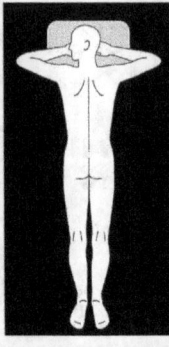 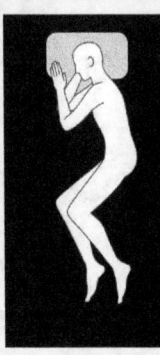 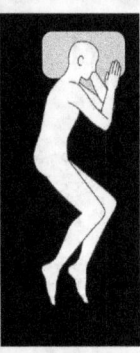

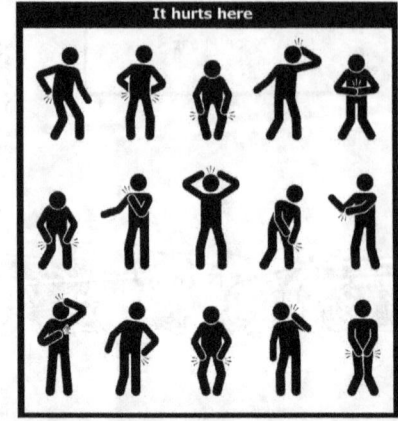

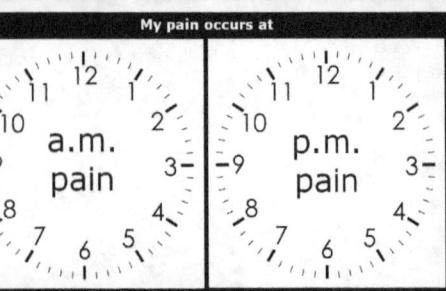

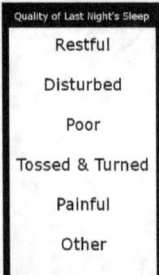

Quality of Last Night's Sleep
- Restful
- Disturbed
- Poor
- Tossed & Turned
- Painful
- Other

My pain is
Hot
Burning
Cold
Stabbing
Throbbing
Fixed
Moving Traveling
Constant
On & Off

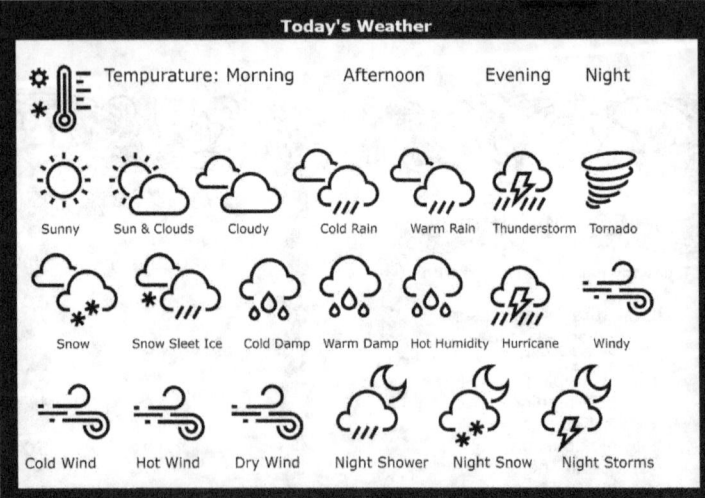

Breakfast

Lunch

Dinner

Snacks

Alcohol

Food Allergy Triggers

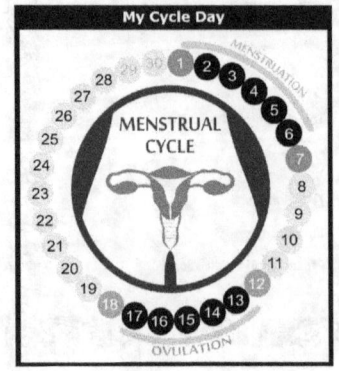

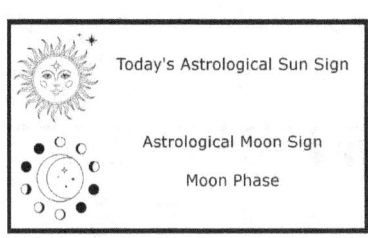

Today's Astrological Sun Sign

Astrological Moon Sign

Moon Phase

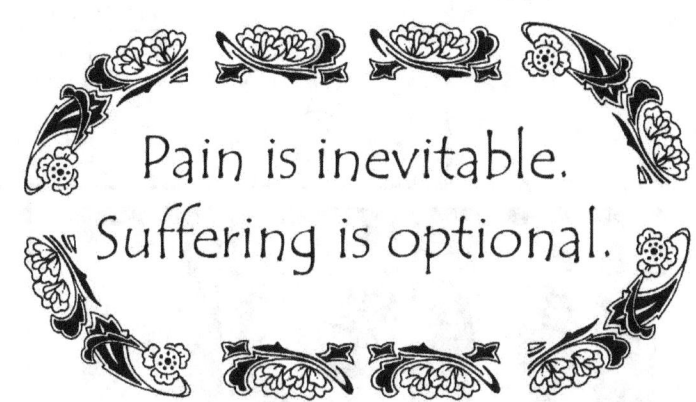

Pain is inevitable.
Suffering is optional.

Notes

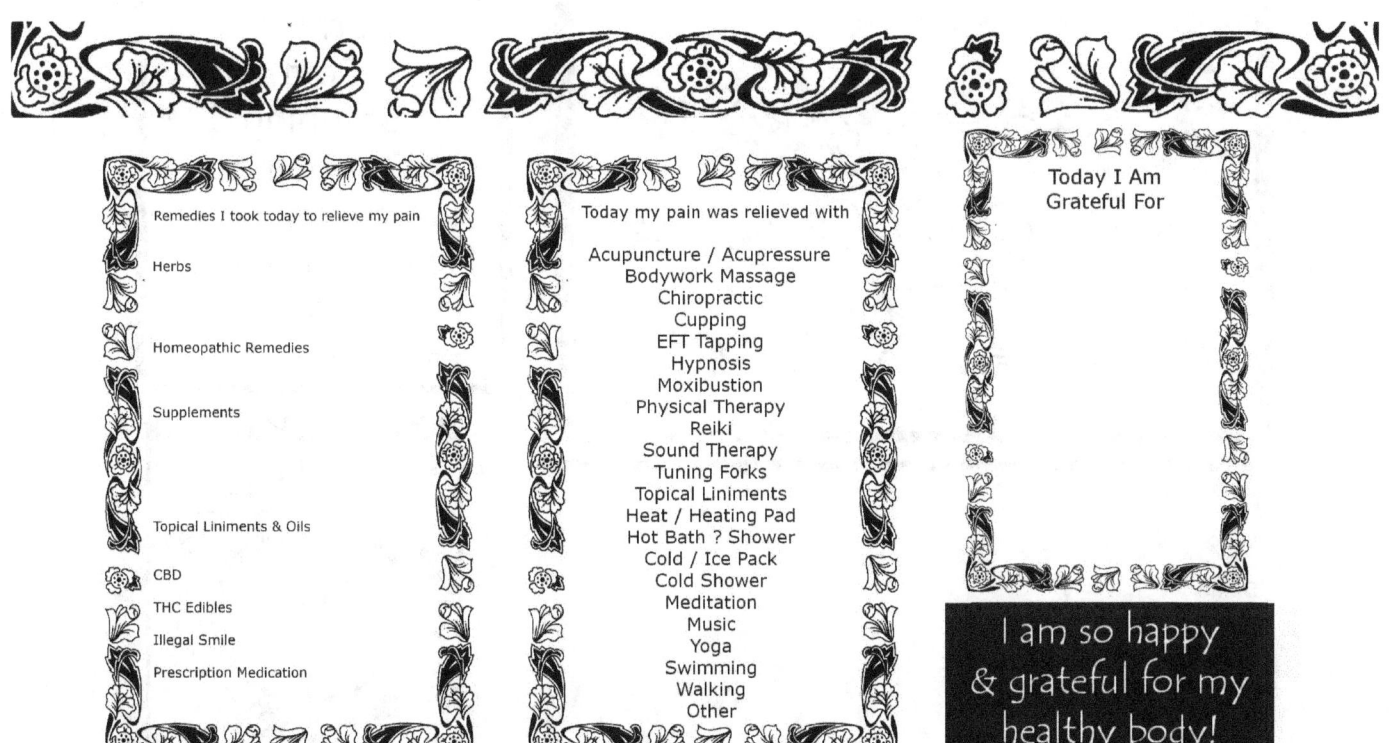

Remedies I took today to relieve my pain

Herbs

Homeopathic Remedies

Supplements

Topical Liniments & Oils

CBD
THC Edibles
Illegal Smile
Prescription Medication

Today my pain was relieved with

Acupuncture / Acupressure
Bodywork Massage
Chiropractic
Cupping
EFT Tapping
Hypnosis
Moxibustion
Physical Therapy
Reiki
Sound Therapy
Tuning Forks
Topical Liniments
Heat / Heating Pad
Hot Bath ? Shower
Cold / Ice Pack
Cold Shower
Meditation
Music
Yoga
Swimming
Walking
Other

Today I Am Grateful For

I am so happy & grateful for my healthy body!

Today's Day & Date

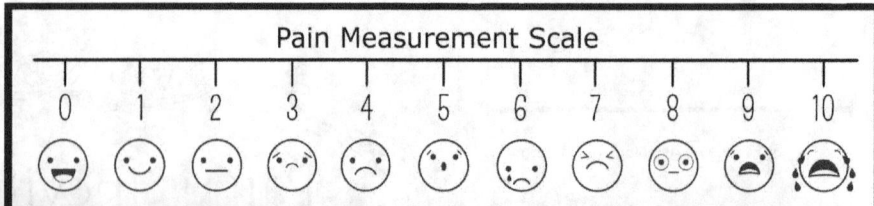

Highlight All Painful Areas

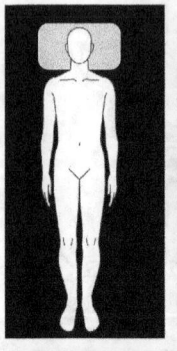 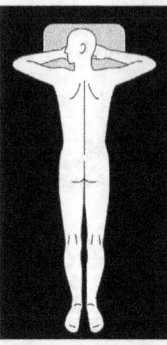 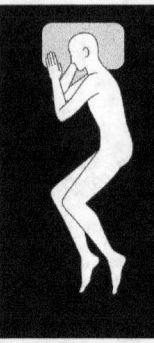 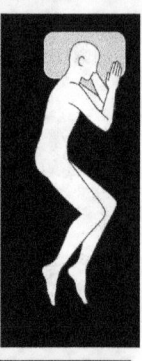

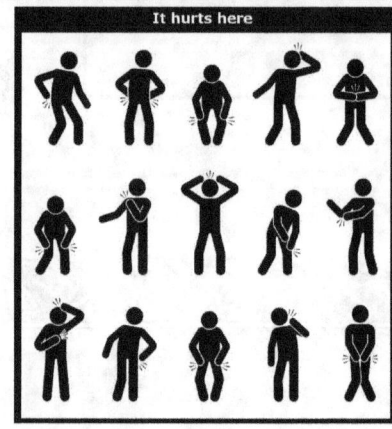
It hurts here

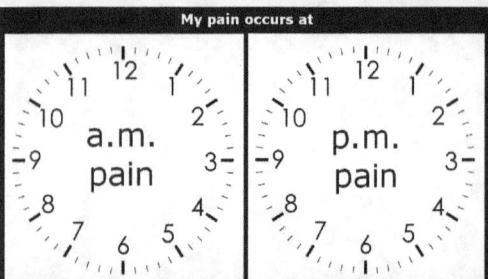
My pain occurs at — a.m. pain / p.m. pain

Quality of Last Night's Sleep
- Restful
- Disturbed
- Poor
- Tossed & Turned
- Painful
- Other

My mood today

My pain is

Hot
Burning
Cold
Stabbing
Throbbing
Fixed
Moving Traveling
Constant
On & Off

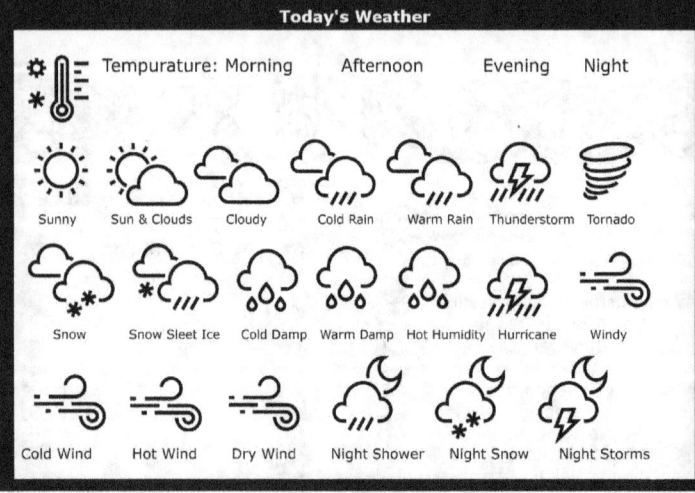
Today's Weather — Tempurature: Morning, Afternoon, Evening, Night

Breakfast

Lunch

Dinner

Snacks

Alcohol

Food Allergy Triggers

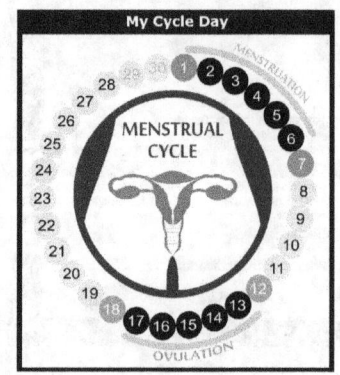
My Cycle Day

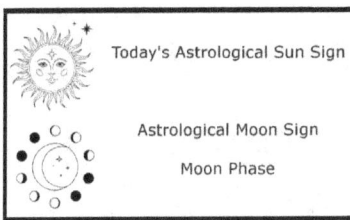

Today's Astrological Sun Sign

Astrological Moon Sign

Moon Phase

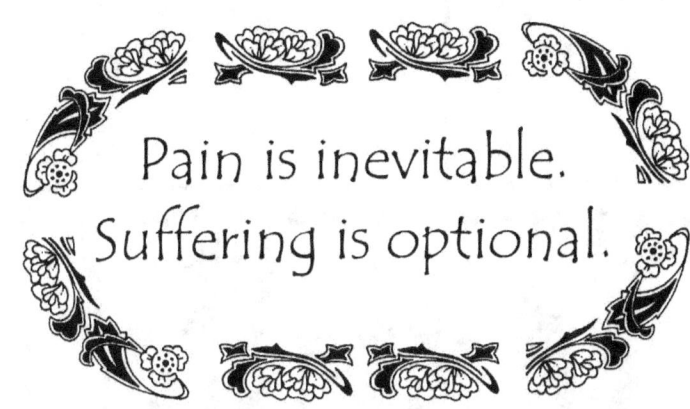

Pain is inevitable. Suffering is optional.

Notes

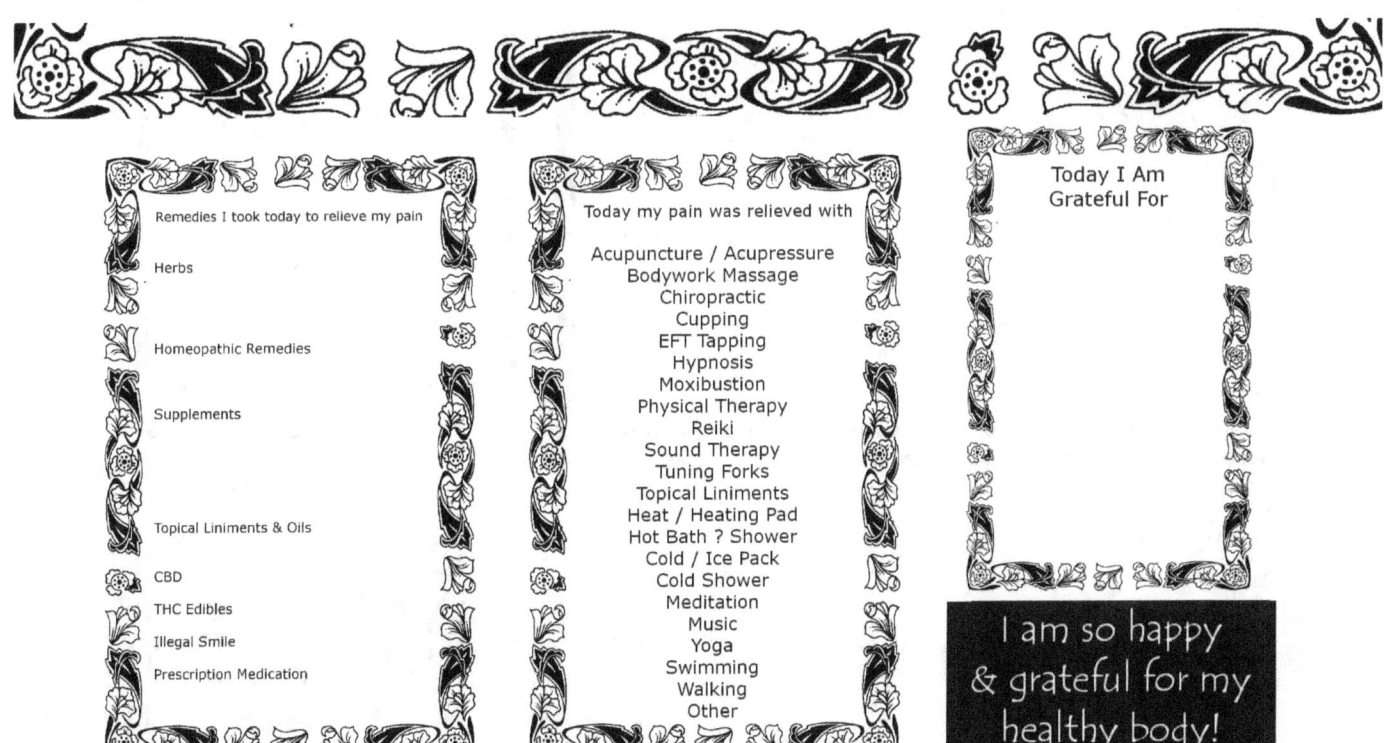

Remedies I took today to relieve my pain

Herbs

Homeopathic Remedies

Supplements

Topical Liniments & Oils

CBD

THC Edibles

Illegal Smile

Prescription Medication

Today my pain was relieved with

Acupuncture / Acupressure
Bodywork Massage
Chiropractic
Cupping
EFT Tapping
Hypnosis
Moxibustion
Physical Therapy
Reiki
Sound Therapy
Tuning Forks
Topical Liniments
Heat / Heating Pad
Hot Bath ? Shower
Cold / Ice Pack
Cold Shower
Meditation
Music
Yoga
Swimming
Walking
Other

Today I Am Grateful For

I am so happy & grateful for my healthy body!

Today's Day & Date

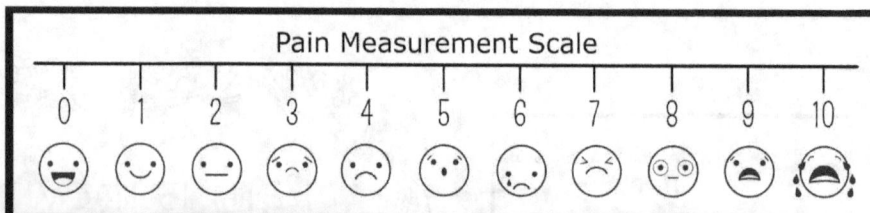

Highlight All Painful Areas

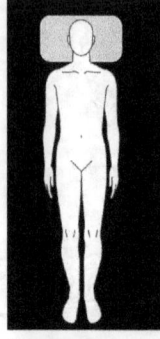 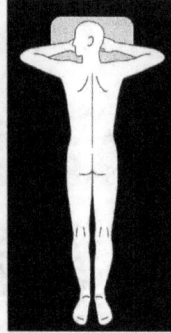 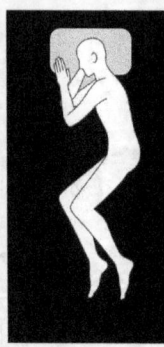 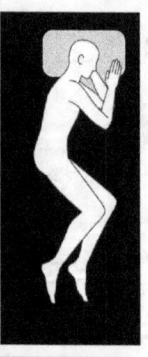

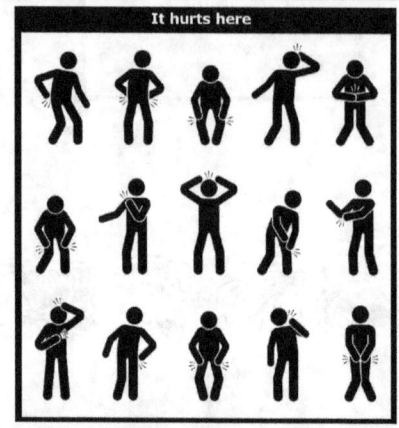
It hurts here

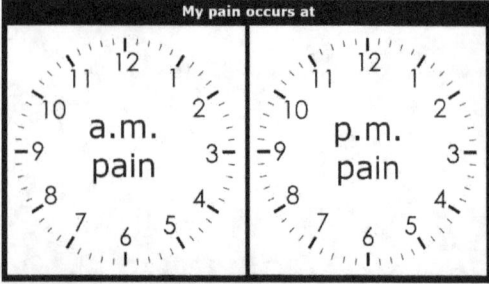
My pain occurs at — a.m. pain / p.m. pain

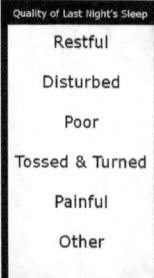
Quality of Last Night's Sleep
- Restful
- Disturbed
- Poor
- Tossed & Turned
- Painful
- Other

My mood today

My pain is
Hot
Burning
Cold
Stabbing
Throbbing
Fixed
Moving Traveling
Constant
On & Off

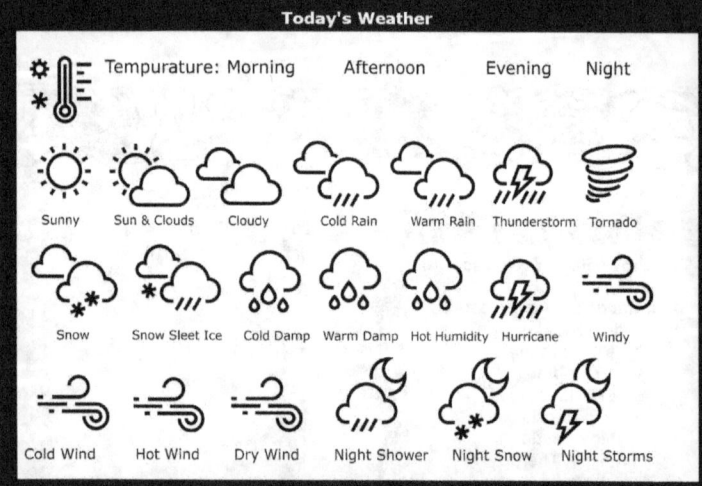
Today's Weather — Temperature: Morning, Afternoon, Evening, Night

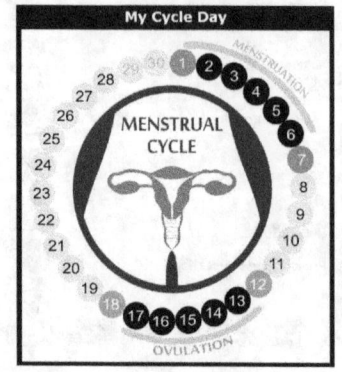
My Cycle Day

Breakfast

Lunch

Dinner

Snacks

Alcohol

Food Allergy Triggers

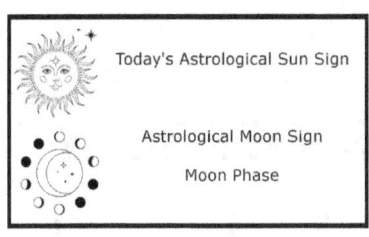

Today's Astrological Sun Sign

Astrological Moon Sign

Moon Phase

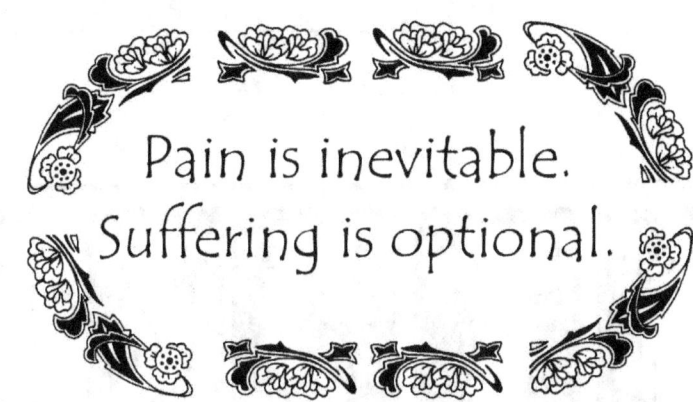

Pain is inevitable.
Suffering is optional.

Notes

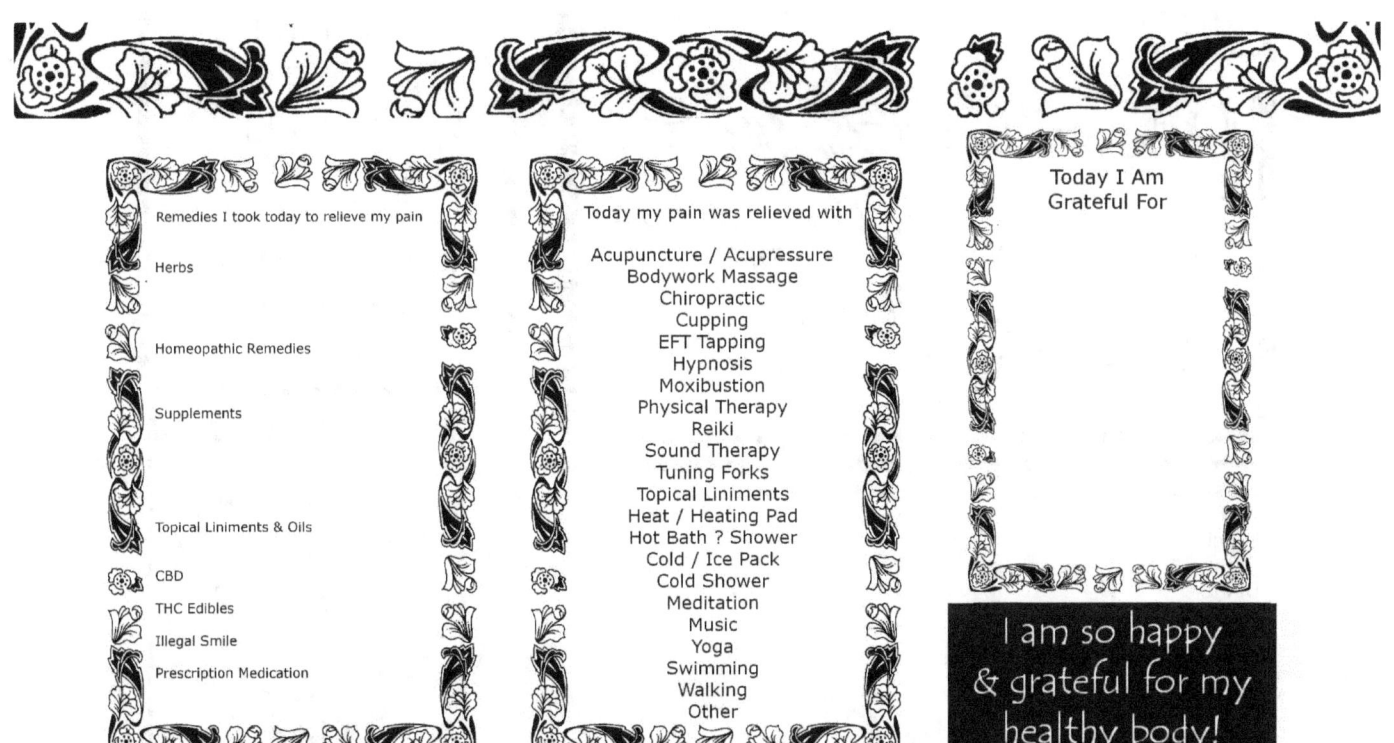

Remedies I took today to relieve my pain

Herbs

Homeopathic Remedies

Supplements

Topical Liniments & Oils

CBD

THC Edibles

Illegal Smile

Prescription Medication

Today my pain was relieved with

Acupuncture / Acupressure
Bodywork Massage
Chiropractic
Cupping
EFT Tapping
Hypnosis
Moxibustion
Physical Therapy
Reiki
Sound Therapy
Tuning Forks
Topical Liniments
Heat / Heating Pad
Hot Bath ? Shower
Cold / Ice Pack
Cold Shower
Meditation
Music
Yoga
Swimming
Walking
Other

Today I Am Grateful For

I am so happy & grateful for my healthy body!

Today's Day & Date

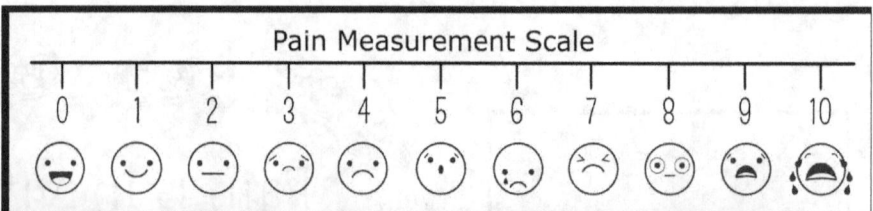

Highlight All Painful Areas

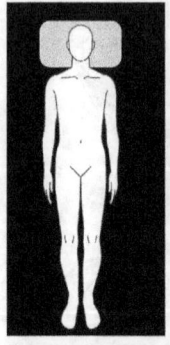 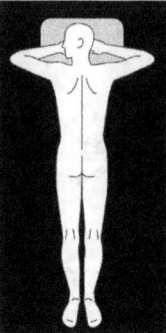 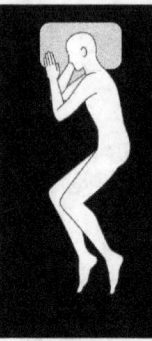 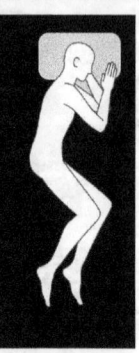

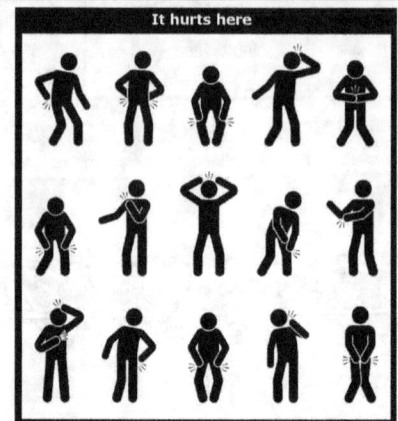
It hurts here

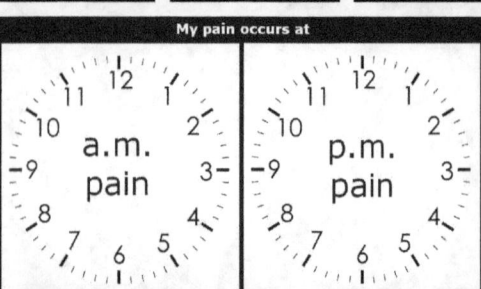
My pain occurs at — a.m. pain / p.m. pain

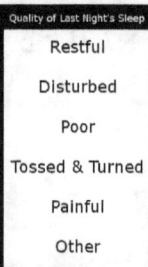

Quality of Last Night's Sleep
- Restful
- Disturbed
- Poor
- Tossed & Turned
- Painful
- Other

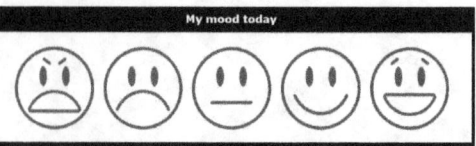
My mood today

My pain is
Hot
Burning
Cold
Stabbing
Throbbing
Fixed
Moving Traveling
Constant
On & Off

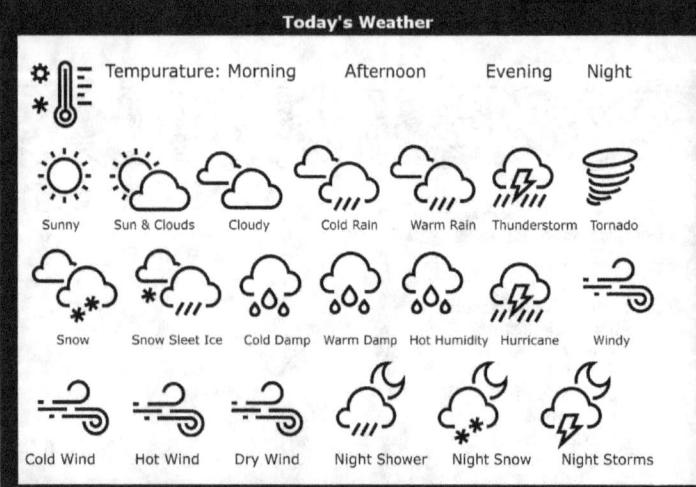
Today's Weather — Temperature: Morning, Afternoon, Evening, Night
Sunny, Sun & Clouds, Cloudy, Cold Rain, Warm Rain, Thunderstorm, Tornado
Snow, Snow Sleet Ice, Cold Damp, Warm Damp, Hot Humidity, Hurricane, Windy
Cold Wind, Hot Wind, Dry Wind, Night Shower, Night Snow, Night Storms

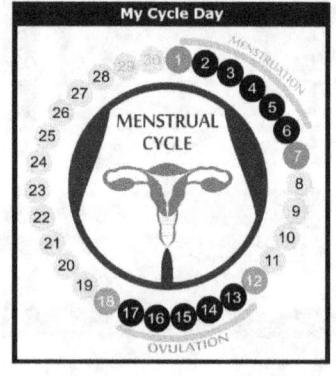
My Cycle Day

Breakfast

Lunch

Dinner

Snacks

Alcohol

Food Allergy Triggers

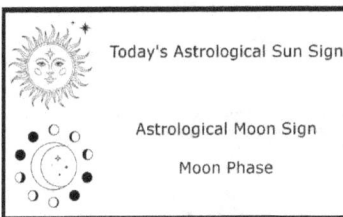

Today's Astrological Sun Sign

Astrological Moon Sign

Moon Phase

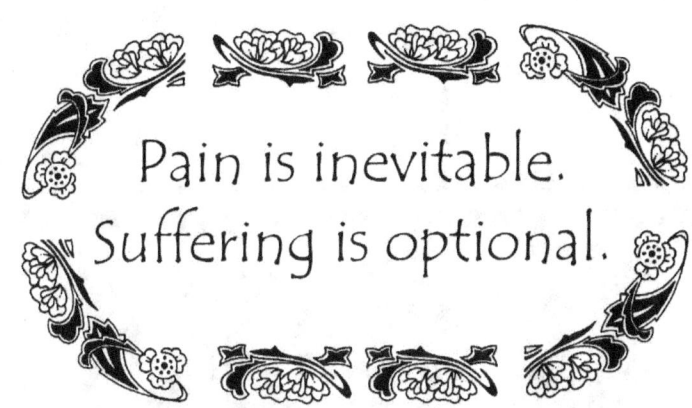

Pain is inevitable.
Suffering is optional.

Notes

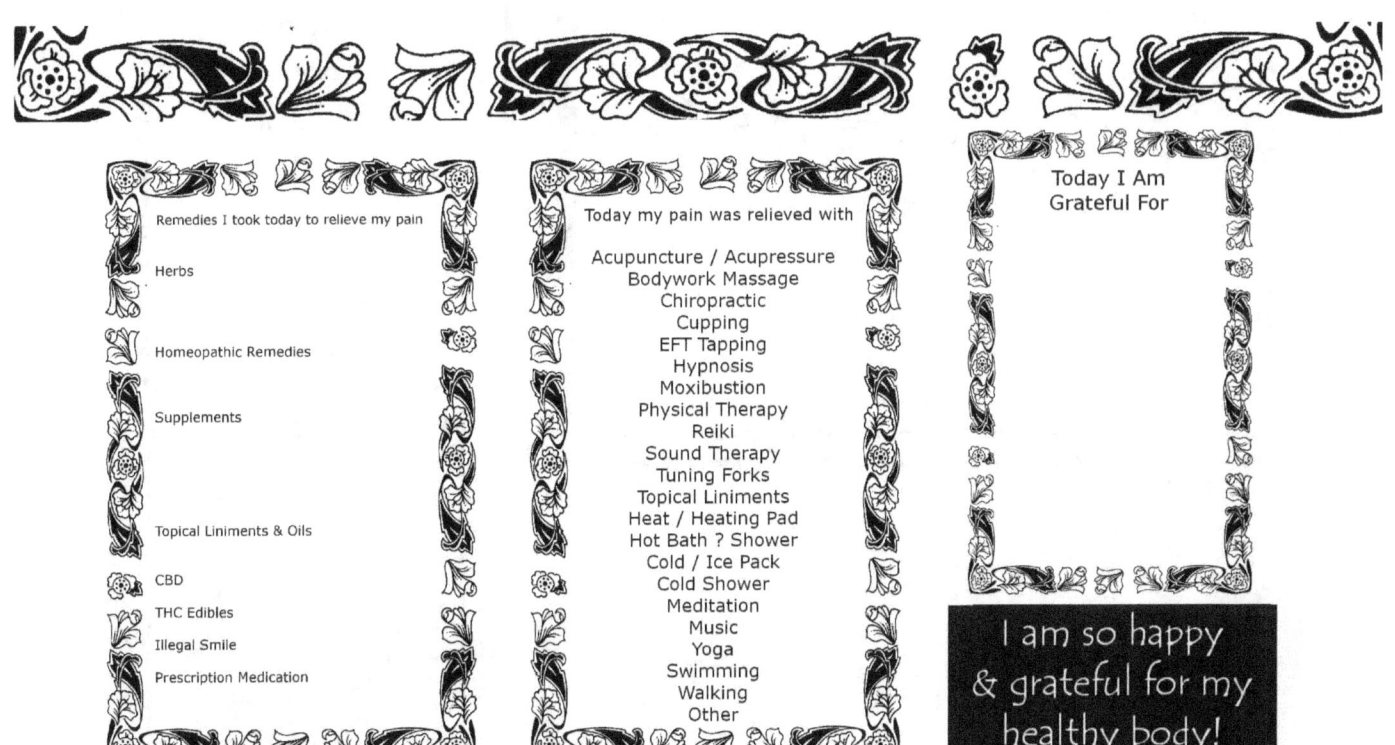

Remedies I took today to relieve my pain

Herbs

Homeopathic Remedies

Supplements

Topical Liniments & Oils

CBD

THC Edibles

Illegal Smile

Prescription Medication

Today my pain was relieved with

Acupuncture / Acupressure
Bodywork Massage
Chiropractic
Cupping
EFT Tapping
Hypnosis
Moxibustion
Physical Therapy
Reiki
Sound Therapy
Tuning Forks
Topical Liniments
Heat / Heating Pad
Hot Bath ? Shower
Cold / Ice Pack
Cold Shower
Meditation
Music
Yoga
Swimming
Walking
Other

Today I Am Grateful For

I am so happy & grateful for my healthy body!

Today's Day & Date

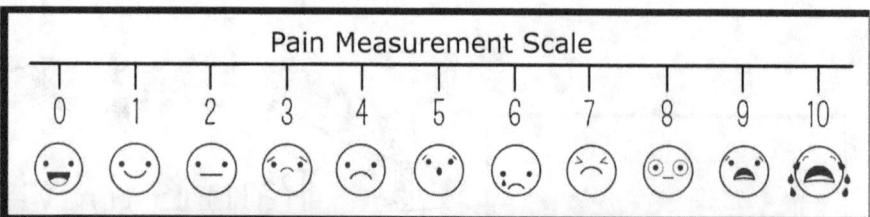

Highlight All Painful Areas

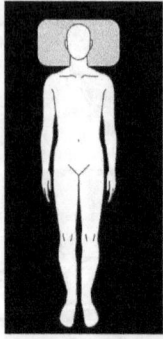 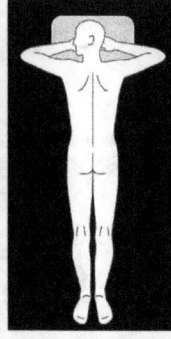 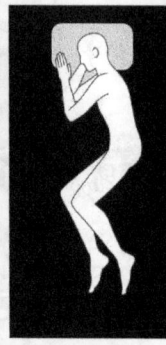 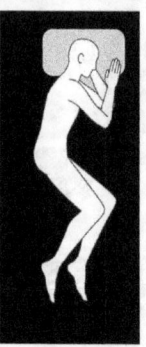

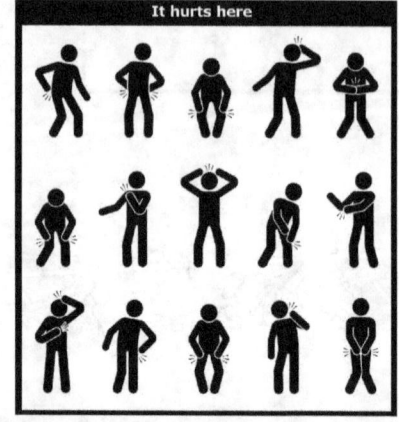
It hurts here

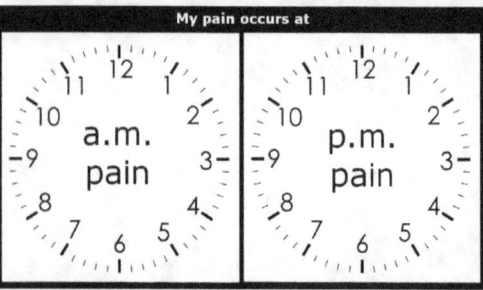
My pain occurs at — a.m. pain / p.m. pain

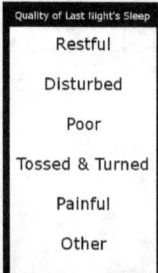
Quality of Last Night's Sleep
- Restful
- Disturbed
- Poor
- Tossed & Turned
- Painful
- Other

My mood today

My pain is
Hot
Burning
Cold
Stabbing
Throbbing
Fixed
Moving Traveling
Constant
On & Off

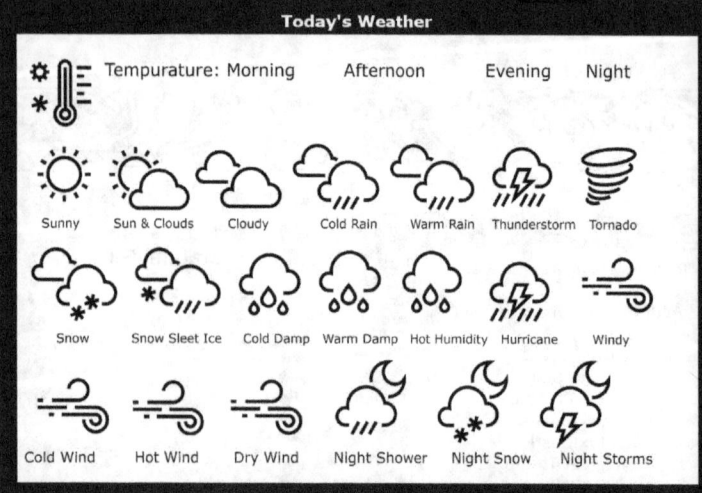
Today's Weather — Temperature: Morning, Afternoon, Evening, Night
Sunny, Sun & Clouds, Cloudy, Cold Rain, Warm Rain, Thunderstorm, Tornado
Snow, Snow Sleet Ice, Cold Damp, Warm Damp, Hot Humidity, Hurricane, Windy
Cold Wind, Hot Wind, Dry Wind, Night Shower, Night Snow, Night Storms

Breakfast

Lunch

Dinner

Snacks

Alcohol

Food Allergy Triggers

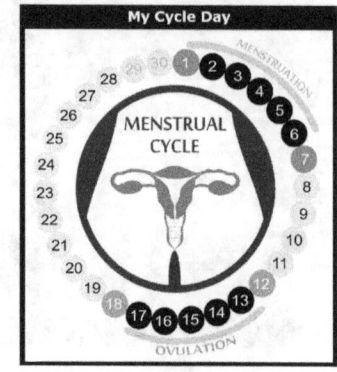
My Cycle Day

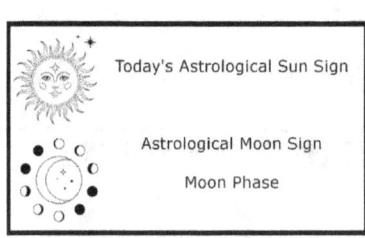

Today's Astrological Sun Sign

Astrological Moon Sign

Moon Phase

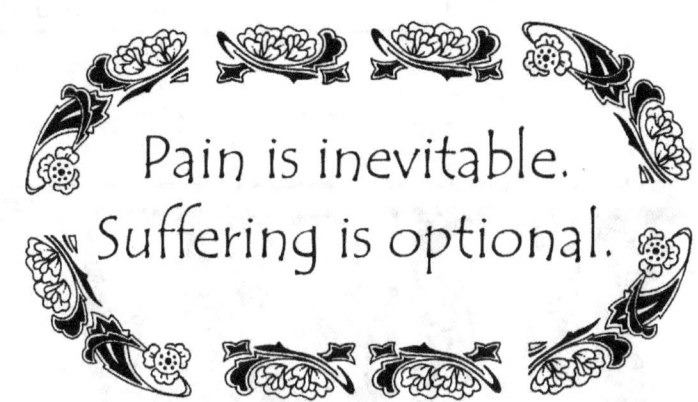

Pain is inevitable. Suffering is optional.

Notes

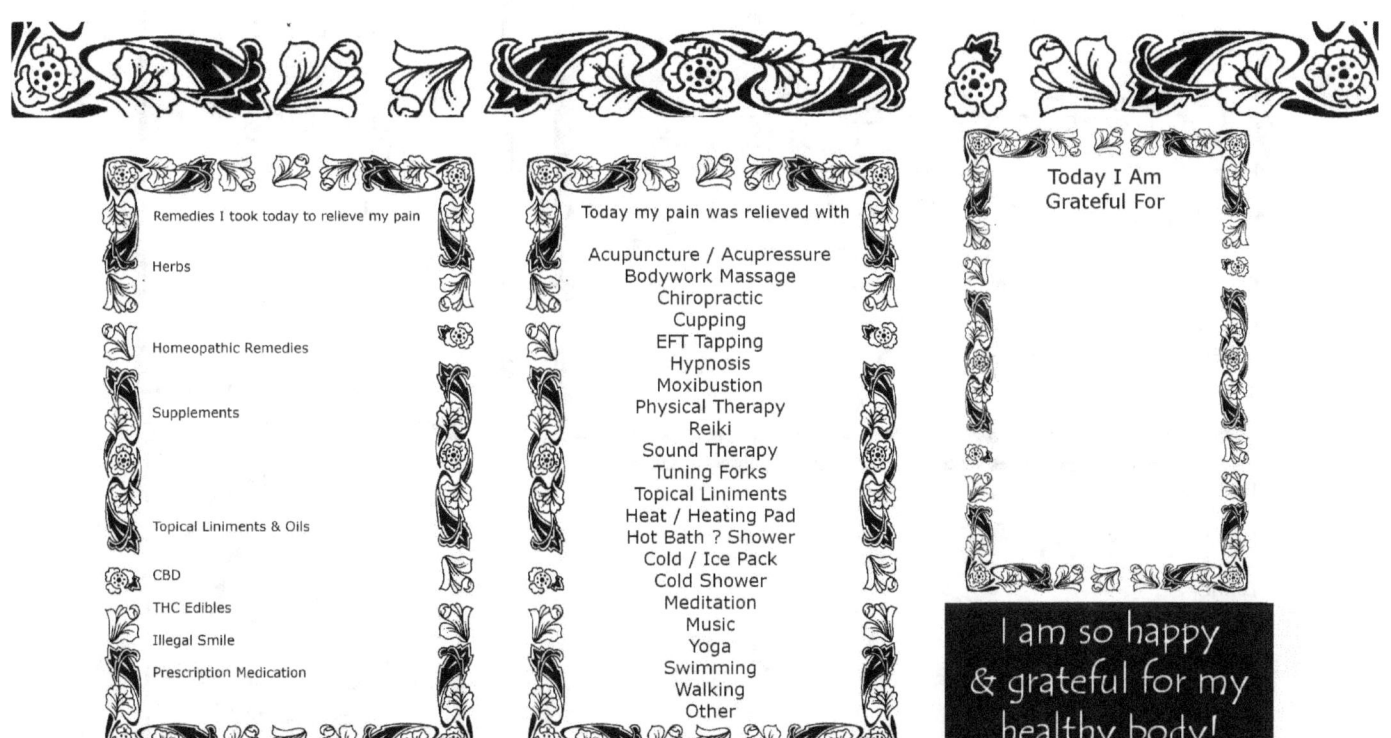

Remedies I took today to relieve my pain

Herbs

Homeopathic Remedies

Supplements

Topical Liniments & Oils

CBD
THC Edibles
Illegal Smile
Prescription Medication

Today my pain was relieved with

Acupuncture / Acupressure
Bodywork Massage
Chiropractic
Cupping
EFT Tapping
Hypnosis
Moxibustion
Physical Therapy
Reiki
Sound Therapy
Tuning Forks
Topical Liniments
Heat / Heating Pad
Hot Bath ? Shower
Cold / Ice Pack
Cold Shower
Meditation
Music
Yoga
Swimming
Walking
Other

Today I Am Grateful For

I am so happy & grateful for my healthy body!

Today's Day & Date

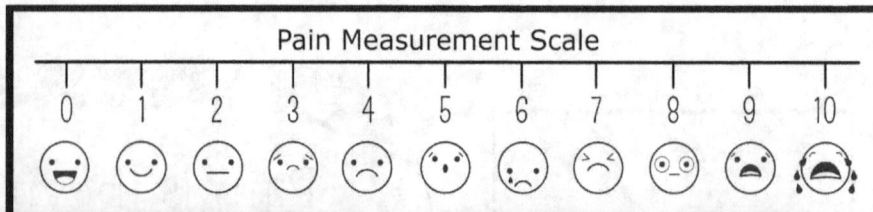

Highlight All Painful Areas

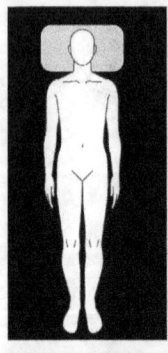 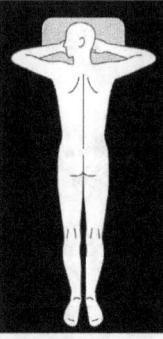 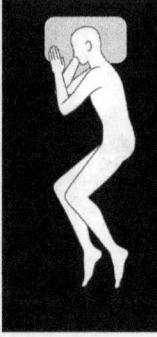 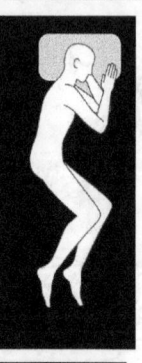

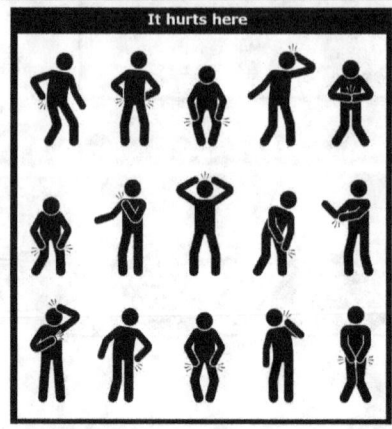
It hurts here

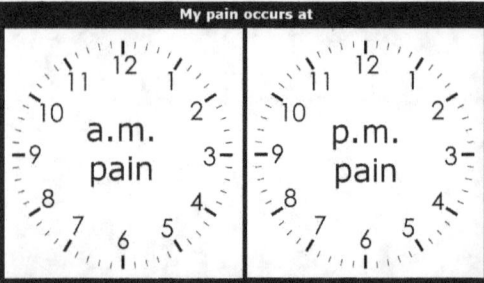
My pain occurs at — a.m. pain / p.m. pain

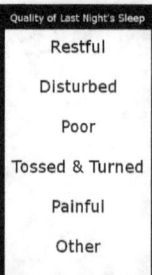
Quality of Last Night's Sleep
- Restful
- Disturbed
- Poor
- Tossed & Turned
- Painful
- Other

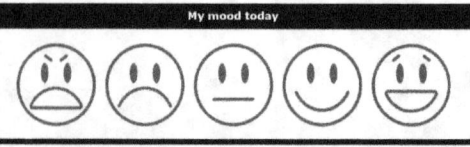
My mood today

My pain is
Hot
Burning
Cold
Stabbing
Throbbing
Fixed
Moving Traveling
Constant
On & Off

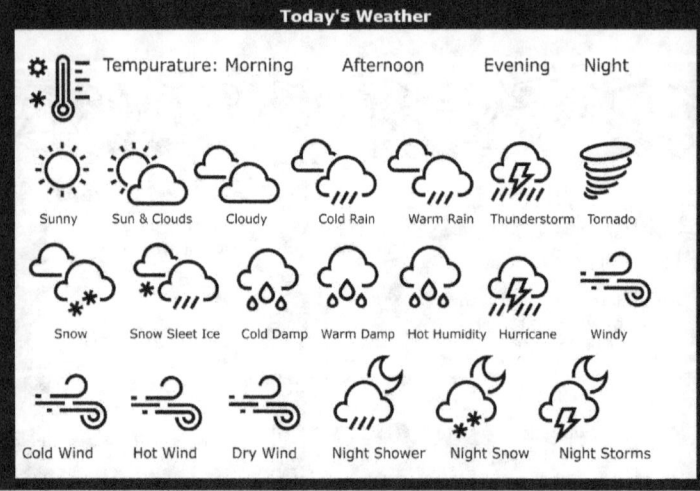
Today's Weather — Temperature: Morning, Afternoon, Evening, Night

Sunny, Sun & Clouds, Cloudy, Cold Rain, Warm Rain, Thunderstorm, Tornado
Snow, Snow Sleet Ice, Cold Damp, Warm Damp, Hot Humidity, Hurricane, Windy
Cold Wind, Hot Wind, Dry Wind, Night Shower, Night Snow, Night Storms

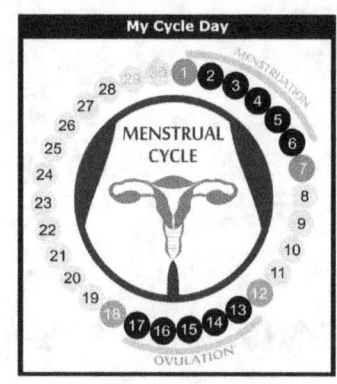
My Cycle Day

Breakfast

Lunch

Dinner

Snacks

Alcohol

Food Allergy Triggers

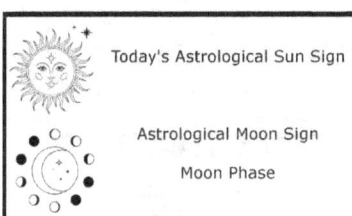

Today's Astrological Sun Sign

Astrological Moon Sign

Moon Phase

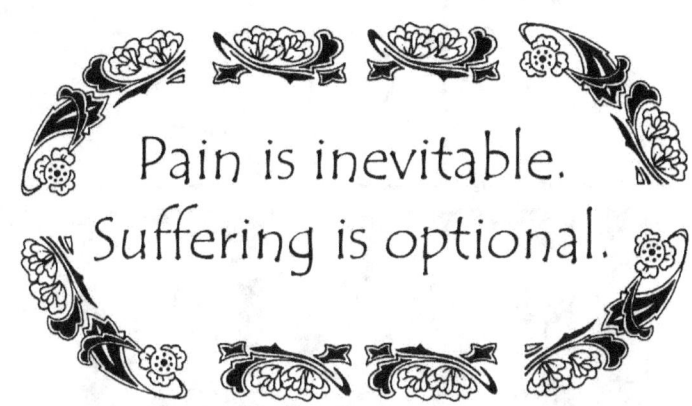

Pain is inevitable. Suffering is optional.

Notes

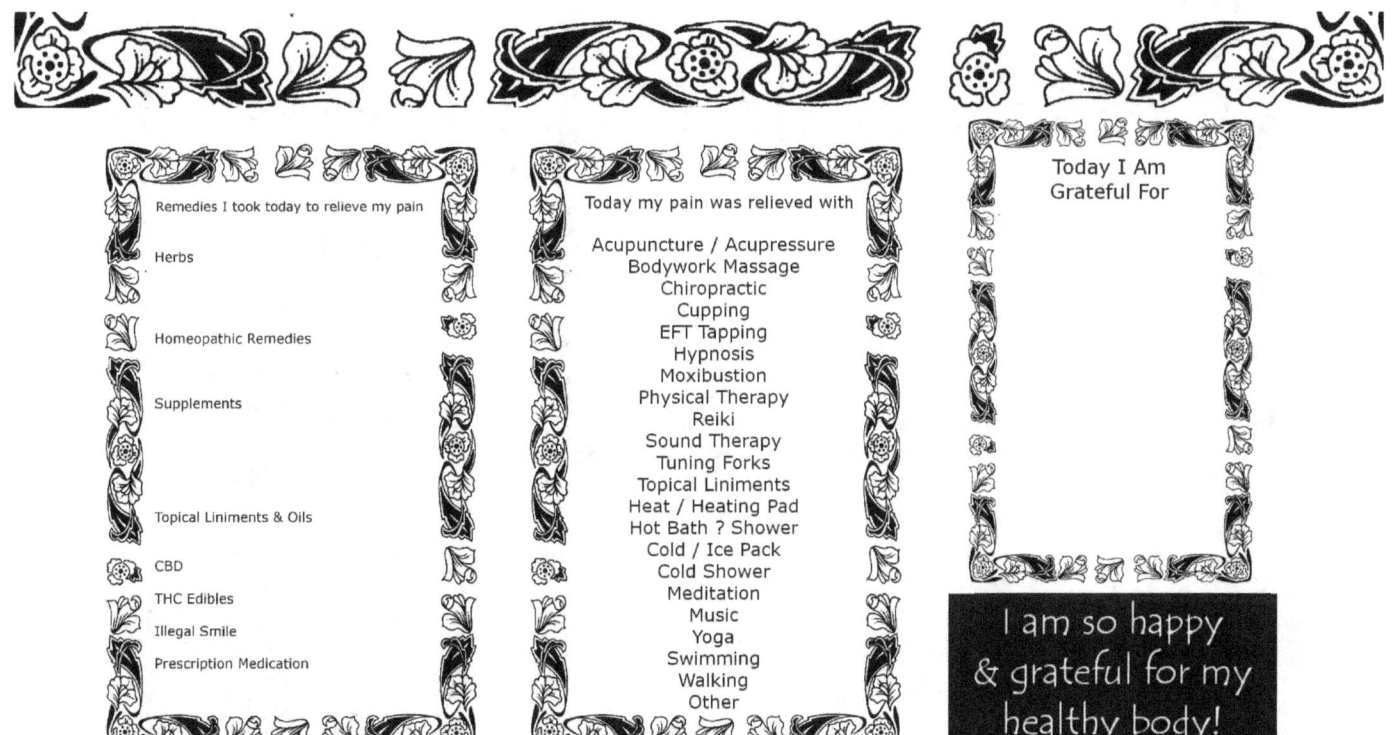

Remedies I took today to relieve my pain

Herbs

Homeopathic Remedies

Supplements

Topical Liniments & Oils

CBD
THC Edibles
Illegal Smile
Prescription Medication

Today my pain was relieved with

Acupuncture / Acupressure
Bodywork Massage
Chiropractic
Cupping
EFT Tapping
Hypnosis
Moxibustion
Physical Therapy
Reiki
Sound Therapy
Tuning Forks
Topical Liniments
Heat / Heating Pad
Hot Bath ? Shower
Cold / Ice Pack
Cold Shower
Meditation
Music
Yoga
Swimming
Walking
Other

Today I Am Grateful For

I am so happy & grateful for my healthy body!

Today's Day & Date

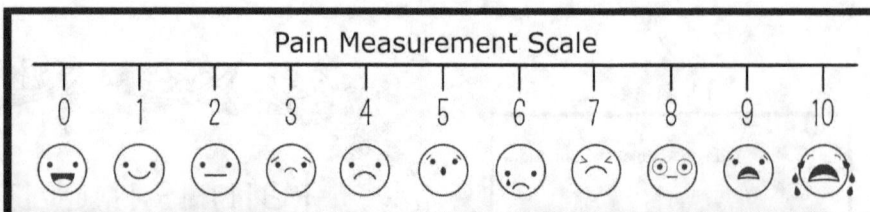

Highlight All Painful Areas

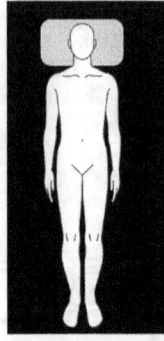 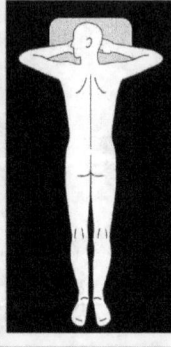 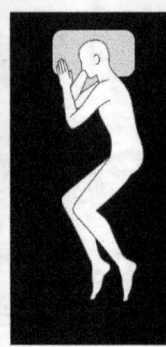 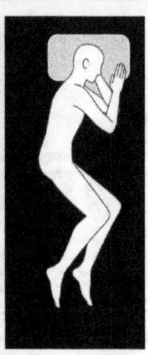

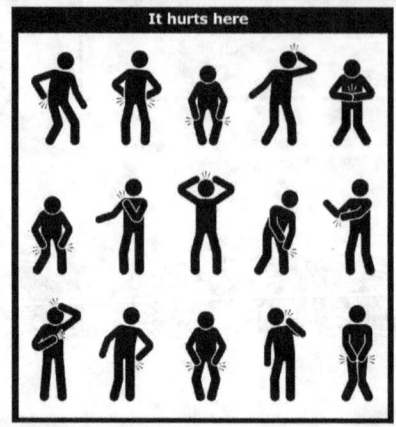
It hurts here

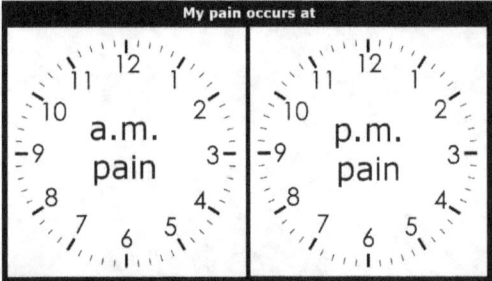
My pain occurs at — a.m. pain / p.m. pain

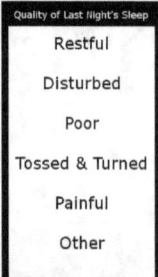

Quality of Last Night's Sleep
- Restful
- Disturbed
- Poor
- Tossed & Turned
- Painful
- Other

My mood today

My pain is
Hot
Burning
Cold
Stabbing
Throbbing
Fixed
Moving Traveling
Constant
On & Off

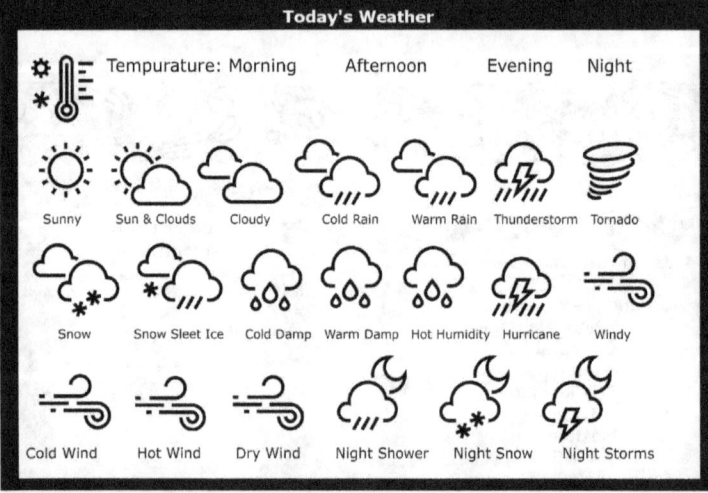
Today's Weather — Tempurature: Morning, Afternoon, Evening, Night

Breakfast

Lunch

Dinner

Snacks

Alcohol

Food Allergy Triggers

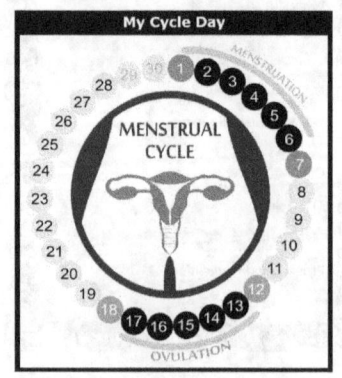
My Cycle Day

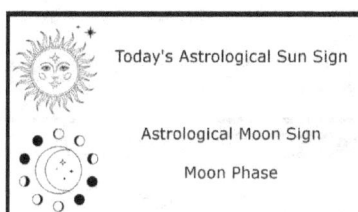

Today's Astrological Sun Sign

Astrological Moon Sign
Moon Phase

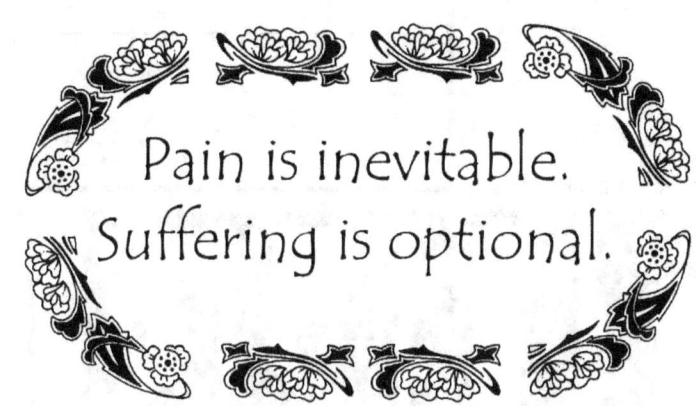

Pain is inevitable.
Suffering is optional.

Notes

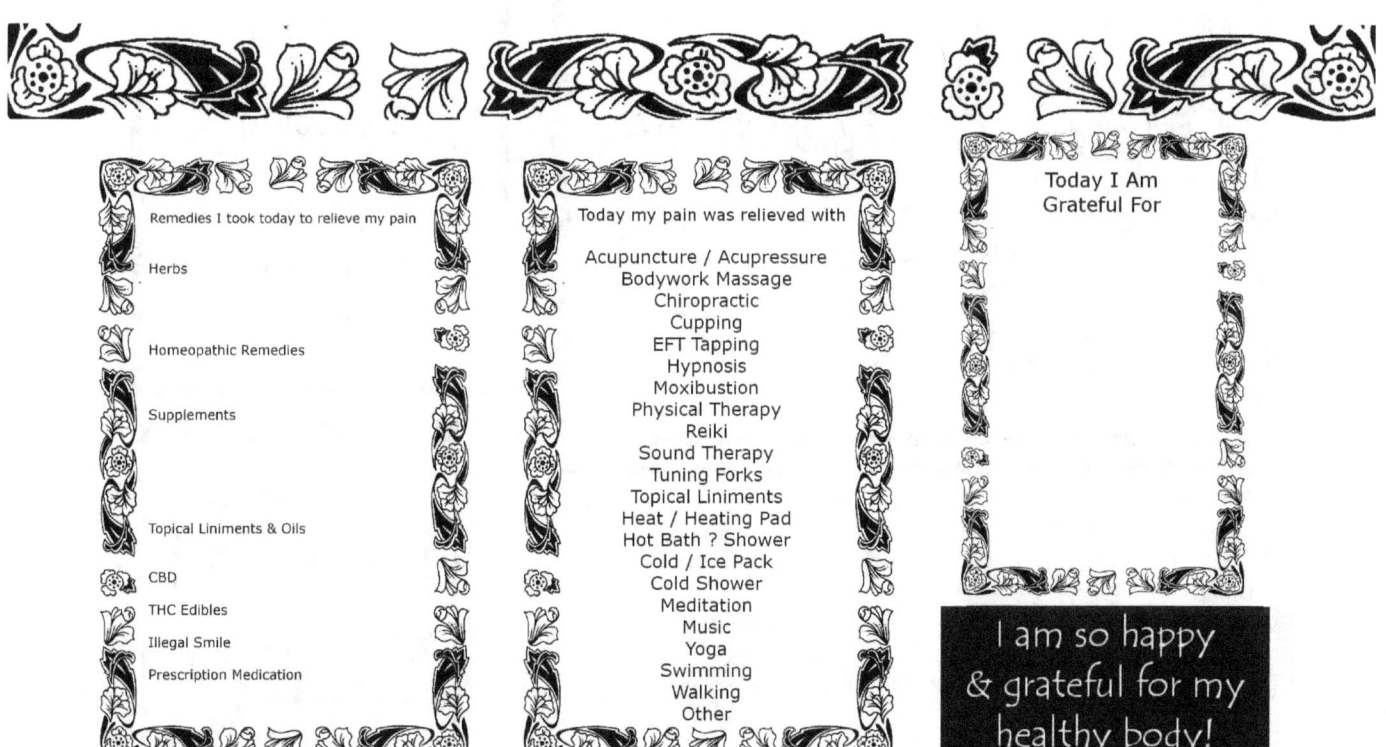

Remedies I took today to relieve my pain

Herbs

Homeopathic Remedies

Supplements

Topical Liniments & Oils

CBD
THC Edibles
Illegal Smile
Prescription Medication

Today my pain was relieved with

Acupuncture / Acupressure
Bodywork Massage
Chiropractic
Cupping
EFT Tapping
Hypnosis
Moxibustion
Physical Therapy
Reiki
Sound Therapy
Tuning Forks
Topical Liniments
Heat / Heating Pad
Hot Bath ? Shower
Cold / Ice Pack
Cold Shower
Meditation
Music
Yoga
Swimming
Walking
Other

Today I Am Grateful For

I am so happy & grateful for my healthy body!

Today's Day & Date

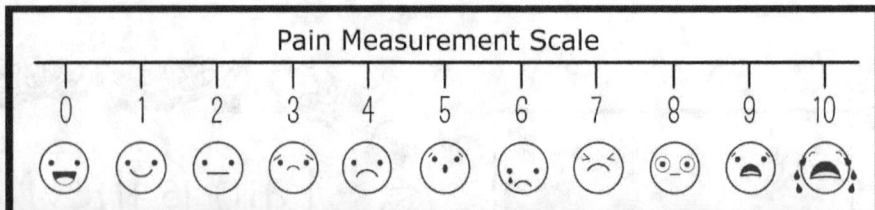

Highlight All Painful Areas

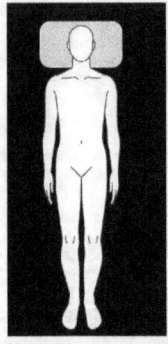 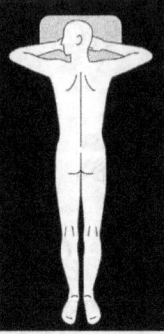 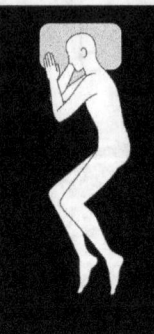 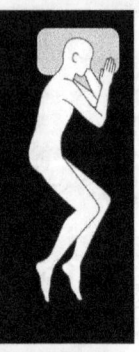

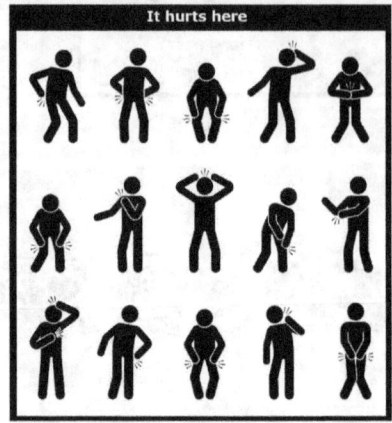
It hurts here

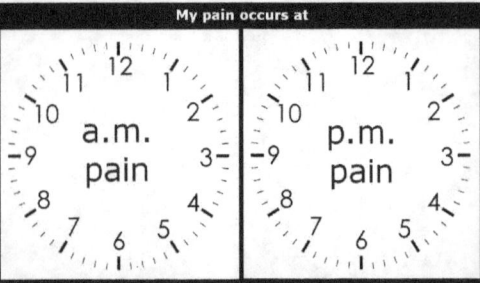
My pain occurs at — a.m. pain / p.m. pain

Quality of Last Night's Sleep
- Restful
- Disturbed
- Poor
- Tossed & Turned
- Painful
- Other

My mood today

My pain is
Hot
Burning
Cold
Stabbing
Throbbing
Fixed
Moving Traveling
Constant
On & Off

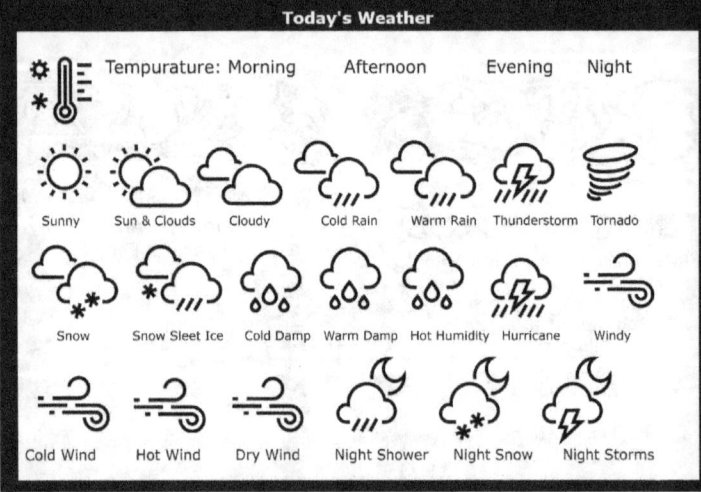
Today's Weather — Temperature: Morning, Afternoon, Evening, Night

Breakfast

Lunch

Dinner

Snacks

Alcohol

Food Allergy Triggers

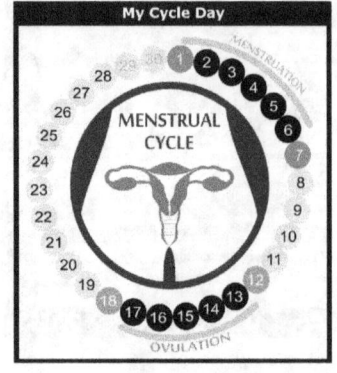
My Cycle Day

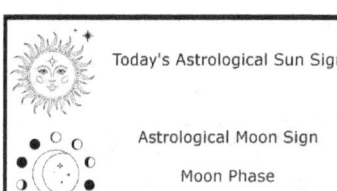

Today's Astrological Sun Sign

Astrological Moon Sign

Moon Phase

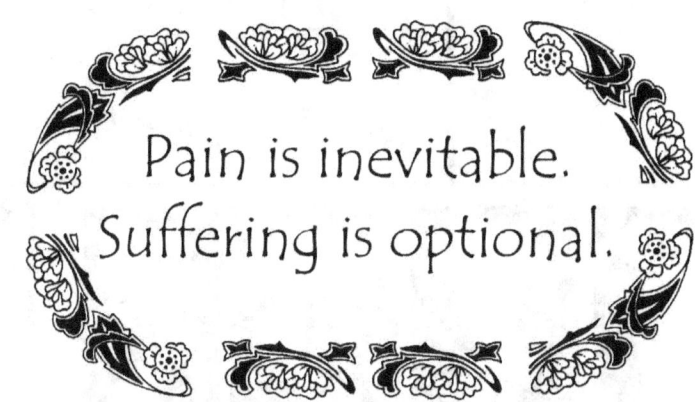

Pain is inevitable.
Suffering is optional.

Notes

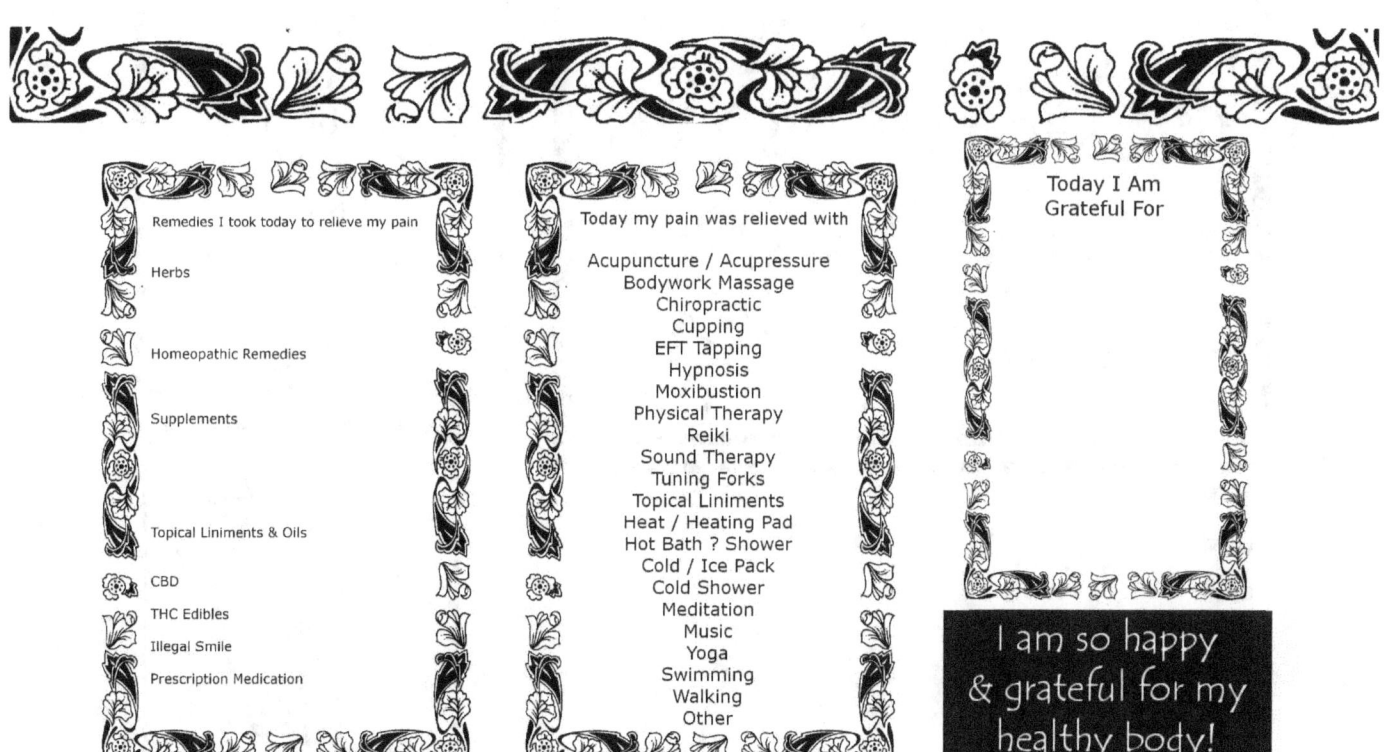

Remedies I took today to relieve my pain

Herbs

Homeopathic Remedies

Supplements

Topical Liniments & Oils

CBD

THC Edibles

Illegal Smile

Prescription Medication

Today my pain was relieved with

Acupuncture / Acupressure
Bodywork Massage
Chiropractic
Cupping
EFT Tapping
Hypnosis
Moxibustion
Physical Therapy
Reiki
Sound Therapy
Tuning Forks
Topical Liniments
Heat / Heating Pad
Hot Bath ? Shower
Cold / Ice Pack
Cold Shower
Meditation
Music
Yoga
Swimming
Walking
Other

Today I Am Grateful For

I am so happy & grateful for my healthy body!

Today's Day & Date

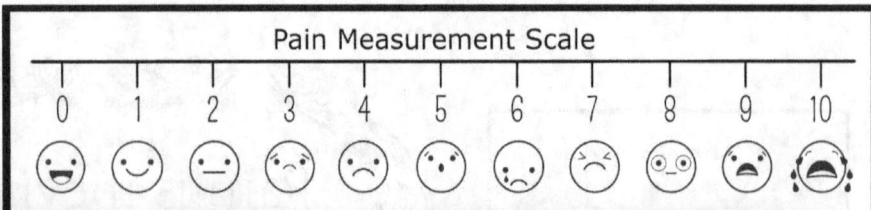

Pain Measurement Scale

Highlight All Painful Areas

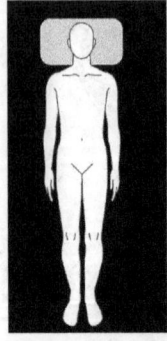 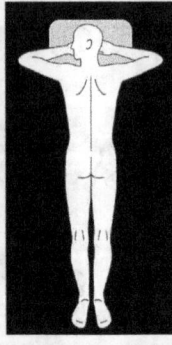 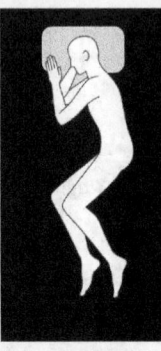 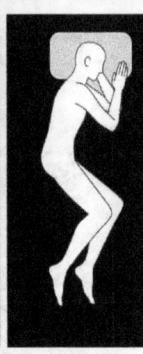

It hurts here

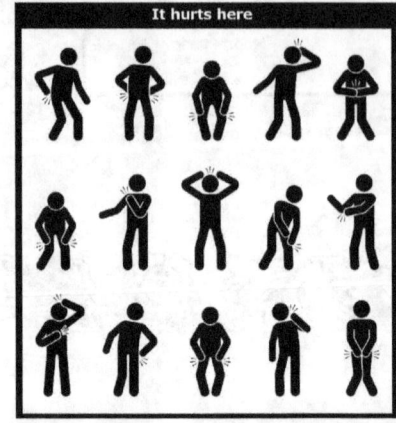

My pain occurs at

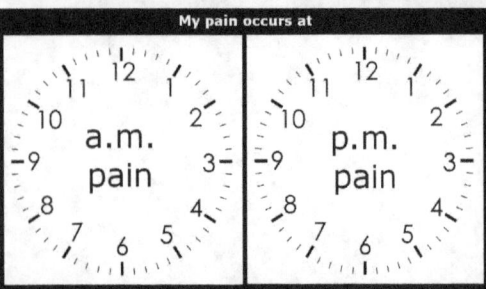

a.m. pain / p.m. pain

Quality of Last Night's Sleep
- Restful
- Disturbed
- Poor
- Tossed & Turned
- Painful
- Other

My mood today

Today's Weather

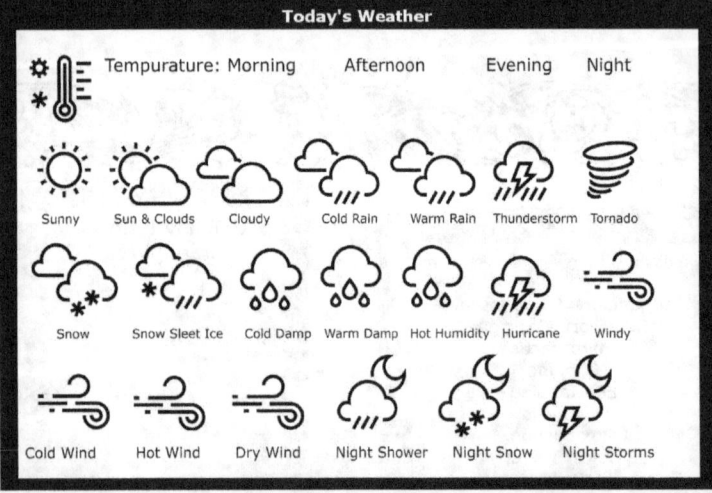

Tempurature: Morning Afternoon Evening Night

Sunny, Sun & Clouds, Cloudy, Cold Rain, Warm Rain, Thunderstorm, Tornado
Snow, Snow Sleet Ice, Cold Damp, Warm Damp, Hot Humidity, Hurricane, Windy
Cold Wind, Hot Wind, Dry Wind, Night Shower, Night Snow, Night Storms

My pain is
Hot
Burning
Cold
Stabbing
Throbbing
Fixed
Moving Traveling
Constant
On & Off

My Cycle Day

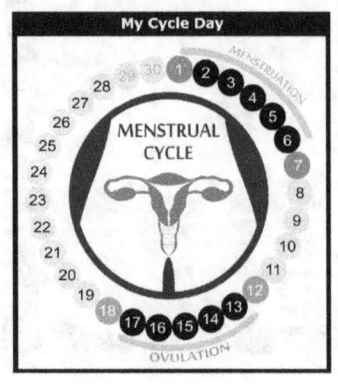

Breakfast

Lunch

Dinner

Snacks

Alcohol

Food Allergy Triggers

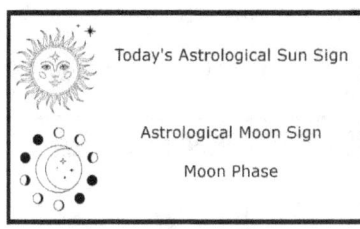

Today's Astrological Sun Sign

Astrological Moon Sign

Moon Phase

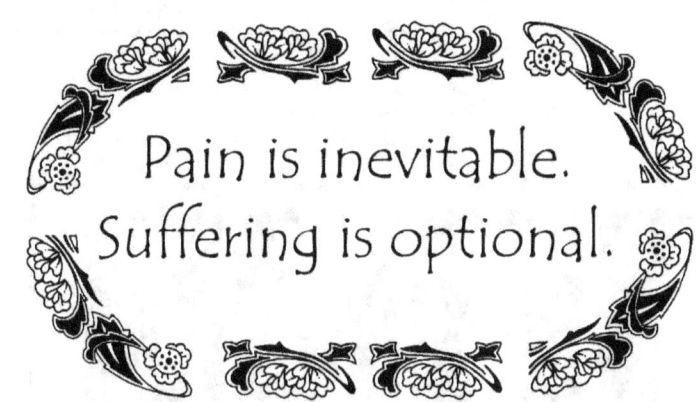

Pain is inevitable.
Suffering is optional.

Notes

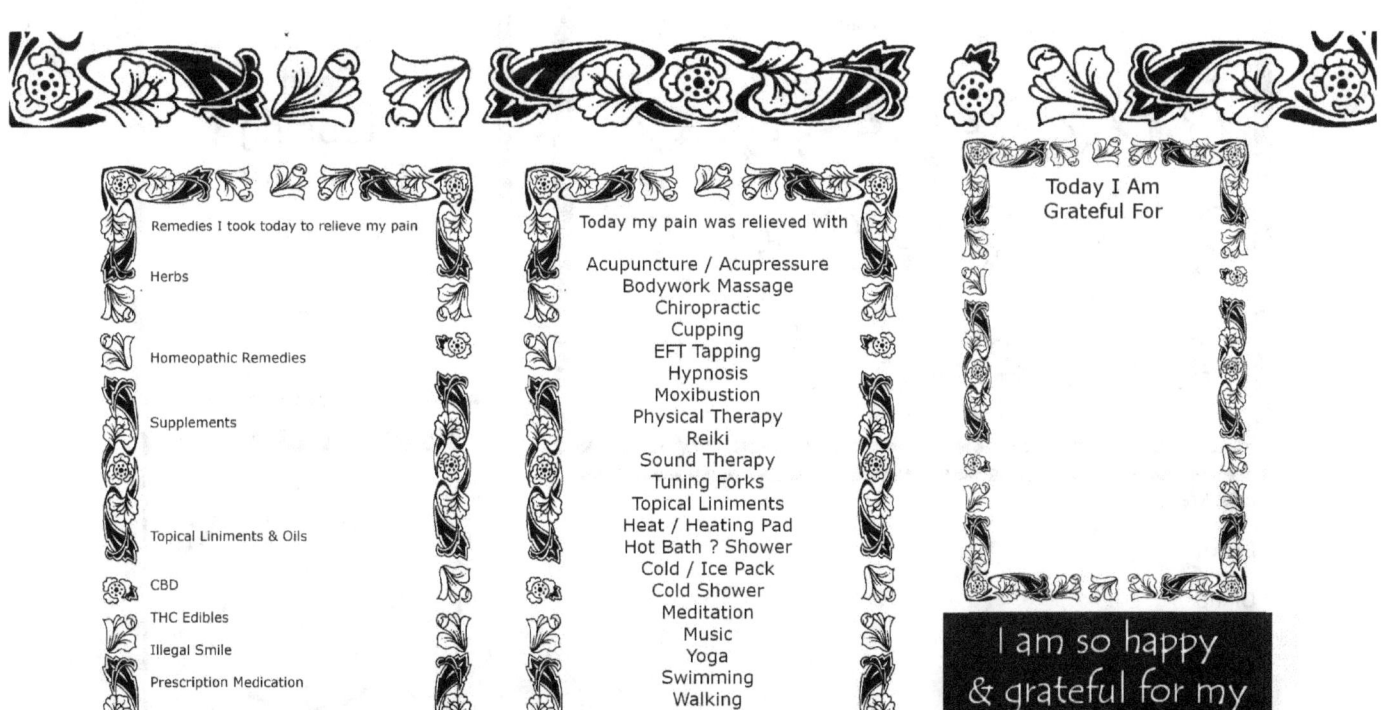

Remedies I took today to relieve my pain

Herbs

Homeopathic Remedies

Supplements

Topical Liniments & Oils

CBD

THC Edibles

Illegal Smile

Prescription Medication

Today my pain was relieved with

Acupuncture / Acupressure
Bodywork Massage
Chiropractic
Cupping
EFT Tapping
Hypnosis
Moxibustion
Physical Therapy
Reiki
Sound Therapy
Tuning Forks
Topical Liniments
Heat / Heating Pad
Hot Bath ? Shower
Cold / Ice Pack
Cold Shower
Meditation
Music
Yoga
Swimming
Walking
Other

Today I Am Grateful For

I am so happy & grateful for my healthy body!

Today's Day & Date

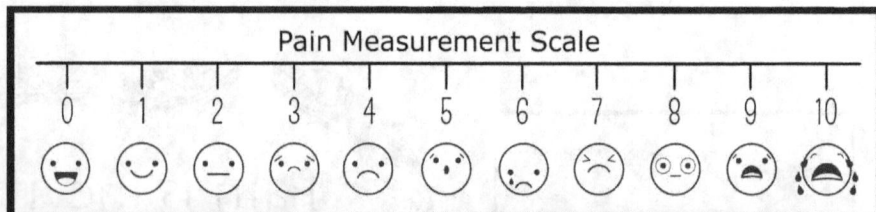

Highlight All Painful Areas

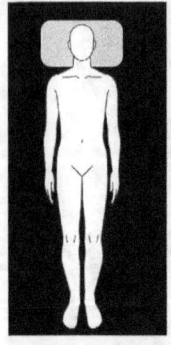 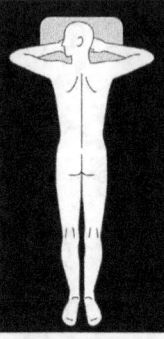 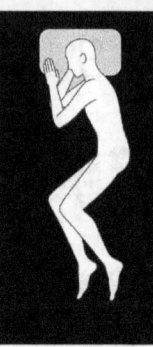 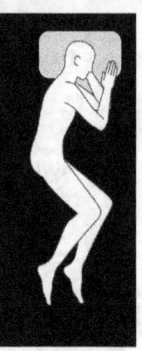

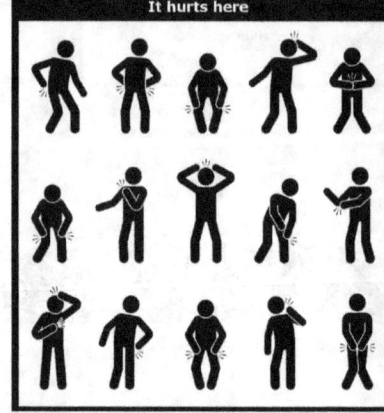
It hurts here

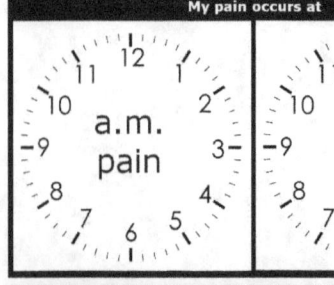
My pain occurs at — a.m. pain / p.m. pain

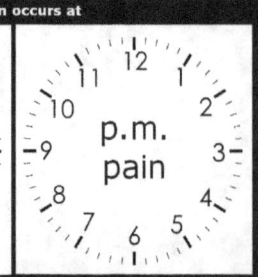
Quality of Last Night's Sleep
- Restful
- Disturbed
- Poor
- Tossed & Turned
- Painful
- Other

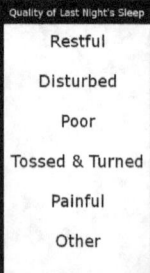
My mood today

My pain is
Hot
Burning
Cold
Stabbing
Throbbing
Fixed
Moving Traveling
Constant
On & Off

Today's Weather

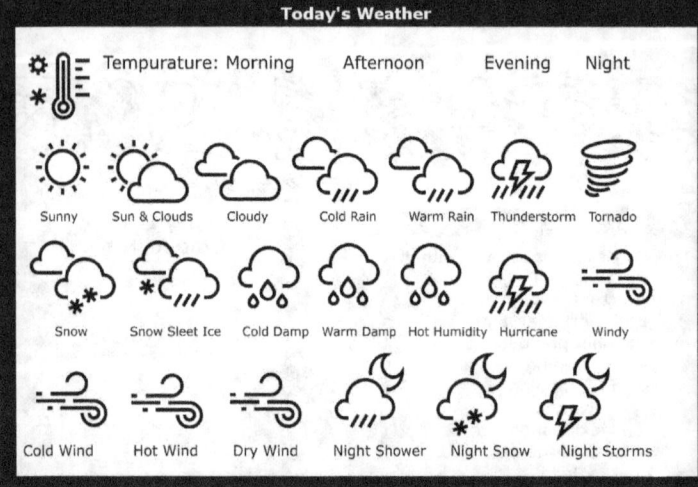

Tempurature: Morning   Afternoon   Evening   Night

Sunny | Sun & Clouds | Cloudy | Cold Rain | Warm Rain | Thunderstorm | Tornado
Snow | Snow Sleet Ice | Cold Damp | Warm Damp | Hot Humidity | Hurricane | Windy
Cold Wind | Hot Wind | Dry Wind | Night Shower | Night Snow | Night Storms

Breakfast

Lunch

Dinner

Snacks

Alcohol

Food Allergy Triggers

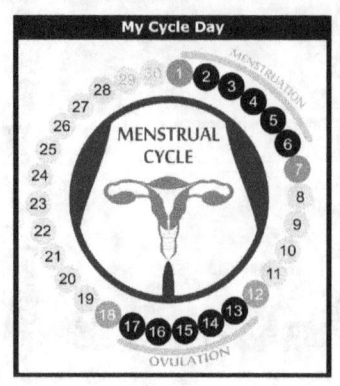
My Cycle Day

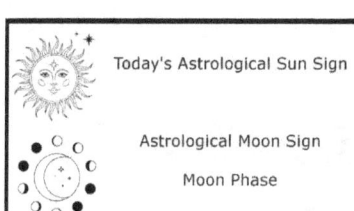

Today's Astrological Sun Sign

Astrological Moon Sign

Moon Phase

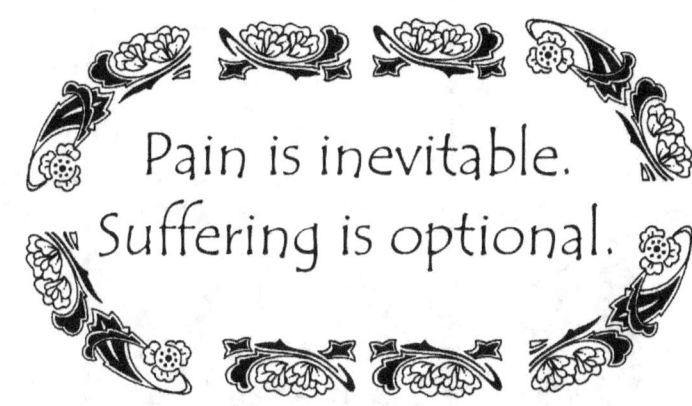

Pain is inevitable.
Suffering is optional.

Notes

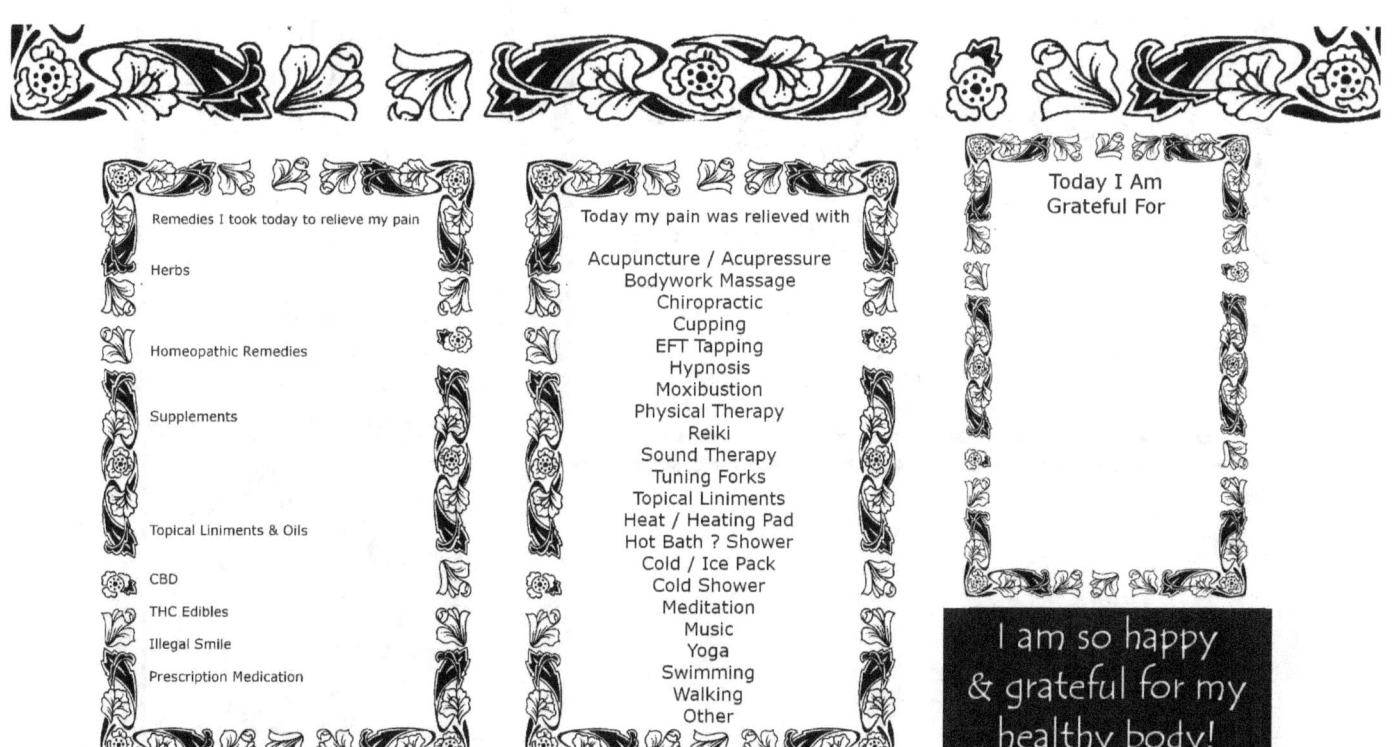

Remedies I took today to relieve my pain

Herbs

Homeopathic Remedies

Supplements

Topical Liniments & Oils

CBD

THC Edibles

Illegal Smile

Prescription Medication

Today my pain was relieved with

Acupuncture / Acupressure
Bodywork Massage
Chiropractic
Cupping
EFT Tapping
Hypnosis
Moxibustion
Physical Therapy
Reiki
Sound Therapy
Tuning Forks
Topical Liniments
Heat / Heating Pad
Hot Bath ? Shower
Cold / Ice Pack
Cold Shower
Meditation
Music
Yoga
Swimming
Walking
Other

Today I Am Grateful For

I am so happy & grateful for my healthy body!

Today's Day & Date

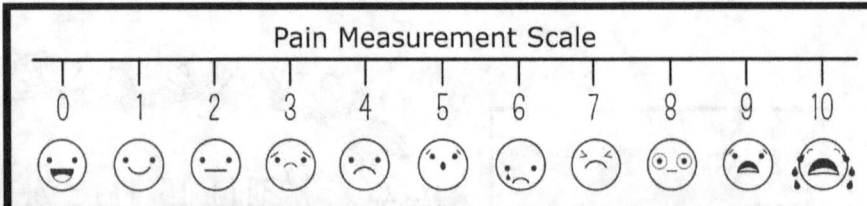

Highlight All Painful Areas

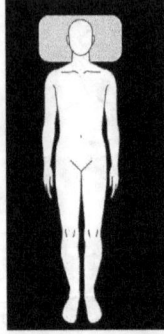 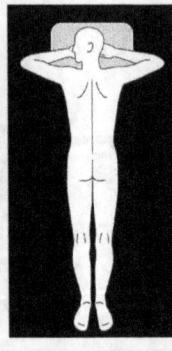 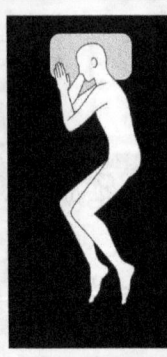 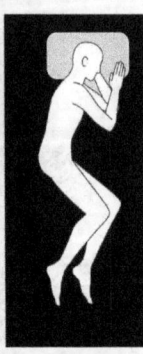

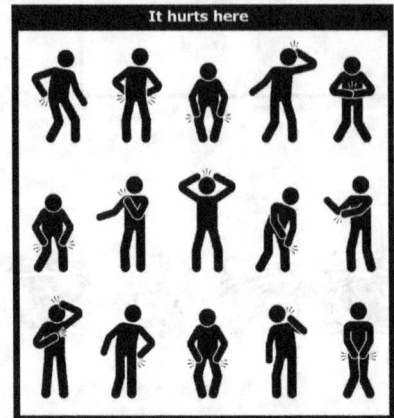

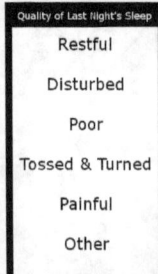

My pain occurs at — a.m. pain / p.m. pain

Quality of Last Night's Sleep
- Restful
- Disturbed
- Poor
- Tossed & Turned
- Painful
- Other

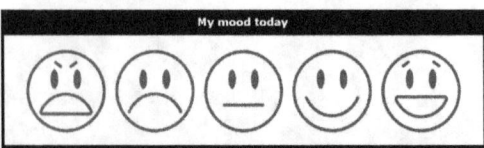

My pain is

Hot
Burning
Cold
Stabbing
Throbbing
Fixed
Moving Traveling
Constant
On & Off

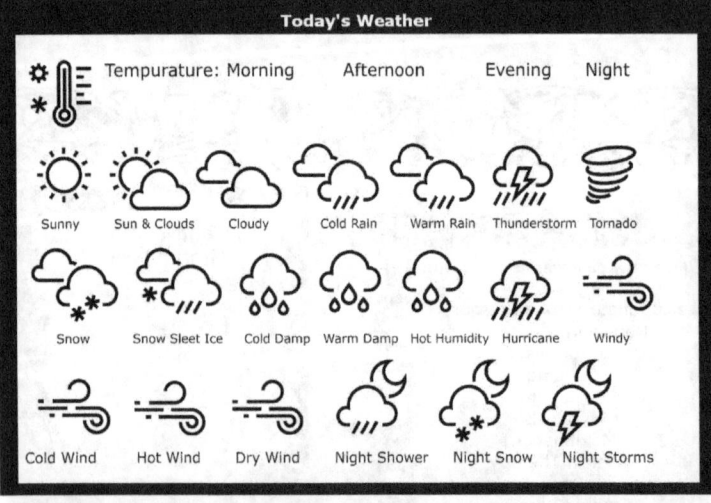

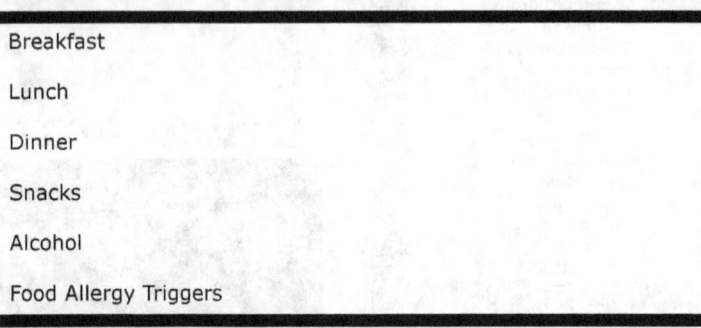

- Breakfast
- Lunch
- Dinner
- Snacks
- Alcohol
- Food Allergy Triggers

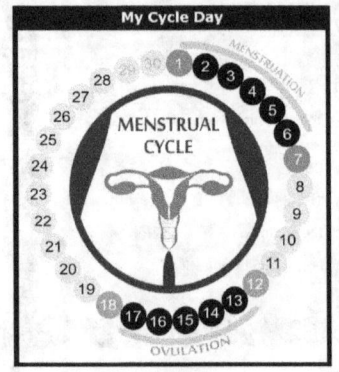

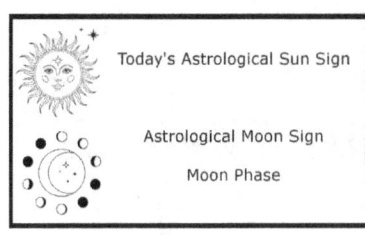

Today's Astrological Sun Sign

Astrological Moon Sign

Moon Phase

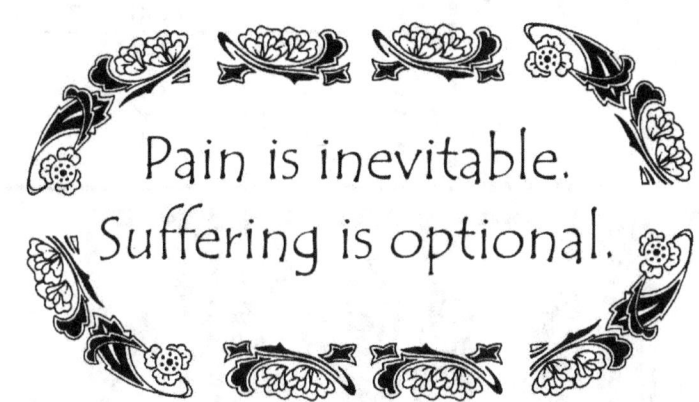

Pain is inevitable.
Suffering is optional.

Notes

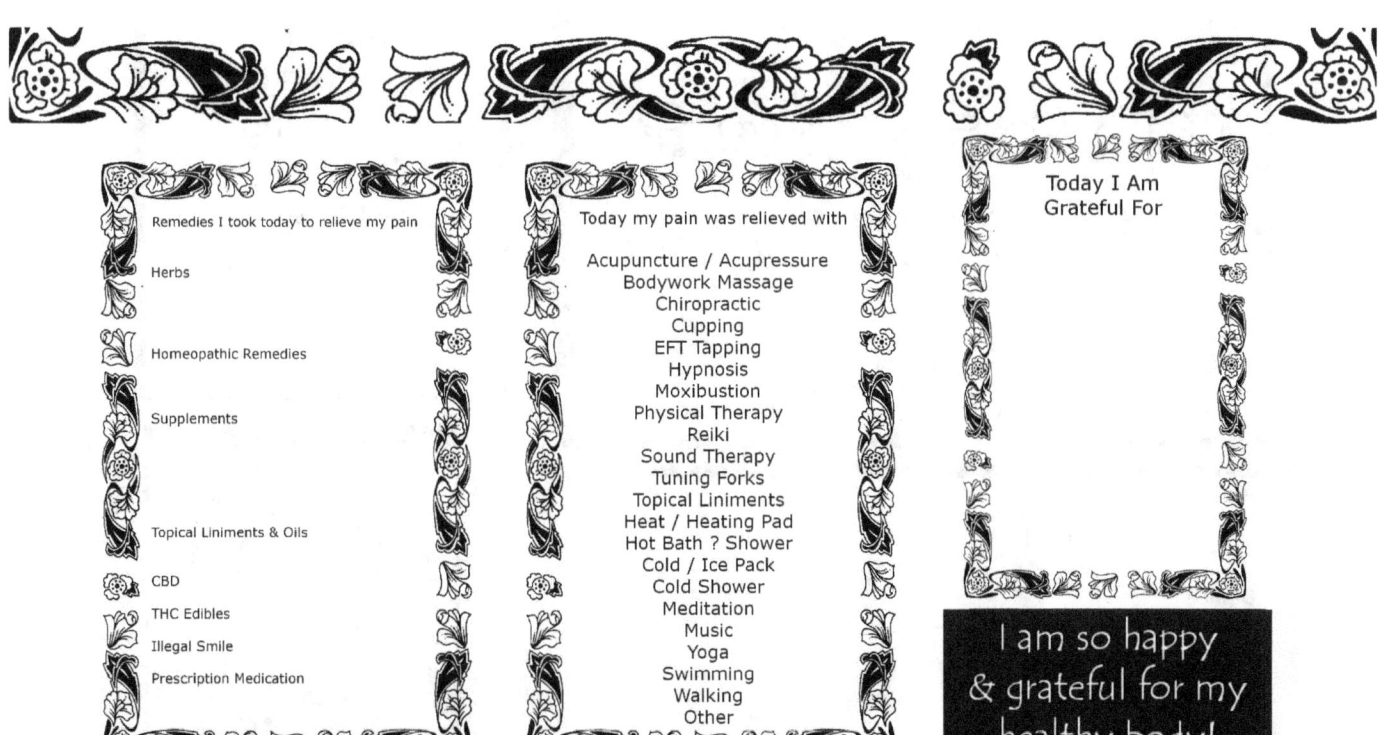

Remedies I took today to relieve my pain

Herbs

Homeopathic Remedies

Supplements

Topical Liniments & Oils

CBD
THC Edibles
Illegal Smile
Prescription Medication

Today my pain was relieved with

Acupuncture / Acupressure
Bodywork Massage
Chiropractic
Cupping
EFT Tapping
Hypnosis
Moxibustion
Physical Therapy
Reiki
Sound Therapy
Tuning Forks
Topical Liniments
Heat / Heating Pad
Hot Bath ? Shower
Cold / Ice Pack
Cold Shower
Meditation
Music
Yoga
Swimming
Walking
Other

Today I Am
Grateful For

I am so happy
& grateful for my
healthy body!

Today's Day & Date

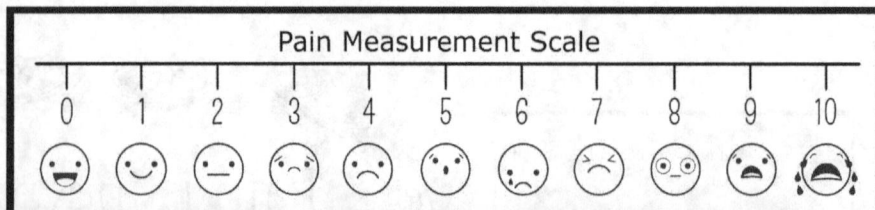

Highlight All Painful Areas

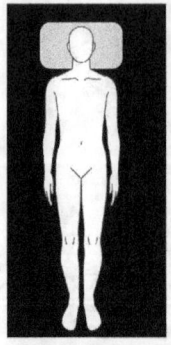
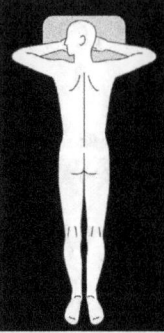
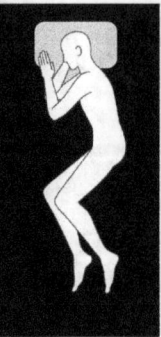
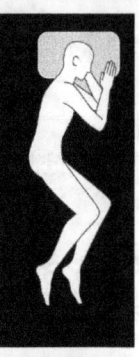

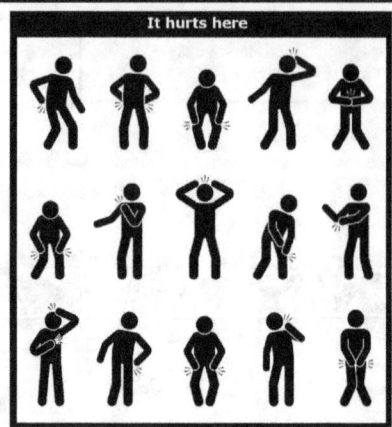

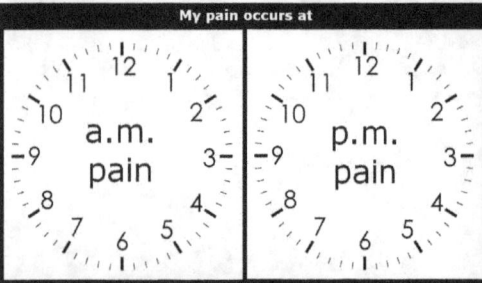
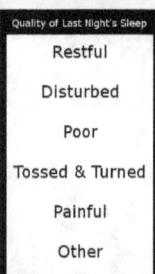

Quality of Last Night's Sleep
- Restful
- Disturbed
- Poor
- Tossed & Turned
- Painful
- Other

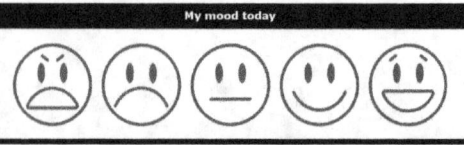

My pain is
Hot
Burning
Cold
Stabbing
Throbbing
Fixed
Moving Traveling
Constant
On & Off

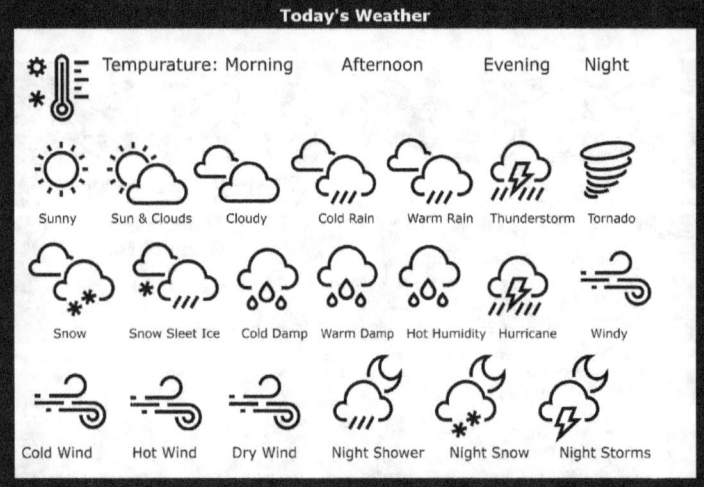

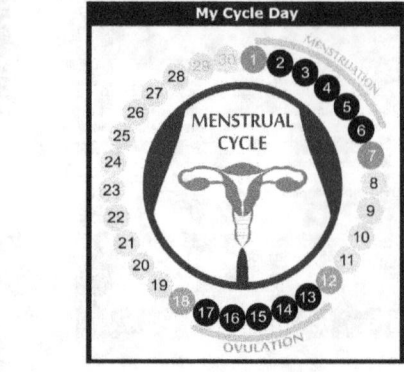

Breakfast

Lunch

Dinner

Snacks

Alcohol

Food Allergy Triggers

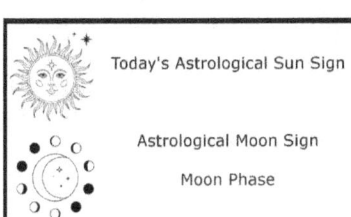

Today's Astrological Sun Sign

Astrological Moon Sign

Moon Phase

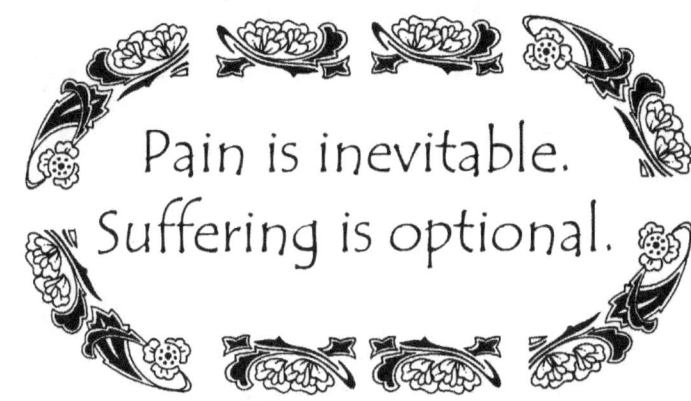

Pain is inevitable. Suffering is optional.

Notes

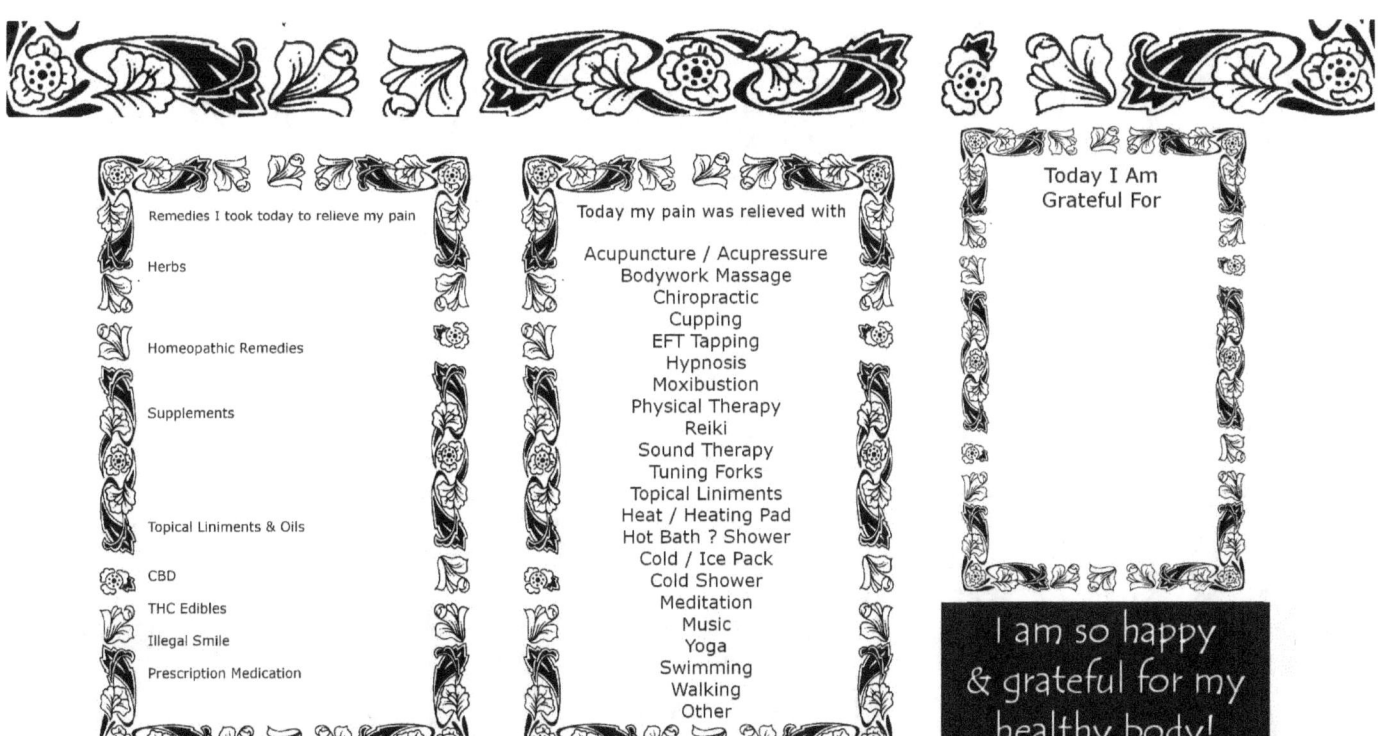

Remedies I took today to relieve my pain

Herbs

Homeopathic Remedies

Supplements

Topical Liniments & Oils

CBD

THC Edibles

Illegal Smile

Prescription Medication

Today my pain was relieved with

Acupuncture / Acupressure
Bodywork Massage
Chiropractic
Cupping
EFT Tapping
Hypnosis
Moxibustion
Physical Therapy
Reiki
Sound Therapy
Tuning Forks
Topical Liniments
Heat / Heating Pad
Hot Bath ? Shower
Cold / Ice Pack
Cold Shower
Meditation
Music
Yoga
Swimming
Walking
Other

Today I Am Grateful For

I am so happy & grateful for my healthy body!

Notes

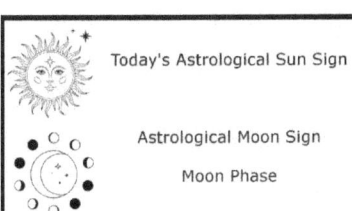

Today's Astrological Sun Sign

Astrological Moon Sign
Moon Phase

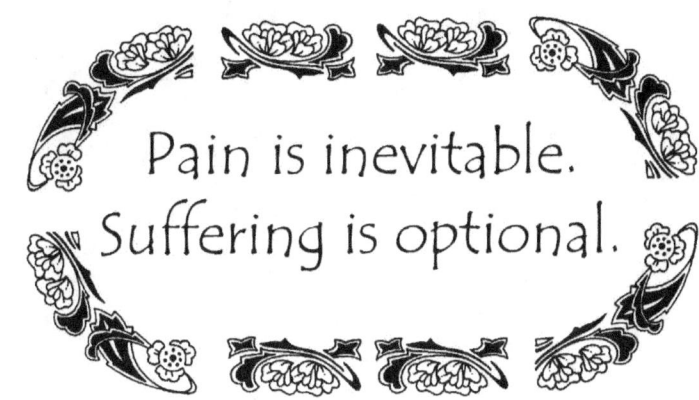

Pain is inevitable.
Suffering is optional.

Notes

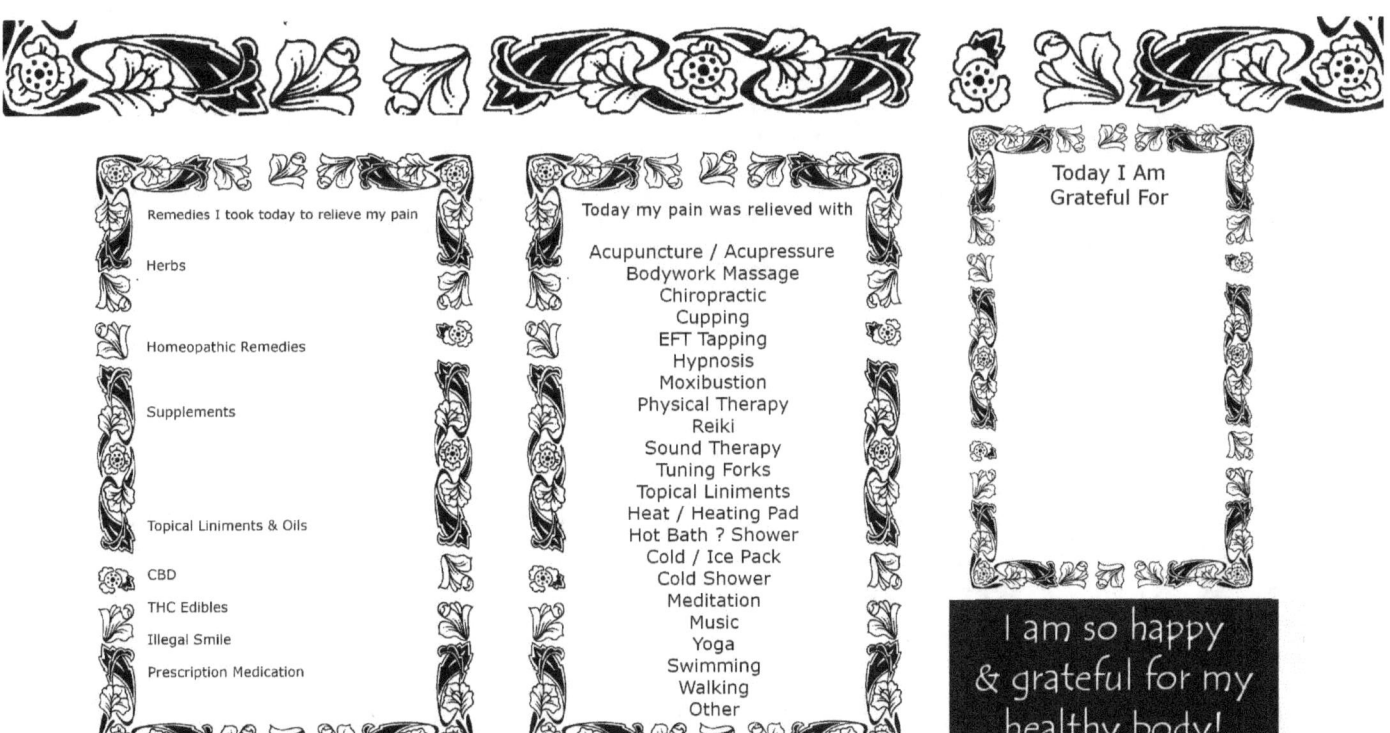

Remedies I took today to relieve my pain

Herbs

Homeopathic Remedies

Supplements

Topical Liniments & Oils

CBD
THC Edibles
Illegal Smile
Prescription Medication

Today my pain was relieved with

Acupuncture / Acupressure
Bodywork Massage
Chiropractic
Cupping
EFT Tapping
Hypnosis
Moxibustion
Physical Therapy
Reiki
Sound Therapy
Tuning Forks
Topical Liniments
Heat / Heating Pad
Hot Bath ? Shower
Cold / Ice Pack
Cold Shower
Meditation
Music
Yoga
Swimming
Walking
Other

Today I Am Grateful For

I am so happy & grateful for my healthy body!

Notes

Notes

Notes

Notes